Deaf People and Society

Deaf People and Society incorporates multiple perspectives related to the topics of psychology, education, and sociology, including the viewpoints of deaf adults themselves. In doing so, it considers the implications of what it means to be deaf or hard of hearing and how deaf adults' lives are impacted by decisions that professionals make, whether in the clinic, the school, or when working with family. This second edition has been thoroughly revised and offers current perspectives on the following topics:

- Etiologies of deafness and the identification process
- The role of auditory access
- Cognition, language, communication, and literacy
- Bilingual, bilingual/bimodal, and monolingual approaches to language learning
- Educational, legal, and placement aspects
- Childhood psychological issues
- Psychological and sociological viewpoints of deaf adults
- The criminal justice system and deaf people
- Psychodynamics of interaction between deaf and hearing people

Each chapter begins with a set of objectives and concludes with suggested readings for further research. This edition contains ten new and original case studies, including ones on hearing children of deaf adults, sudden hearing loss, a young deaf adult with mental illness, and more. Written by a seasoned deaf/hearing bilingual team, this unique text continues to be the go-to resource for students and future professionals interested in working with deaf and hard-of-hearing persons.

Irene W. Leigh is Professor Emerita of Psychology at Gallaudet University, Washington, DC, and has an extensive record of research, publications, and presentations in the areas of depression, psychosocial adjustment, parenting, attachment, identity, and cochlear implants.

Jean F. Andrews is Professor Emerita of Deaf Studies/Deaf Education at Lamar University, Beaumont, Texas, where she has taught and conducted research in language and literacy for deaf students across the lifespan.

Deaf People and Society

Psychological, Sociological, and
Educational Perspectives

Second Edition

Irene W. Leigh and Jean F. Andrews

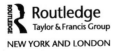

Routledge
Taylor & Francis Group

NEW YORK AND LONDON

Second edition published 2017
by Routledge
711 Third Avenue, New York, NY 10017

and by Routledge
2 Park Square, Milton Park, Abingdon, Oxon, OX14 4RN

Routledge is an imprint of the Taylor & Francis Group, an informa business

© 2017 Taylor & Francis

First edition published 2004 by Pearson Education Inc.

Library of Congress Cataloging-in-Publication Data
Names: Leigh, Irene, author. | Andrews, Jean F., author.
Title: Deaf people and society : psychological, sociological and educational
    perspectives / Irene W. Leigh and Jean F. Andrews.
Description: New York, NY : Routledge, 2016. | Includes bibliographical references
    and index.
Identifiers: LCCN 2016013402 | ISBN 9781138908130 (hbk : alk. paper) |
    ISBN 9781138908147 (pbk : alk. paper) | ISBN 9781315473819 (ebk)
Subjects: LCSH: Deaf. | Deafness—Psychological aspects. | Deaf—Means
    of communication. | Deaf—Education.
Classification: LCC HV2380 .L35 2016 | DDC 305.9/082—dc23
LC record available at https://lccn.loc.gov/2016013402

ISBN: 978-1-138-90813-0 (hbk)
ISBN: 978-1-138-90814-7 (pbk)
ISBN: 978-1-315-47381-9 (ebk)

Typeset in Goudy
by Apex CoVantage, LLC

Contents

4   Cognition, Language, and the Mind   62

5   Educational Aspects of Deaf Education   88

6   Language Learning and Language Teaching Approaches   108

7   Psychological Issues in Childhood   130

Preface

People take their sense of hearing for granted, at least until they encounter someone who has trouble hearing them, or who communicates differently because they do not hear, or who wears hearing aids or cochlear implants. And there are more of these individuals than one might realize. Actually, hearing loss is increasingly common. Recent statistics indicate that there are approximately 48 million Americans with hearing loss (Lin, Niparko, & Ferrucci, 2011). This represents a significant increase when one considers that only a decade earlier, almost 28 million Americans were identified with hearing loss. Most of them fall into the hard-of-hearing category or the ever-increasing category of late-deafened due to genetics, noise-induced hearing loss, infections, drugs, head injuries, as well as the aging process. You've seen persons with hearing issues all around you. Indeed, they are everywhere. You may have elderly family members who wear hearing aids and use amplifiers on their telephones. Or you may have a neighbor with a noise-induced hearing loss from playing loud music constantly. You may even have friends with deaf family members. Possibly you have seen a deaf actress in a movie or a commercial or seen a sign language interpreter in an emergency warning session or in your college classroom. Or you may be deaf or hard of hearing yourself. Such encounters, ranging from superficial to significant, are bound to stimulate thoughts or raise questions, questions we hope to address in this revised book with updated information. As we attempt to answer these questions, our intent is also to focus on the unique issues surrounding what it means to be deaf. We hope these questions will stimulate discussion among our readers and the next generation of students as well as propel future teachers and researchers to explore these issues in their classrooms and research laboratories. We present a sampling of questions to whet your appetites.

What causes hearing to change? Is it always a good idea to "fix it"? Are hearing aids or cochlear implants really effective? Genetic engineering is happening. Is it a good idea to use genetic manipulation to stimulate hearing? Can deaf persons read lips? How well does sign language convey information? Should deaf children go to special schools or mainstream public schools that supposedly provide appropriate services? Just what are appropriate services? How do deaf children think and learn? How do they learn to read without being able to hear words? Are deaf people stuck at low levels educationally? Are they able to get the jobs they want? Is there such a thing as a medical doctor who is deaf? How do deaf people wake up in the morning or know when someone is ringing their doorbell? What kind of visual assistive devices are there? What does it mean for a deaf person to be monolingual, bilingual, or even trilingual? What is Deaf culture all about? Do deaf people consider themselves bicultural or multicultural? Is there a "deaf" personality that differentiates deaf people from hearing people? Do deaf communities isolate deaf people from the hearing world? What does "hearing world" really mean? Does being deaf cause mental illness? How do deaf parents parent their children? Is the Internet accessible to deaf people? What kind of life does an elderly deaf person have—one of isolation or of community? If deaf individuals have a cognitive disability, a learning disability, or vision loss, how do they cope in our society?

So many people wonder how deaf individuals manage their lives and what society does for them. Perhaps you wonder as well? We have thought about the responses to all these questions and have attempted to address these inquiries, thereby adding to your awareness and understanding of issues that arise from being deaf or hard of hearing.

What is this book about? Essentially, it is about trying to understand what it means to be deaf. This is based on our own years of study and experiences working in the fields of psychology and deaf education. Historians, philosophers, and scientists have pondered what it means to be deaf for centuries. Deaf people have fascinated psychologists, who have studied their behaviors, personalities, and intelligence. More recently, linguists have analyzed the structure of signed languages. Developmental psychologists, cognitive scientists, and sociolinguists have studied how deaf children acquire, learn, and remember languages. Teachers experiment with recently suggested ways to encourage student learning, hopefully based on applied research results. Anthropologists and sociologists have investigated Deaf culture and how deaf communities[1] in the United States and throughout the world are formed and change over time. Geneticists and biologists explore hereditary causes of hearing loss and map the different genes involved in hearing. Speech pathologists and audiologists have researched the impact of different auditory input on the acquisition of speech. Deaf artists have created visual media, and deaf writers have composed stories, poems, plays, skits, and histories about the deaf experience.

Portrayal of deaf people in the media has highlighted public awareness of the issues they face. After years of arguing that hearing actors should not assume roles as deaf persons, deaf actors are now increasingly in the limelight. The TV series *Switched at Birth* has deaf main characters played by deaf actors; these characters show what deaf people can do. The film *Through Deaf Eyes*, a panorama of the history of Deaf people, has been broadcast on PBS. Irene Taylor produced and directed *Hear and Now*, a documentary about her deaf parents' experiences as they went through the process of getting cochlear implants to get a sense of what hearing means, a film that garnered multiple awards and an Oscar nomination. A storm of controversy was created by the use of the fake sign language interpreter who stood feet away from heads of government attending Nelson Mandela's funeral. This unfortunate incident served to publicize the importance of qualified sign language interpreters for prominent interpreting roles. Former New York City Mayor Michael Bloomberg had a sign language interpreter who was televised and became a star overnight while interpreting Mayor Bloomberg's report about the dangers of Hurricane Sandy in 2012, illustrating the importance of access to emergency information for deaf people. And ABC News on March 27, 2014, reported on a deaf couple who received an apology from American Airlines after they objected to the airline's use of "Deaf and Dumb" on a note attached to their lost luggage, showing how deaf people are using advocacy to counter negatively toned attitudes and educate the public.

How do these varied insights of different disciplines, personal histories, and media stories mesh together? Although many books have been written that cover a breadth of issues concerning the development of deaf, hard-of-hearing, and DeafBlind people throughout the life span, there have been few books that have looked under the surfaces of these issues related to the deaf experience from a more culturally Deaf perspective. In this book, more so than in others, the focus is on what they *can* do: grow, think, learn, create, and become contributing members of society. This book explains how being deaf affects people's lives, not only from the professional perspective, but also from the adult deaf persons' viewpoint.

The deaf experience is a reflection of people who do not hear and who by virtue of this fact have to adjust to life in different ways. Experiences, interpersonal relationships, and ways of communication are altered. Auditory experiences are not a given. All too often, there may be cognitive and linguistic deprivation, not because of diminished hearing, but because of a society that creates environments without ensuring visual or auditory access to language and communication. Understanding these causes and consequences as well as healthy ways to facilitate optimal development has fallen under the purview of a broad range of disciplines: psychology, linguistics, sociology, anthropology, and education, all of which are covered in this book.

Although the lives of a significant number of people who are deaf do not necessarily center on access to auditory experiences, we will not ignore this issue as it has profound meaning for many others. Hearing levels range on a continuum from mild to profound, and an increasing number of deaf individuals do benefit from advances in auditory technology (digital hearing aids, cochlear implants, and other assistive devices). Nor can we ignore the medical aspects. Many of the varied etiologies of hearing loss, whether congenital or adventitious, also result in health problems such as ear infections, heart malfunctions, psychiatric issues, and cognitive and behavioral difficulties, among others. These warrant medical attention, treatment, and special services.

Special services are also warranted for another group, specifically the population of Deaf-Blind individuals. This population deals with issues related to diminishing vision and hearing, that is, if they are not born completely DeafBlind. Special considerations are needed, such as mobility, technology access, vocational and employment training, counseling, transportation, housing, literacy, life-skills, and interpreter services.

Far too many people think that once medical and/or auditory fixes take place for the deaf person, all will end well. But understanding the deaf or hard-of-hearing person goes beyond that level. This is where the authors of this book, one deaf and one hearing, enter the picture. The deaf author has experienced what it means to be deaf in a multitude of ways. She is the consequence of what professional advice was given to her hearing parents at the time her deafness was identified. She has grown up with auditory amplification. She is the product of special education and mainstream systems, and in the process, she has explored different communication and language parameters. She has interacted with deaf individuals from different walks of life and with different ways of adapting. She is part of the deaf community and intimately aware of Deaf culture. The hearing author is also intimately aware of Deaf culture, having immersed herself in the deaf community and participated in Deaf culture activities. She has encouraged deaf people to enter training programs and achieve professional status in the deaf education field. She has observed the development of deaf children in a wide variety of educational settings and noted the need of attention to children from diverse cultural backgrounds, including the increasing number of deaf immigrants who bring their sign languages and Deaf cultures to the U.S. The information and life experiences of people who are deaf that are presented in this book have been filtered through our eyes.

The concept of *Deaf culture* has strongly impacted the way deaf persons are viewed by the societies around them and how they view themselves. For many, Deaf culture provides a pathway for achieving a healthy psychosocial development and adjustment to life. Deaf culture has the potential both to prevent and limit social isolation, contrary to what a number may think if they view deaf people as being isolated from the world around them. Deaf culture allows for a shared experience and a sense of commonality among deaf people that they find hard to experience in the majority hearing society. Many deaf people use American Sign Language (ASL) and its contact variations (Lucas & Valli, 1992).[2] Not only does this permit easy communication through vision, gestures, and movement unfettered by speech that becomes difficult to produce without clear access to auditory feedback, but it also strengthens the bonding within the deaf community.

So, what are the perspectives we emphasize in this book? Here they are:

- Historical perspective of Deaf people and psychology
- The deaf community as a diverse entity
- Etiologies of deafness and the identification process
- The role of auditory access

- Cognition, language, communication, and literacy
- Bilingual and monolingual approaches to language learning
- Educational, legal, and placement aspects
- Childhood psychological issues
- Psychological viewpoints of deaf adults
- Sociological viewpoints of deaf adults
- The criminal justice system and deaf people
- Psychodynamics of interaction between deaf and hearing people
- Future thoughts

Each of these topics represents puzzle pieces that, when arranged together, form a coherent whole through which you, the reader, can better understand deaf people and their experiences. In the last decade, significant changes have taken place in many of the areas we cover, particularly in deaf education, linguistics related to ASL and English bilingualism, Deaf culture perspectives, neuroscience, and evolving access to new technology that has transformed the lives of many deaf and hard-of-hearing individuals at home, in schools, and at work, and awareness of psychological aspects. This book aims to address these changes.

A word about terminology: In common parlance, people tend to use the word *deaf* in a narrow sense to mean persons who cannot hear, and who may be mute. Many audiologists and medical professionals are also reluctant to use the word *deaf* due to misinterpretations of the word as it can imprint in one's mind a sense of discomfort based on association of the word *deaf* with a person isolated and apart from the world, unable to communicate. As mentioned earlier in this Preface, the airline personnel at American Airlines who wrote "Deaf and dumb" on a note attached to a deaf person's luggage illustrates the subtle attitude of "dumb," and in turn "deaf," thereby reinforcing what many see as a stigmatized perception. Deaf people may struggle to achieve academically because of limitations in environmental access, but there are deaf individuals who have become, for example, financial analysts, restaurant owners, lawyers, medical doctors, and small plane pilots. As a matter of fact, in July 2014, legislation was introduced for consideration by the House Armed Service Committee in the U.S. Congress to the effect that qualified deaf individuals be allowed to serve in the Air Force as part of a pilot program (www.military.com/daily-news/2014/08/11/new-bill-would-open-air-force-to-deaf.html). So "deaf and dumb" is clearly a problematic description of deaf people.

Deaf people vary in their ability to speak clearly or to use whatever level of residual hearing they have, depending on a multitude of factors that we elaborate on in this book. Often, audiologists and medical professionals may be shortsighted in counseling parents or deaf people themselves as they try to translate audiogram information into lay terms. They may on some level unintentionally mislead parents about realistic limitations on optimal use of auditory aids for everyday communication in noisy classroom situations, for example. In this kind of situation, as movingly illustrated in *El Deafo*, a children's book about a deaf girl by Cece Bell (2014), it often turns out that these children end up not understanding everything and feeling lonely and different even with the best of intentions, though many do manage to have active social lives. While parents may understand that cochlear implants will enable their deaf baby to hear beyond what hearing aids can provide, they may not realize that cochlear implants are imperfect ears, thus necessitating intensive auditory training for optimal use. Simply putting amplification on a child and expecting the child to function as a typically hearing child, without additional spoken language and auditory training or visual support services, can jeopardize the child's academic progress, emotional adjustment, and social relationships. In this book, we describe educational programs that build on all the strengths the child has, including both auditory and visual access. Many parents dream of deaf children hearing and speaking, but again, the reality is that there is much variability in a deaf child's abilities to speak and hear. Professionals would do well to remember this and communicate the special and unique nature of the child to parents, rather than imply that all deaf people can talk, hear, speechread, and read.

We acknowledge the pride that culturally Deaf people have when it comes to the term *deaf*. They prefer to use the term *Deaf* to represent them, even if some of them are audiologically hard of hearing. These individuals proudly identify themselves as being *culturally Deaf*. To culturally Deaf people, the term *hearing impaired* is offensive, implying as it does that something is wrong with them. In contrast, they view themselves as fully functioning human beings, able to learn, work, play, and love. Those Deaf people who consider themselves as part of that culture are identified as *Deaf* with the uppercase *D* letter, whereas those who are not affiliated with Deaf culture are viewed as being just *deaf*, with the lowercase letter *d*. This distinction is important and respected in Deaf culture but not known by most of the general population. This uppercase *Deaf* and lowercase *deaf* terminology reflects fundamentally different ways of coping with and feeling about hearing loss.

Our intended readership is a wide range of undergraduate and graduate students, parents, and professionals interested in working with deaf and hard-of-hearing persons, including psychologists, linguists, social workers, medical personnel, educators and administrators, special educators, artists, anthropologists, sociologists, and other interested persons. We hope that researchers will be stimulated by our efforts to raise and examine key issues that puzzle us all in terms of the Deaf/deaf experience and its implications on how we think, socialize, learn, behave, and acquire languages, whether we hear or not.

We use the term *deaf* in a positive manner to mean a person who does not necessarily rely on audition for everyday conversations but can also benefit from the use of visual means of communication in relating with the people around them. We use the term *hard of hearing* to mean a person who can use audition to understand speech but who can also make use of visual forms of communication and support services. Our use of the words *deaf* and *hard of hearing* also encompasses the positive values of identity and inclusion in a vital support group—the Deaf culture and the deaf community. Most Deaf Americans would like physicians, other medical personnel, audiologists, and speech-language pathologists to learn about their Deaf culture and to share this information with parents and other professionals. We also hope that deaf and hard-of-hearing people and their families will be interested in comparing their own personal experiences with what we present in this book.

Notes

1 The lowercase *d* reflects the inability to hear, whereas a capital *D* is frequently used to represent a group of people who share a signed language and culture.
2 Contact signing in the Deaf community is that kind of signing that results from the contact between ASL and English and exhibits features of both languages (Lucas & Valli, 1992, p. xiv).

Acknowledgments

This book reflects the observations and knowledge culled from lifetimes of experience. It also reflects a collective endeavor, and we gratefully acknowledge the help of those who contributed in bringing this book to completion.

In the process of producing a book, precision is enhanced by those who help to ensure accuracy in content and editing. We start with expressions of appreciation to the anonymous reviewers who helped us focus on what we needed to add in this book. Martha Sheridan, Ph.D., of Gallaudet University contributed the case studies featured in this book and thereby brought critical issues facing deaf people to life. We appreciate the support of Kathleen Arnos, Ph.D., and Robert Pollard, Ph.D., both of whom wrote in-depth articles on their relevant topics (genetics and psychology, respectively), as we drew much information from these articles for the book. Dr. Arnos also provided additional documentation to support the reference base for the chapter. James G. Phelan, Au.D., made sure that the information in the Audiology Appendix was accurately and impeccably presented. Marc Charmatz of the National Association for the Deaf Law Center cast an eagle eye over the forensic chapter, as did Talila Lewis and Michele LaVigne. David Martin, Ph.D., graciously agreed to provide helpful suggestions for the cognition chapter. Michael John Gournaris provided information on the current status of mental health services for deaf individuals that confirmed current trends in the field. We also thank Chauman Sieben for his editorial assistance. Special thanks go to our editor, Georgette Enriquez and editorial assistant Xian Gu, who provided encouragement and logistical support as we proceeded with our writing.

Gallaudet University graduate research assistant Erica Wilkins ably contributed to the organization of the reference list and resource list in final forms. She also assisted in creating some of the figures in this book. We appreciate her assistance. We also thank the children, parents, and teachers who allowed us to use their photographs.

Both of us have taught university undergraduate and graduate students. The inspiration for our work came from our students, who challenged us to teach them using the most recent knowledge. We are also inspired by the desire to impart to all students our dedication to the training of new generations of professionals working with deaf children, youth, and adults. To these students, we give profound thanks. We know that our students, both deaf and hearing, are our future. We hope this book stimulates them to question traditional practices, look critically and thoughtfully at our varied perspectives, and add to our research base in their future work.

Even though one of us is deaf and the other is hearing, we both know in our own ways what it means to be deaf and how deaf people live their lives in different ways. Our perceptions are not always in agreement, because we come from divergent backgrounds. But these perceptions definitely have been enlarged by our varied experiences with the deaf community and Deaf culture. Without knowing the deaf community, our lens would have had a much more narrow focus, and finding common ground would have been more arduous. We thank the deaf community for enriching us with their zest for life, their worldviews, and their confidence in their own abilities to assert themselves in the face of a world that is not always accommodating.

Irene W. Leigh would like to express appreciation to the Department of Psychology at Gallaudet University for providing her with an extremely supportive home base and professional stimulation as she continued her professional development and research work there, and for allowing her access to resources as needed. She also thanks the mental health staff at the Lexington School for the Deaf/Center for the Deaf in New York City, where she originally worked as an early career psychologist, who enriched her growth as a psychologist working with deaf people. Without her friends in the Chicago, New York City, and Washington, DC, deaf communities, her understanding of the deaf community and Deaf culture would have been that much less.

Jean F. Andrews would like to thank the Department of Deaf Studies and Deaf Education under the leadership of M. Diane Clark, Ph.D., who allowed her to use departmental resources. She also expresses respect and admiration for her former professors, McCay Vernon, Ph.D., and Hugh Prickett, Ed.D., who introduced her to Deaf culture and bilingualism as did her Deaf classmates, Eugene LaCosse and Tom Bastean, while she was a graduate student at McDaniel College (formerly Western Maryland College) and for Stephan M. Nover, Ph.D., who introduced her to the intricate workings of ASL/English bilingualism through the Star School project at the New Mexico School for the Deaf.

Last, but not least, both of us express our love and appreciation for those on the home front who patiently endured our lengthy sessions at the computer. The support of these loved ones motivated us all through the hours as we worked to find the words to convey to the readers of this book what it means to be deaf and to live Deaf lives.

1 Historical Perspectives of Deaf People and Psychology[1]

Study the past if you would define the future.

Confucius (551 BC–479 BC)

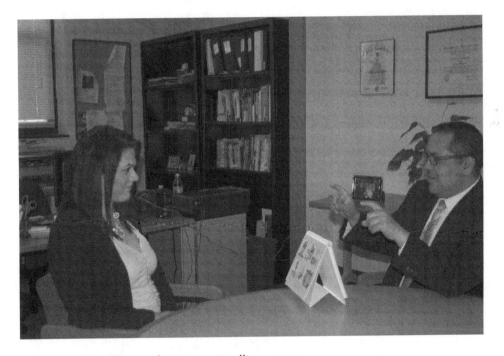

Figure 1.1 Dr. Gabriel Lomas administers an intelligence test
Source: Courtesy of Dr. Gabriel Lomas. Used with permission.

A 1943 book about deaf people had the following inscription for its dedication:

> To Deaf People:
> The most misunderstood among the sons of men,
> But the gamest of all

(Best, 1943, with apologies for gender)

It took centuries for deaf people to break out of the shackles of misunderstanding. And even today, there continues to be misunderstanding, notwithstanding the fact that deaf people more than ever are achieving their potential in education, communications (thanks to ever-evolving technology), theater, law, and many other areas and can psychologically move on in their efforts to live productive and happy lives. This progress has come about as a consequence of the presence of a more enlightened era and populace that understand diversity and multiculturalism. Within the domains of psychology, sociology, anthropology, linguists, education, and mental health, psychologists, social workers, mental health counselors, sociologists, neuroscientists, anthropologists, linguists, educators, psychiatrists, and allied mental health professionals have served as catalysts that propelled the changes we see today.

Chapter Objectives

In this chapter, we describe historical highlights that played significant roles in facilitating the mental health and well-being of deaf people with primary focus starting in the 1950s and onward. We review critical court decisions in the areas of education and mental health access that have played prominent roles in these historical changes. We also review the impact of the use of sign language by professionals in mental health settings. Readers will learn about the way in which professionals highlighted and tied together American Sign Language (ASL), Deaf culture, and the positive nature of the deaf community, thereby enhancing the quality of service delivery to deaf individuals in need of psychological/mental health services.

Before 1950

Just prior to the 1950s, there were fewer than ten psychologists and no psychiatrists in the United States with full-time commitment to the mental health of deaf and hard-of-hearing people (Levine, 1977). The few available psychologists were located in residential schools for deaf children that had been established in the United States, starting in the 1800s. During those early decades, most of these schools utilized sign language as a vehicle for educating deaf children. Despite the fact that these schools existed to provide deaf children with skills needed to manage their lives, general nineteenth-century perceptions about deaf people's abilities reflected the belief that because deaf persons had problems with speaking and relied on signing, their intellectual functioning was limited and they were educationally deficient (Pollard, 1992–1993).

In the late 1800s and early 1900s, there were individuals who demonstrated the fallacy of this belief system, starting with William James, a well-known philosopher/psychologist. James encountered two deaf men who demonstrated to him through personal correspondence that abstract cognition could exist even without the mastery of spoken words, explaining how they thought even before starting school and learning language (James, 1893, as cited in Pollard, 1992–1993). For the first time, this upended the belief that language was required prior to abstract cognition. However, it would be decades before cognitive psychologists confirmed the possibility that the existence of thought was not necessarily dependent on internalized language.

In the meantime, the pendulum was swinging towards the use of spoken language, encouraged by Alexander Graham Bell (1847–1922), most popularly known as the inventor of the telephone. With the advent of behaviorism and the stimulus-response theory of learning, psychologists were beginning to focus on how language acquisition was impacted by the inability to hear. Rudolph Pintner (1884–1942) and Donald Paterson (1892–1961) (1915, as cited in Pollard, 1992–1993) were in the forefront of psychologists who noted the unfairness of linguistic requirements in IQ tests used to evaluate the intelligence of deaf children. As an interesting aside, during that time, psychologists not only were testing deaf people but were also testing immigrants at Ellis Island with the ultimate goal of evaluating the use of IQ tests and other psychological instruments with different populations. In many cases, they gave verbal IQ tests in English to both groups, thinking that was appropriate and, as a result, inappropriately classified many individuals as mentally retarded (currently referred to as having an intellectual disability).

Pintner went on to develop a variety of performance-based psychological tests for deaf students, including primary and preschool intelligence tests, a test of educational achievement, as well as research projects focusing on tests to measure deaf children's personalities and psychosocial functioning. Together with a group of psychologists, he also took a lead in recommending the development of tests covering intellectual abilities and academic achievement that would be standardized with deaf people. Additional recommendations included studies of deaf children's psychosocial and emotional development within different educational approaches and parenting styles. Finally, the need to research approaches to deal with adult psychopathology was acknowledged (National Research Council, 1929, as cited in Pollard, 1992–1993).

Unfortunately, despite a spate of studies following these recommendations, these studies contradicted each other to the point of creating dissension (Levine, 1977). This was primarily due to limited familiarity with deaf people and their communication needs as well as problematic validity of the measures used with deaf subjects. Reviewing the progress in 1941, after a decade of research, Pintner, Eisenson, and Stanton (1941) concluded that, while variability in IQ scores existed, deaf children on average scored lower compared to hearing peers. This conclusion was to stand until McCay Vernon (1928–2013) (1969) reviewed 21 studies involving IQ results and found that, contrary to popular opinion, if nonverbal performance-type tests were used, the IQs of deaf and hearing children did not significantly differ. This had a significant impact on how schools for the deaf perceived the intellectual functioning of deaf students.

Pintner and colleagues also cautioned that the use of personality measures developed for hearing children would unduly pathologize deaf children. As a matter of fact, this is exactly what happened. Prior to 1950, for example, there had been only 18 studies on behavioral aspects of deafness, all done on children (Vernon & Andrews, 1990). Most of these investigations involved the use of grossly inappropriate psychological tests, many of which were verbal or based on the knowledge of English, which many deaf children were unfortunately deficient in, or behavioral checklists with many items that were biased against deaf youth. The results seemed to demonstrate that multiple types of pathology were present. It took decades to show that many of these studies have been proven false by subsequent, more valid types of testing and assessment (see Chapter 8 for further details). It seems that what was left out of the equation was the lack of awareness that deaf children were in difficult communication situations to which they reacted and that of course reflected different types of adjustment, some of which were pathological. It was not the deaf aspect that was the issue; rather it was the inaccessible environment and the negative attitudes to deaf children that all too often prevailed.

Sadly, between that time and the 1950s, no formal research was done on deaf adults because psychologists working with deaf individuals tended to be employed in schools where they essentially functioned as psychometrists, with the primary responsibility of administering IQ tests to incoming students in order to identify those with low IQs or severe behavior problems. The intention was to exclude from school enrollment those with mental retardation, the label used at the time (currently labeled as intellectual disability) or severe mental illnesses and to refer them to hospitals. Although the state hospitals serving individuals with mental illness or mental retardation were required by law to accept these deaf patients, these deaf patients were not offered access to treatment nor were the hospital staffs trained to provide treatment to deaf inpatients or to communicate with them in sign language (Levine, 1977).

This unfortunate state of affairs had two negative consequences. First, deaf people with mental illness or mental retardation (intellectual disability) got, at best, what was essentially antitherapeutic custodial care, or in other words, they were "warehoused" with no treatment. The second consequence of this dearth of psychologists and psychiatrists was a lack of any quality research into the ways being deaf influenced psychological functioning. That was to change starting in the 1950s.

After 1950

Starting in the 1950s, interest in the implications of being deaf began to increase, partly as the outgrowth of audiological training in response to the influx of World War II veterans returning home with hearing loss. Helmer Myklebust (1910–2008) was a well-known psychologist who did research on deaf children and young adults that exemplifies research done up to 1960. For example, he did work on diagnosing aphasia in deaf youth and wrote on educating aphasic children. He also conducted personality studies using the Minnesota Multiphasic Personality Inventory (MMPI, 1960), a verbal-based psychological instrument, with deaf participants, for which he was vilified because of the inappropriateness of using such a verbally loaded measure that resulted in a negative personality picture of deaf youth. Even though much of his research was not supported by later findings, in part because of the inappropriate use of existing instrumentation at the time, he was a psychological pioneer in the effort to understand the psychological functioning of deaf people. His work and that of his students at Northwestern University were important stages in the process of this effort. In particular, Myklebust (1964) was among the first to emphasize that there might be functionally different ways in which deaf children interact with the world compared with hearing peers. This of course has implications for psychological development. Current neuropsychological research demonstrates this phenomenon, meaning that deaf children function differently, but not in inferior ways compared with hearing peers.

Edna Simon Levine (1910–1992), a contemporary of Myklebust, was for many years a psychologist at the Lexington School for the Deaf in New York City, at that time a prominent school that focused on spoken language for deaf children, and later became a professor at New York University. In the latter role, she conducted research projects on the personalities of deaf children and on children who were deaf due to rubella (popularly known as German measles) that affected their mothers during the first trimester of pregnancy. Most importantly, she was among the first to suggest that the environment was a critical factor in the development of the deaf child, and therefore its influence required critical study (Levine, 1981). In addition to these contributions, Levine also was a major factor in the establishment of the National Theater of the Deaf in 1966, which enhanced the careers of deaf actors. She also authored a fictional story about a deaf child—*Lisa and Her Soundless World* (1974), which oriented hearing children to what it meant to be deaf.

Psychopathology and Mental Health

Most importantly, Levine played an influential role in determining federal policies impacting deaf children and adults. She spearheaded efforts to develop research and treatment programs for deaf people with mental health problems by taking advantage of some of the funding opportunities created by post-World War II rehabilitation legislation (Levine, 1977). How was this accomplished?

In the early 1950s, Edna Levine and Boyce Williams (1910–1998), the Rehabilitation Services Administration (RSA) administrator, who happened to be deaf, approached Franz Kallman, M.D. (1897–1965), a psychiatrist affiliated with Columbia University in New York City who had done genetic and schizophrenia research with deaf persons, to discuss the establishment of such a program (Vernon & Andrews, 1990). Funding was obtained for the establishment of the first outpatient psychiatric treatment program for the deaf at the New York State Psychiatric Institute in New York City as well as for an inpatient unit at Rockland State Hospital located north of the city. Together with psychiatrists John Rainer, M.D., and Ken Altshuler, M.D., Kallman published the first significant research projects on psychopathology and its identification and treatment in deaf people (Vernon & Daigle-King, 1999).

This has to be considered groundbreaking, as prior to the mid-1950s, there was only one research study on the psychopathology of deaf people to appear in the psychiatric literature, done by a late-deafened Danish psychiatrist, V. C. Hansen (1929). In Denmark, he gathered data on 36 deaf patients in psychiatric hospitals and reported that his numbers represented a 10 times greater prevalence of deaf inmates than would be expected based on the prevalence of deafness in Denmark. He also found deaf patients to be significantly more chronic than hearing patients, with hospital stays being 20 years on average. Almost one-third (31 percent) of the deaf patients were undiagnosed. This is understandable, considering that there was no hospital staff able to communicate with them in sign language, that is, if the patients themselves even knew sign language. It is possible that some had no language.

The work done by the New York State Psychiatric Institute was in the forefront of other research and clinical projects that began shortly afterwards. These projects were located at St. Elizabeth Hospital in Washington, DC; Langley Porter Psychiatric Institute in San Francisco, California; Michael Reese Hospital in Chicago, Illinois; and John Denmark's psychiatric program in England. The results of their research projects as well as later studies are reported in some detail in a 1999 paper (Vernon & Daigle-King, 1999). They were landmark studies that have had a profound impact on our knowledge of deaf people and mental health as well as on the care these patients receive.

A major finding was that, when deaf patients with mental health issues are placed within a general hospital population and provided no staff or therapists who can communicate with them in sign language, their stays are much longer than those of hearing patients. More recent studies (Daigle, 1994; Trumbetta, Bonvillian, Siedlecki, & Haskins, 2001) indicate that, when provided care by psychologists, psychiatrists, social workers, and nursing staff who can sign and/or when provided round-the-clock sign language interpreting services, deaf patients who know sign language are no more chronic than their hearing counterparts. It is this access to sign language and professional staff knowledgeable about deafness that has been legislated by the Americans with Disabilities Act of 1990 (ADA, amended in 2008) and other civil rights laws. Unfortunately, such services have been provided in only a minority of states. Consent decrees, which involve a settlement of a lawsuit in which hospitals agree to take specific actions without admitting guilt, have had to be used to force compliance when hospitals are sued for lack of access (Katz, Vernon, Penn, & Gillece, 1992).

Even though deaf people generally have not been well served by the mental health system, deaf members of minority ethnic backgrounds have been even more poorly served (Pollard, 1994). In the psychiatric studies reported in the literature, minimal attention has been paid to the relationship between ethnic background and diagnostic categorization for these individuals (Leigh, 2010). However, in these studies, it is important to note that one conclusion was generally agreed upon. The limited availability of American Sign Language (ASL) in the schools and the difficulties deaf people experience when communicating with hearing people, including family members as well as outsiders, were partially responsible for both the type and amount of psychopathology seen in deaf patients and in the educational retardation and lack of general knowledge found in these individuals (Vernon & Daigle-King, 1999).

Much of that literature also suggests that, while the publications of the 1950s and early 1960s on the mental health of deaf adults reflected focus on those who had psychiatric diagnoses, the implication that their pathology was caused in part by their being deaf continued to be perpetuated. In these studies, they were perceived as being concrete thinkers, emotionally immature, and egocentric and having problematic relationships and a tendency to act out. These results permeated general perspectives of the general, nonpsychiatric deaf population, thanks to the "spread" effect.

The only psychiatrist to do a significant amount of research with deaf children was Hilde Schlesinger, who worked together with sociologist Kay Meadow to conduct studies of deaf children and their families (Schlesinger & Meadow, 1972). Their clinical research focused on three primary areas—language acquisition, using sign language, and mother/child interaction comparing deaf and hearing children—in addition to a comparative study of deaf children whose parents were deaf with those deaf children having normally hearing parents. Among their conclusions was that the controversy then raging over methods of communication (spoken versus signed) was detrimental to the mental health of the children involved. They recommended that a combination of signed communication and speech/speechreading be used. This recommendation predates what is being implemented today in the bilingual programs within the educational setting with the focus on ASL and English, as indicated in Chapter 6.

Schlesinger and Meadow (1972) also found that when families used sign language with their young deaf children, acquisition generally paralleled milestones in spoken language acquisition. Knowledge of sign language did not interfere with speech acquisition. Instead, spoken words and speechreading facility increased with sign language acquisition. In addition, the level of communication frustration was decreased in the families they observed who used both spoken and signed communication in combination. Among their other findings were the distinct advantages deaf children with deaf parents enjoyed versus deaf children with hearing parents. The difference manifested in areas such as educational achievement, family climate, maturity, and a number of other variables.

Finally, it is important to note that, even though inpatient and outpatient services have increased in the United States and Europe over the last few decades, most of the significant and relevant research was done more than two decades ago (Vernon & Daigle-King, 1999). However, this has changed, with an emerging number of new research data as described in Chapter 9.

Influence of Psycholinguistics

You will note the frequent references to the role of sign language in working with deaf mental health clients. How has this role emerged, considering the fact that many schools for the deaf were geared towards the use of spoken language? Prior to the 1960s, the typical professional perspective of sign languages was that of an unsophisticated communication system or a crude visual representation of English. There were many deaf people who endorsed this view, feeling that mastery of spoken English was the ideal in order to interact with hearing society.

Then along came William Stokoe's (1960) assertion that there were structural elements in American Sign Language (ASL), meaning that it was a bona fide language. This was a revolutionary concept, causing significant controversy at the time considering that ASL had typically been framed as a degenerate form of English. As time passed, the recognition of ASL as a formal language became the foundation of Deaf culture and its legitimacy in the eyes of many hearing people, including those in the mental health field, as well as deaf people. Psychologists' earlier, negative views of the linguistic, intellectual, and psychological characteristics of deaf people were profoundly affected such that there was more consideration of how language impacted these characteristics and how ASL needed to be incorporated in research projects. As Pollard (1992–1993, p. 40) states, "Stokoe made the premise of deaf psychological health a far more viable one than it had ever been before."

Subsequently, the literature showed more evidence of studies evaluating the use of ASL in school classrooms as well as investigations into the appropriate use of psychological assessments. McCay Vernon, mentioned earlier, was a pioneer in this effort with his seminal publications on the importance of nonverbal assessment methods to demonstrate that in fact the distribution of intelligence scores among deaf testees approximated that of hearing peers, countering the heretofore prevailing notion of deaf intellectual inferiority.

The first major psychology texts reflecting the impact of Stokoe's work appeared in the early 1970s (Mindel & Vernon, 1971; Schlesinger & Meadow, 1972, mentioned earlier). The focus of these publications was on the importance of early parent-child communication in the development of healthy cognitive and emotional functioning in deaf adults. This notion fed into the increasing attention to the environment as a significant influence on the psychosocial functioning of the deaf child/adult, whether healthy or pathological.

Hans Furth (1920–1999) personifies the advent of psycholinguistics into the field. He, together with Vernon, was ahead of their times in challenging the notion that thought was possible only with internalized language. Through his research, he noted that deaf individuals, even those with no formal language system, sign or otherwise, still were capable of successful problem-solving strategies similar to those of hearing peers (Furth, 1966). Additionally, at that time, the noted Ursula Bellugi of the Salk Institute in La Jolla, California, together with her linguist husband Edward Klima, confirmed the true language nature of ASL, complete with grammar and syntax (Klima & Bellugi, 1979). Later studies run under her purview at the Salk Institute demonstrated that ASL is processed by parts of the brain that also processes spoken language, contradicting the belief that ASL is solely right-hemisphere based (Poizner, Klima, & Bellugi, 1987). The work of these early psycholinguists has contributed to today's understanding of ASL as a rich, complex, and evolving language, similar to many other languages in this regard. These earlier studies also laid the groundwork for current research in neurosciences and neurolinguistics that uses brain-imaging technology to substantiate findings published by Bellugi and her colleagues related to how ASL is processed in the brain (Campbell, MacSweeney, & Waters, 2008; MacSweeney, Capek, Campbell, & Woll, 2008).

The Role of Court Decisions and Legislation

Despite the advances in the psychological understanding of deaf people, they continued to be viewed as a burden to society, with their civil rights hardly taken into account. As mentioned earlier, in the 1950s, Levine had to work with the RSA to get the first significant governmental involvement in the mental health needs of deaf people. It was not until the 1970s when court decisions and congressional legislation began to positively affect the lives of deaf people, specifically, two major court decisions and a series of laws enacted by Congress from the 1970s onward. The court decisions were the *Pennsylvania Association for Retarded Citizens v. Commonwealth of Pennsylvania* (1972) and *Mills v. Board of Education* (1972), both of which represented a victory for children with disabilities, including those children with IQs below 70, behavior disorders, or multiple physical disabilities, who had previously been denied access to public education. These court decisions laid the foundation for the 1975 Education of All Handicapped Children Act (Public Law 94–142), which brought changes to educational programming by requiring free and appropriate public education for all children with disabilities. In 1990, this law was renamed the Individuals with Disabilities Act of 1990 (IDEA); it added the mandate that an individual family service plan be developed for each child, required that children with disabilities be educated with nondisabled children to the greatest extent possible, and stated that parents have an active role in the decisions related to their children's educational plan.

Unfortunately, the concept that children with disabilities be educated with nondisabled children to the greatest extent possible can result in potential harm to children who are deaf when less than ideal communication access is provided. In 2000, the 11th Circuit Court provided the largest single award in special education history to date, approximately $2.5 million to two deaf children who were placed in a generic special education setting for children with multiple disabilities without the benefit of communication access, the services of a professional teacher of the deaf, or related services (Easterbrooks, Lytle, Sheets, & Crook, 2004; National

Association of the Deaf, 2014a). The impact on the social, emotional, communication, and academic development and earning potential of the students was catastrophic. To this day, the right to a free, appropriate public education, particularly one that is accessible, remains unrealized by a considerable number of deaf and hard-of-hearing children who are in mainstream settings.

What does this have to do with psychology? The influx of multiply disabled children, particularly after the rubella epidemic in the early 1960s that caused neurological and behavioral difficulties as well as hearing loss created a demand for psychological services. By 1977, 178 people were working as school psychologists with deaf children, based on a survey by Cantor and Spragins (1977). However, only 9 percent of these persons were credentialed as school psychologists. Of these, none had any special training in working with deaf children. Not only that, the research base regarding assessment methods appropriate for this population was still inadequate. Edna Levine (1977) deserves most of the credit for highlighting the need for trained psychologists and what the training and professional expectations should be. She organized what came to be known as the acclaimed 1975 Spartanburg Conference on the Functions, Competencies, and Training of Psychological Service Providers to the Deaf.

In response to this obvious need for qualified professionals, starting in 1972, Gallaudet University established a social work program to prepare social workers to work with deaf and hard-of-hearing children. In 1979, programs were established to prepare both school psychologists and school counselors for work with these children. As graduates of these and other programs have gone out into the field, a nucleus of well-qualified social workers, educational psychologists and school counselors now exists, although there is no information on these professionals currently employed. These trained individuals are providing direct services, some are doing research, and a number have gone on to complete doctoral work and serve on university faculties. One such individual, Dr. Jeffrey Braden (1994), formerly a school psychologist, has also researched the intellectual functioning of deaf people. His treatise on the implications of being deaf for IQ differences between groups represents a significant contribution to the literature.

As the supply of psychologists increased, it reached a level that would have been sufficient to meet the needs of deaf children who were in state and private residential and day schools for the deaf. However, since the early 1950s, the trend is for deaf children to be placed in local public school settings. This accelerated as part of the least restrictive environment for children with disabilities as mandated in PL 94–142 and a series of court dates based on it, which has favored the placement of deaf children in their home school districts (though some have argued that limited access to language and communication in the classroom make this a more restrictive environment compared to specialized schools). As we discuss further in this book, there may be only one or a few students with profound hearing losses in an entire school system. In these situations, psychologists, teachers, and administrators who have little or no experience with deaf children and who may not always be able to communicate with them are making critical decisions regarding these deaf children. In such situations, the results potentially may be catastrophic for the child, both educationally and psychologically. There have been challenges to this practice both in the courts and in the literature, but stronger test cases such as the ones mentioned earlier in this section need to be brought to court before this practice can be stopped. It has been suggested that instead of setting up school-based counseling for students who are deaf, the school counselor in the public school might contact an outside agency that provides counseling services by school counselors or social workers who are knowledgeable about what it means to be deaf. In this way, deaf students could have their needs met by a provider who is working collaboratively with the public school counselor. Another suggestion is to have school-based counseling in sign language available to all students via a signing counselor hired by the centralized deaf education program (Andrews, Shaw, & Lomas, 2011).

Since it has been argued that early identification of deaf children is critical to facilitate the development of language and communication, Congress passed the Newborn Infant Hearing Screening and Intervention Act of 1990. This law provided for funding for state grants for newborn hearing screening and intervention programs (Joint Committee on Infant Hearing, 2013). Considering that children typically were identified as deaf or hard of hearing at ages 2, 3, or even later, the implications for earlier access to language are significant.

Section 504 of the Rehabilitation Act of 1973 mandated that institutions receiving federal funding could no longer deny services based on physical disability. As a consequence, deaf students were increasingly able to access higher education institutions that received federal funding, and deaf patients could now access public mental health programs for the same reason. The presence of those deaf individuals stimulated further growth in psychological research and service activity.

The Americans with Disabilities Act (ADA) was signed into law in 1990 and amended in 2008 to provide more clarity. This Act served the purpose of expanding the provisions of Section 504 to the private sector, since Section 504 covered only entities receiving federal support. This law also gave deaf persons the right to greater access to public accommodation, transportation, employment, and telecommunications. More details are provided in Chapter 9, including an examination of the true benefits and difficulties related to the ADA that have sociological and psychological implications.

Suffice it to say that, overall, considering the need for court cases and legislation, all too often education and mental health service providers and policymakers generally have little understanding of the complex language and communication needs of this population and the implications for program design and service delivery. This leads us to a consideration of the human right to health that is recognized and protected by international rules (García & Bravo, 2015). Case in point, the International Convention on the Rights of Persons with Disabilities was approved by the United Nations General Assembly. It incorporates the right to enjoy the highest attainable standard of health without discrimination as part of the general purpose of ensuring the full and equal enjoyment of human rights and fundamental freedoms by all persons with disabilities. The importance of recognizing limitations in equal access needs to be acknowledged in order to facilitate action in providing equitable services.

Professional Training

In addition to its accredited programs to prepare school psychologists (1979), social workers (1989), and counselors (1986) at the master's level to work in schools with deaf children, Gallaudet University now has an accredited doctoral program in clinical psychology, started in 1990 (Brice, Leigh, Sheridan, & Smith, 2013). Rochester Institute of Technology, which houses the National Technical Institute for the Deaf, has a master's program in school psychology. Few other specialized programs exist.

Increasingly, in part thanks to legislation mandating access to public services, more and more deaf students are attaining graduate degrees in psychology, counseling, and social work at other universities offering accredited programs. An increasing number of deaf social workers (250; Sheridan, White, & Mounty, 2010), mental health counselors (approximately 200; Kendra Smith, personal communication, December 6, 2014), and doctoral level psychologists (80+; Carolyn Corbett, personal communication, December 8, 2014) with deaf-related knowledge and experience among others are currently working in mental health and counseling centers and hospitals, thereby addressing the ongoing shortage of qualified professionals. There is a new specialization: Certified Peer Support Specialist, which refers to individuals who have experienced mental health issues being trained to provide counseling and support services (Gournaris, 2016). These developments facilitate the slowly burgeoning improvement in services, particularly for adult deaf patients using these facilities. However, there are too few facilities that specialize in working with deaf people. This reflects the ongoing marginalization of this low-incidence population in the planning of services and programs that meet their needs. The number of hospital inpatient units specializing in deaf patients can be counted on one hand, if not more, thanks to cost-cutting measures. The situation for adolescents with serious mental illnesses requiring inpatient care is dire as there is an almost total lack of adequate, appropriate inpatient care (Willis & Vernon, 2002). One has to search long and hard throughout the country to find inpatient psychiatric wards for deaf children. This of course limits training sites for deaf trainees who rely on sign language interpreters. Alternatively, they occasionally find it difficult to gain entry to training positions at various agencies because of concerns about the role of sign language interpreters and how clients might feel about having trainees and interpreters in the room. When training programs work closely with these agencies and hospitals to lay the groundwork for collaboration, training experiences have for the most part been positive.

All too often, however, professionals will get their specialized training and take additional coursework or a certificate program for the deaf component (Brice et al., 2013). Nonetheless, we continue to find professionals who lack expertise or training but still perceive themselves to be sufficiently competent to work with deaf or hard-of-hearing clientele. Because of this, as Leigh and Gutman (2010) noted, "Quality mental health services for deaf clients have only recently become an aspiration rather than an oxymoron" (p. 3). Overall, bilingual (ASL and English) mental health professionals continue to be in short supply despite recent improvements, considering the dire need for such professionals to work in the field of mental health with deaf clients (Steiner, 2015).

Professional Associations

In the 1970s, psychologists within the American Psychological Association (APA), the premier organization of psychologists in the United States, began advocating for more attention to disabilities issues, including issues pertinent to deafness (Pollard, 1992–1993). This also included improving accessibility for deaf psychologists within the organization. Their work led to the development of a task force on psychology and handicaps that eventually recommended the formation of the Committee on Disabilities and Handicaps. This committee, now labeled the Committee on Disability Issues in Psychology, met for the first time in 1985 and is currently a standing committee within the APA's Public Interest Directorate. A deaf, sign-fluent, or hard-of-hearing individual has been a member of the committee since its inception, and three deaf individuals have chaired it: Tovah Wax, Allen Sussman, and Irene W. Leigh. Their focus has been that of influencing the APA's sensitivity to people with disabilities as part of the diversity spectrum. APA conferences have included sign language interpreter services, thus creating access for deaf, signing psychologists. Outside of governance, the APA's Division 22 (Division of Rehabilitation Psychology), historically much more involved with mobility and central nervous system (CNS) impairments than sensory disabilities, became home to a special interest section on deafness in 1990 that has also given recognition to psychologists who have contributed to the field through biennial awards. Increasingly, papers on deaf-related issues are appearing in the association's journals and convention programs.

As for psychiatry, in the 1970s, a similar transformation occurred in the American Psychiatric Association when seminal papers dealing with psychiatric issues of deaf individuals written by prominent psychiatrists, including those affiliated with the New York State Psychiatric Institute project mentioned earlier, were published. A coterie of psychiatrists working with deaf people exists within the American Psychiatric Association. American Psychiatric Association journals and other psychiatric journals will occasionally publish articles related to psychopathology in deaf people.

In the 1970s, a group of deaf social workers in what was then the American Society of Deaf Social Workers (founded by Sanremi LaRue, Steven Chough, Bernice Hooper, Martha Sheridan, Barbara White, and William Ortega) decided to attend the national convention of the National Association of Social Workers (NASW). They had requested sign language interpreters for conference presentations, but the organization did not provide enough interpreters to meet requests for service. The ADA of 1990 was the catalyst that impelled NASW to improve interpreter services for their conferences (B. White, personal communication, October 22, 2014). With interpreter access provided, deaf social workers now participate in the Council on Social Work Education annual program meetings to ensure accreditation for training programs and provide a pathway for deaf students in social work. This only happened when the Council on Disability and People with Disabilities had members, including deaf social workers such as Barbara White, Martha Sheridan, and Elizabeth Moore, who worked together to ensure that the annual program meetings were accessible to all (M. Sheridan, personal communication, October 22, 2014).

According to Kendra Smith (personal communication, November 9, 2014), the responses to requests for sign language interpreters as part of the American Counseling Association (ACA) conferences have unfortunately been mixed, usually poor, even though this organization does, in a limited way, understand its obligation to provide access. This organization has in fact requested that all deaf attendees go to the same presentations to reduce interpreting costs, thereby limiting the concept of functional equivalence (meaning that everyone has the freedom to attend whatever sessions they select). However, to their credit, the ACA governance has provided special funds to meet the communication needs of deaf and hard-of-hearing attendees in professional development activities hosted by the District of Columbia Counseling Association. In contrast, the American Mental Health Counseling Association (AMHCA) is more accommodating in providing interpreters for whatever sessions are chosen. No deaf counselors have been involved in the governance of both organizations thus far. The American School Counseling Association (ASCA) has been most accommodating of the needs of deaf counselors in terms of interpreting access (Linda Lytle, personal communication, November 7, 2014; Cheryl Wu, personal communication, November 10, 2014). Dr. Cheryl Wu (personal communication, November 10, 2014) is spearheading a project to adapt ASCA's national model of comprehensive school counseling for school counseling programs in deaf education settings, considering the need for awareness of unique needs and issues, including communication access.

Deaf Culture: Its Impact

Over the last few decades, an interesting psychological dynamic has arisen. Today, some deaf constituencies have had a strong reaction to the perception of deaf as pathology. This is the result of a number of influences. One was the all-too-common repression, exclusion, and denigration of deaf people by the majority hearing society (e.g., Branson & Miller, 2002; Burch, 2002). For example, historically, deaf people were all too often denied the right to use American Sign Language. They were not permitted to teach ASL in most schools for the deaf, and if they were permitted, it was usually to teach vocational trades (Andrews & Franklin, 1997; Vernon, 1970). Only a few managed to attain lower-level administrative jobs, and there were no deaf educators serving as heads of schools up until the last few decades. Deaf applicants were refused admission into teacher-training programs and graduate schools, even at what was known then as Gallaudet College (now Gallaudet University), an institution of higher learning for deaf students. The rationale for this discrimination was that deaf people would not be able to emphasize articulation (speech) training because they could not hear (Winefield, 1987). Irene W. Leigh herself remembers that, in the 1960s, when a contingent of teacher trainers observed her teaching a class of deaf preteens, they remarked on her ability to correct speech despite the fact she was deaf, not on her ability to teach content, thus illustrating the ongoing focus on speech training at the time. According to Deaf scholars Cripps and Supalla (2012), spoken language has dominated the landscape of Deaf education and consequently sign language has been relegated to the back door. Today this is changing, with attention now being directed to ASL/English bilingual methods and with qualified deaf applicants being accepted into teacher-training programs throughout the country, including Gallaudet University.

Another current development that has occurred is the increase of Deaf professionals who successfully earn doctoral degrees and now are joining the ranks of professors at community colleges and universities. Staff at hearing universities with Deaf faculty are finding that while they have in place support services for Deaf college students they do not necessarily have in place services or due processes for Deaf professors (Smith & Andrews, 2015). There has been at least one case, a costly lawsuit. In 2011, a Lubbock county jury provided a $500,000 award to Dr. Michael Collier, a Deaf professor at Texas Tech University who faced discrimination, having been dismissed without due process (Carver, 2011).

Across all types of jobs and professions, the pervasive implication of "deaf can't" psychologically means that deaf people had to either develop an inferior sense of self or believe in themselves and fight against society's limitations on their dreams. After Stokoe's seminal work on the recognition of ASL as a bona fide language, deaf people took the lead in arguing for the existence of a Deaf culture with roots in ASL. Carol Padden, currently dean of the Division of Social Sciences at the University of California San Diego, was a Deaf linguist who in 1980 wrote a seminal article arguing for the existence of an American Deaf culture (Padden, 1980). Her thoughts about this culture were further elaborated in two books co-authored with Tom Humphries: *Deaf in America: Voices from a Culture* (1988) and *Inside Deaf Culture* (2005). Other deaf scholars such as Benjamin Bahan, Barbara Kannapell, and Paddy Ladd also created anthropologically based scholarly work that focused on the importance of language and culture within the deaf community. (See Chapter 2 for further elaboration of the deaf community and Deaf culture. Note also that the lowercase *d* reflects the inability to hear, whereas a capital *D* typically represents a group of people who share a signed language and culture.) Bahan (2008) in particular emphasizes that Deaf people are "people of the eye," a term that has been attributed to George Veditz back in 1912 when he, as president of the National Association of the Deaf, wrote in his President's message: "The deaf are . . . first, last, and all the time the people of the eye" (Lane, Pillard, & Hedberg, 2011, p. vii). The point being made here is that these deaf people are reliant on their eyes to access and interact with their environments, using a visual language (sign language) that brings them together. This phrase contrasts with the term Deaf. Even though this term formally refers to Deaf culture, people who hear the word "Deaf" will often immediately associate it with inability to hear. Using "people of the eye" shifts that focus to one that centers on vision. However, "Deaf" and not "people of the eye" is what deaf people are more likely to use as a self-reference descriptor. Additionally, this term is problematic for individuals who are DeafBlind and feel connected to Deaf culture.

The concept of Deafhood is far more recent. Paddy Ladd (2003) initiated discussion of this concept, defining it as a Deaf consciousness that incorporates the processing and reconstructing of Deaf ways of being, and thereby becomes a way of actualizing oneself as a Deaf person. This process is continually changing, depending on the type of situation the person is in, whether hearing or deaf, and is usually framed in a positive sense. Because it is always changing, Ladd sees it as ensuring the flexibility of membership within the culture of Deaf people. However, there are multiple perceptions of what Deafhood means, and some have broadened this concept to include all the diverse ways of being deaf, not just in the cultural Deaf sense. Kusters and De Meulder (2013) write that, even though the Deafhood concept is very wide and vague, that is a strength. They see the focus as being on the self-exploration of *deaf* (italics in original) individuals and groups and the various ramifications of this self-exploration. Ladd (2015) has further expanded Deafhood in a global sense, in terms of "valorizing the process of searching for global Deaf commonalities while identifying and respecting Deaf diversity" (p. 284).

The deaf pioneers of the Deaf culture, the "people of the eye," and Deafhood concepts have also been supported by hearing professionals, including most notably Harlan Lane, a specialist in the psychology of language and linguistics and a recipient of a MacArthur fellowship. Dr. Lane has written extensively about the literature under the rubric of "psychology of the deaf" (e.g., Lane, Hoffmeister, & Bahan, 1996). He lambasted studies that encouraged the perception of deaf people as deviant, deficient, and pathological—studies that were too often based on questionable methodology and that did not sufficiently take into account numerous factors that might have differentially influenced study results. His work has focused on the importance of sloughing off negative perceptions of deaf people and negative research information about deaf people based on faulty psychological measures. His goal was to get professionals to recognize their detrimental attitudes towards deaf people and their tendency to pathologize deaf people instead of analyzing their strengths in addition to their limitations. They now listen more to deaf people while developing research protocols (Mertens, 2014). At this point, psychological research is now focusing more on strengths and what works for deaf people, and courses in psychology and deaf people have as their goal the increased understanding of how deaf people function psychologically.

In recent work, Lane and colleagues (Lane, Pillard, & Hedberg, 2011) have moved beyond Deaf culture and argued for the need to classify deaf people as proud members of an ethnic group in contrast to the perspective of deaf as disability. In their book, *People of the Eye*, they explain that Deaf people do meet the requirements of ethnicity in that Deaf is a collective name representing a certain group of people, with a shared language (a signed language); feelings of community (with Deaf peers); behavior norms (based on Deaf cultural expressions); distinct values, cultural knowledge, and customs; social/organization structures such as Deaf organizations, Deaf churches, Deaf conventions, etc.; arts that show the Deaf experience (in literature, paintings, sculpture, and so on); a shared history; and a sense of kinship based not necessarily in the same geographic place but rather on a sense of human connection and solidarity related to the use of vision for language and communication. They also add the biological argument that genetic factors cause people to be deaf, therefore supporting the ethnicity perspective.

Considering that deaf people also identify themselves as members of the ethnic groups they are born into, whether they can claim a separate ethnicity as a deaf person is an intriguing and controversial point. Lennard Davis (2008), a hearing son of deaf parents and a distinguished professor of liberal arts and sciences, argues that the biological aspect typically refers to race rather than dysfunctional ears or genetic causes for deafness. Additionally, people tend to be born into ethnic groups, but not necessarily into Deaf culture if they have hearing parents, as a large majority do (see Chapter 2). If their life circumstances include exposure to Deaf culture, they may choose to be enculturated into this culture.

To get around this biological point, Eckert (2010) coined the term *Deafnicity*. Its source is the ancient Greek concept of *ethnos*, which he defines as community of origin, community of language, and community of religion. Community of origin commonly assumes a biological or blood relationship, but Eckert argues that it can encompass the notion that Deaf people are part of a community of culture and education. The fact that culturally Deaf people share languages that are signed and visual supports the concept of a community of language. And finally, community of religion does not refer to the typical concept of religion. Rather, this concept derives from the ancient Greek meaning of religion as based on a collective consciousness of a Deaf worldview. Clearly, this is not the final word on the existence of a Deaf ethnicity, and discussion as to whether Deaf people are an ethnic group or not continues.

From a psychological perspective, all the theoretical frameworks of who and what deaf people are that have emerged in recent years have served to emphasize the point that as a variety of the human race, deaf people are entitled to have their place in the sun as a vibrant group of people and have unique, positive ways of functioning. However, considering the reality that getting to their place in the sun often involves the need for resilience in a world that is not always accommodating of the visual needs of deaf people, Dirksen Bauman (hearing) and Joseph Murray (deaf) (2010; 2014) have expanded the psychological implications of being Deaf to incorporate the notion of gain, using the term *Deaf gain*. In view of the trend towards educational mainstreaming of deaf students and the minimization of Deaf identities, they have written extensively about the areas in which Deaf is a gain, from a cognitive, cultural, and creative diversity perspective, as contrasted with hearing loss and its functional implications. For example, visual ways of being can reinforce visuospatial abilities; the emergence of Deaf space has encouraged an approach to facilitate the use of space not only for deaf people but also for hearing people (Byrd, 2007); and society would become more engaged in the use of eye contact together with visual nuances of communication as these would highlight a broader notion of communication paradigms. Psychologically, this reframing of Deaf as Deaf gain serves to portray what it means to be Deaf in a positive light, and therefore being Deaf can be more positively perceived by society in general rather than being denigrated due to the notion that Deaf is a limitation.

The scholarly work on Deaf culture has resulted in deaf people embracing the notion that they are part of a culture and do experience positive quality of life as Deaf people. Another result is the increased use of ASL in schools and classes as part of a bilingual method of teaching deaf students. The other involves increased opportunities for deaf professionals to become teachers and administrators, bringing with them the knowledge and expertise of optimal visual pathways to learning. Following McDaniel College, the Gallaudet University teacher-training program finally opened its doors to deaf applicants in the early 1960s, at a time when most colleges were still refusing to admit deaf students into their teacher-training programs, in order to provide deaf students with opportunities equal to those of hearing students. Other institutions such as Lamar University followed, thus creating a larger cohort of deaf teachers, deaf administrators, and deaf doctoral level leaders (Andrews & Covell, 2006).

The climatic culmination of all these changes occurred in March 1988, when a late-deafened psychologist, I. King Jordan, was named president of Gallaudet University (Armstrong, 2014; Christiansen & Barnartt, 1995). A week earlier, the Gallaudet University Board of Trustees had selected an "outsider," a hearing woman without expertise in deaf people and with no ability to sign. At that time, this 124-year old college for the deaf had always had hearing presidents, but this time the deaf student body, deaf faculty, and deaf alumni erupted in open rebellion at what they rightly perceived as an outrageous insult to the competency and integrity of deaf people. Considering that, for example, majority African American higher education settings have Black presidents and colleges for women have female presidents, deaf people felt their time had come. After a week of strong protests covered in great detail by national and international television, newspapers, and other media, the trustees backed down and named Dr. Jordan as president. Interestingly, it would be another 20 years before the first "born deaf" president, T. Alan Hurwitz, Ed.D., assumed the presidency of Gallaudet University. During these two decades, the proportion of Deaf faculty, staff, and administrators increased as well (Armstrong, 2014). At the time of this book's publication, we now have another "born deaf" president following President Hurwitz at Gallaudet University, this time a Deaf woman, Roberta "Bobbi" Cordano.

The 1988 Deaf President Now event was a seminal moment in the process of internalizing a sense of Deaf pride and Deaf culture hegemony and recognition that Deaf is a human difference, not a deficiency. As implied earlier, the issue of whether being deaf is a disability has collided with the perception of Deaf as a cultural difference. It is true that many of the cultural dimensions of deafness—such as the use of sign language and facial expressions to communicate, a sometimes lack of subtlety in interpersonal relationships, overt ways of getting the attention of others, and so on, have often been perceived by society and professionals in the field as pathological instead of as human differences that represent effective communication from the perceptions of deaf people themselves. However, there are some aspects in which being deaf is a disability. When it comes down to reality, most deaf people realize this and accept the fact as evidenced by their fight for their rights under the Americans with Disabilities Act of 1990 (amended in 2008), Social Security Disability and Supplementary Income provisions, and the Vocational Rehabilitation Act of 1978.

The point to be made is that the hearing population, including professionals, need to focus on and recognize the assets and positive aspects of deaf people. Psychologically, the pendulum has swung from a time when being deaf was viewed as a pathology that requires eradication to a limitation that can be corrected with current technology that can coexist with a cultural way of being that affirms the desire of deaf people to have their culture respected and the focus placed on their abilities, not limitations.

Conclusions

Psychologists, sociologists, anthropologists, linguists, educators, social workers, psychiatrists, counselors, and allied mental health professionals have played important supporting roles in changing the ways society perceives deaf people and their culture and in facilitating the ability of deaf people to achieve their potential and demanding more equality. In the final analysis, this may be the greatest contribution of these disciplines to the mental health and well-being of those who are deaf and hard of hearing.

Suggested Readings

Bauman, H-D., & Murray, J. (Eds.). (2014). *Deaf gain: Raising the stakes for human diversity*. Minneapolis, MN: University of Minnesota Press.
   This edited book elaborates the changing perspective from deaf as a lack to deaf as a gain. The reader will be exposed to debates from different disciplines about what it means to be human.

Holcomb, T. (2013). *Introduction to American Deaf Culture*. New York, NY: Oxford.
   The focus of this book is on how Deaf people are best understood from a cultural perspective and how they have adapted to today.

Maher, J. (1996). *Seeing language in Sign: The work of William C. Stokoe*. Washington, DC: Gallaudet University Press.

Pollard, R. Q. (1992–1993). 100 years in psychology and deafness: A centennial retrospective. *Journal of the American Deafness and Rehabilitation Association, 26*(3), 32–46.
   This article consists of a comprehensive retrospective of the history of psychology and deafness.

Note

1   Author note: This is an updated version of McCay Vernon, Ph.D.'s chapter on historical perspectives of deaf people and psychology, published in Andrews, J., Leigh, I. W., & Weiner, T. (2004). *Deaf people: Evolving perspectives from psychology, education, and sociology*. Boston, MA: Allyn & Bacon. Robert Pollard, Ph.D., has graciously given permission for the inclusion of additional information from his article: Pollard, R. Q. (1992–1993). 100 years in psychology and deafness: A centennial retrospective. *Journal of the American Deafness and Rehabilitation Association, 26*(3), 32–46.

2 The Deaf Community
A Diverse Entity

Clearly, there is no one typical deaf person, nor a single identity that all deaf people share.

Holcomb (2013, p. 67)

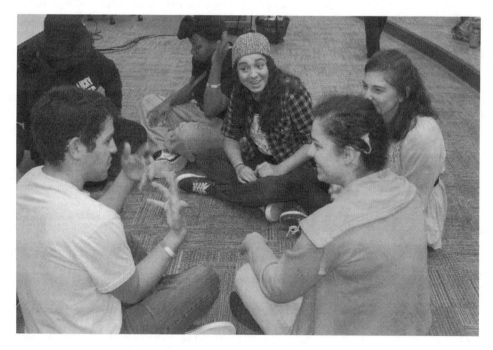

Figure 2.1 Photo of young people on the floor
Source: Used with permission.

The deaf community has a vibrant history. It is rich and diverse, with Deaf people having various backgrounds and experiences. The deaf community is a fluid, evolving community that provides many deaf people with a place they can call "home." We view the deaf community and Deaf culture as valuable resources for professionals in the fields of medicine, hearing health, psychology, the social sciences, and education, as well as for deaf, hard-of-hearing, and hearing parents and their deaf and hard-of-hearing children.

Chapter Objectives

In this chapter, we provide demographics for the deaf and hard-of-hearing population. We examine the medical and cultural models and challenge negative stereotypes of socially isolated and deprived deaf individuals. We then discuss the deaf community's diversity and the transmission of Deaf culture. Our description of Deaf culture—its history and heritage, its art and literature, its customs, values, and collective set of common experiences—focuses on what might be helpful in understanding and working with deaf and hard-of-hearing people.

The Deaf Community: Prelude to Demographics

When people refer to the deaf community, what often comes to mind is the picture of a community of people signing. One way to define the deaf community is to see it as comprising "those deaf and hard-of-hearing individuals who share a common language, common experiences and values and a common way of interacting with each other and with hearing people" (NL Association of the Deaf, n.d.). It is easy to think of this community as a monolithic entity. But in actuality this term represents a very diverse entity with demographic, audiological, linguistic, political, and social dimensions. There are international, national, regional, and local deaf communities that share and work together to achieve common goals (Friedner & Kusters, 2015; Goodstein, 2006; Holcomb, 2013; Moores & Miller, 2009). The deaf community includes deaf children (both spoken and sign language users) of hearing parents, deaf children of Deaf parents, hearing members who participate as parents of deaf children, hearing children of Deaf adults (popularly known as CODAs, which stands for children of deaf adults), marriage or life partners, siblings, and so on (see further description later in this chapter). The term *deaf* is used to denote individuals with hearing differences that preclude the understanding of speech through hearing alone, with or without the use of auditory amplification. In contrast, the term *Deaf culture* refers to individuals within the deaf community who use American Sign Language (ASL) and share beliefs, values, customs, and experiences (Holcomb, 2013). These Deaf individuals are not only deaf offspring of Deaf parents; they are also deaf individuals with hearing family backgrounds who learn about Deaf culture in adolescence or adulthood, if not earlier.

History shows that deaf communities in America have typically emerged where there are deaf schools and deaf religious settings or where there is a critical mass of deaf individuals. Many organizations of the deaf were established during various functions at state schools for the deaf as well as in deaf religious organizations. For example, the New England Gallaudet Association was formed in 1853 during a reunion at the American School for the Deaf in Hartford, Connecticut. Deaf religious leaders, including Reverend James Fair in Beaumont, Texas; Father Tom Coughlin, a Catholic priest; and Rabbi Yehoshua Soudakoff, have played and are playing important roles in providing religious services that bring deaf people together in their communities for religious education and fellowship.

However, unlike earlier deaf generations, recent generations get together less often in person at clubs to exchange news, ideas, signs, and stories. With the proliferation of captioned television and movies, the Internet, electronic mail, smartphones, relay services, and mainstreaming, which facilitates virtual interactions, small regional and local Deaf clubs and settings have diminished in numbers across the country. Yet the preservation and promotion of the psychosocial aspects of the deaf community still exists through alternative means: home entertainment, conferences sponsored by organizations such as Deaf Senior Citizens and the National Association of the Deaf, sports competitions, Deaf festivals, alumni events, and, of course, the Internet. Speaking of the Internet, as one Deaf American stated, "My smartphone is my Deaf-Space. . . . I go there . . . for Deaf people" (Kurz & Cuculick, 2015, p. 225).

Deaf Americans—children and adults—are as ethnically diverse as the general population and reflect changes similar to, for example, the increase in Latino/a and Asian populations (Census, 2010). When we write that Deaf Americans are diverse or multicultural, we mean that they differ, not only in skin color or ethnic heritage, but also in a variety of dimensions: degree, age, extent of hearing difference, etiology, gender, geographic location, country of birth, language use, communication preference, use of vision and technology, educational level, occupation, religion, and socioeconomic background. Many of them have a unique Deaf perspective, based on their backgrounds and experiences.

Demographics

There are no hard and fast data on the number of deaf and hard-of-hearing individuals. The last actual census of deaf people in the United States was done in 1971 (Schein & Delk, 1974). However, we do have estimates, but the caveat is that estimates are approximations, not actual numbers. This is due to the fact it is difficult to get accurate data because there is a lack of uniformity in defining the term *hearing loss*. Different surveys ask for information about hearing levels in different ways. For example, respondents may be asked if they have trouble hearing, and this classification is very broad. Or they may be asked if they are deaf or hard of hearing. And less often, they could be asked about their specific level of hearing loss. Self-reports are not always reliable.

Worldwide, it is estimated that 360 million people (328 million adults and 32 million children) have hearing loss, defined as 40 dB[1] or greater in adults and 30 dB or greater in children, using the better ear (World Health Organization, 2014). In the United States, the numbers differ, depending on which organization provides these and how the estimates are calculated. Blackwell, Lucas, and Clarke (2014) analyzed data from the 2012 National Health Interview Survey and calculated that approximately 35 million, or 15 percent, of American adults age 18 and up report having a little trouble hearing all the way through a lot of trouble hearing or deaf, with women less likely to report hearing issues. Based on National Health and Nutritional Examination Survey data (collected during cycles between 2001 and 2008) of participants whose hearing was tested, Lin, Niparko, and Ferrucci (2011) estimated that 30 million individuals aged 12 or older have hearing loss in both ears (12.7 percent of the population) or 48 million (20.3 percent) when individuals with hearing loss in one ear are added. This is similar to the estimate provided in the Preface, specifically 45 million Americans. In addition to the 30–48 million figure, which does not include children below the age of 12, Lin et al. demonstrated that prevalence nearly doubled with every age decade, with the prevalence rate for those who were aged 80+ being eight times greater than for those aged 12 to 19. Additionally, women and African Americans were significantly less likely to have hearing loss at any age. Blackwell et al. (2014) also indicated that 18 percent of males are likely to have hearing loss compared to 12 percent of females. They report that the numbers of persons over age 65 with hearing loss in the United States currently exceeds 14 million. Percentage-wise, approximately 74 percent of this population has hearing loss compared to approximately 6 percent of those in the 18- to 44-age range. In terms of race (their classification), compared to 16.2 percent of Whites, the African American percentage for those with hearing loss was 10 percent; Asian, 9.7 percent; Hispanic/Latino, 11 percent; and American Indian/Alaska Native, 12. 9 percent. White males were significantly more likely to have hearing loss compared to White females as well as African American males and females. The prevalence is greater for those who are not high school graduates than for college graduates. Looking at poverty status, the poor, near poor, and not poor groups reflected approximately 16 percent with hearing loss overall. Essentially, in reference to family income, the more income there is, the greater likelihood there is for lower incidence of hearing loss. As for sudden deafness, approximately 4,000 new cases occur each year (www. deafandhoh.com/hearing_loss_statistics.html).

Additional data derived from the U.S. Census Bureau (2010; see also Task Force on Health Care Careers for the Deaf and Hard-of-Hearing Community, 2012) support the basic finding that within the population of deaf and hard-of-hearing individuals, incidences of deafness are higher among the White/Latinos who consider themselves White population

(85 percent) compared to African American/Black (7.9 percent), Asian American (2.4 percent), and American Indian/Alaskan Native (1.1 percent) populations. It is common knowledge that Hispanics/Latinos now comprise the largest ethnic/cultural minority group in the United States. Projections indicate that by 2050 that number could approximate 128 million (U.S. Census Bureau, Population Division, 2012). More specifically, 1 in every 8 Americans is Hispanic/Latino now, and in less than 50 years, 1 in every 4 Americans will be Hispanic/Latino. Roughly 15 million are 21 years or younger. In this school-age group, nearly 10,000 are deaf or hard of hearing (www.lifeprint.com/asl101/topics/trilingualism.htm#_Toc155264601155264601). This group of 10,000 represents approximately 28.4 percent of the entire deaf/hard-of-hearing student population in the United States and 40.8 percent of all deaf/hard-of-hearing students in the West (Gallaudet Research Institute, 2013). This certainly reflects the rapid growth of the Hispanic/Latino deaf and hard-of-hearing student population in comparison to Whites and other ethnic/racial student populations.[2] In fact, deaf children of color outnumber White children in Texas, California, and New York. They may become assimilated into Deaf culture when they attend a state or day school for the deaf or, if in the mainstream, later when they connect with other deaf peers either via the Internet or when they join deaf-related organizations. They often have to live in four worlds: the world of their families; the world of the dominant White culture; the world of the dominant Deaf culture; the worlds of Deaf American Latinos, Asians, African Americans, Native Americans; and so on. To meet these challenges, Deaf multicultural Americans have established national organizations to advocate for deaf and hard-of-hearing individuals from culturally diverse communities, as indicated in Chapter 9.

The immigrant population is currently estimated at approximately 41 million, and the number of unauthorized immigrants fluctuates around the 11 million mark (Nwosu, Batalova, & Auclair, 2014). We do not know the percentage of immigrants who are deaf or hard of hearing as these have not been statistically separated within the different ethnic/racial populations. However, it can be surmised that significant numbers of these populations can claim either immigrant status or parental immigration status, considering that nearly a quarter of children under the age of 18 have an immigrant parent (Mather, 2009). Newspaper reports indicate that dating back to 2010 one lawyer has approximately 250 Deaf immigrant clients who have come to the U.S. from Mexico, Guatemala, Honduras, El Salvador, and Colombia and are applying for asylum. Reasons cited for coming to the U.S. include social ostracization and persecution and the lack of advocacy, communication, education, and employment in their home country (Castillo, 2011; Tolan, 2015). Deaf immigrants declaring asylum are not refugees, but they have to prove they are being persecuted by their home country, in particular by being denied access to education and viewed as incompetent, therefore losing their human rights, before they are allowed to proceed on the path to U.S. citizenship (Tolan, 2015).

Children and Youth

Researchers using current data from universal newborn screening programs in the United States have reported aggregated data to be 1.6 babies identified with hearing loss per 1,000 births, ranging from 0 to 4.3 cases per 1,000 screened depending on the state (Center for Disease Control and Prevention, 2014). Statistics for otitis media, commonly known as ear infections, indicate that the incidence is approximately 48 percent at age 6 months, 79 percent at age 1, and 91 percent by age 2 (Donaldson, 2014). Donaldson also reports that poor urban children have a high rate of otitis media, as do Native Americans and Inuit children, while the incidence for African American children appears to be lower than for Whites in the same community. If untreated, otitis media can lead to loss of hearing.

Noise-induced

Approximately 26 million Americans have permanent, irreversible hearing loss that may have been caused or exacerbated by noise (National Institute on Deafness and Other Communication Disorders, 2014a). Additionally, among teenagers aged 12 to 19, as many as 16 percent report some type of hearing loss, perhaps in part from noise, substantiating the possibility that people are losing their hearing earlier in life.

Deaf

Numbers reflecting those who label themselves as deaf, meaning that they cannot hear without assistive devices, have not been consistently disaggregated from the statistics presented earlier. The best estimates we currently have are found in Mitchell's (2005) work. According to Mitchell, 2 to 4 out of 1,000, or close to 1 million, are functionally deaf, half of whom are 65 years or older. Fewer than 1 out of 1,000 became deaf before age 18. For deaf people who use American Sign Language and may identify as culturally Deaf, the estimated number is 375,000, or 19 percent of the population (Mitchell, Young, Bachleda, & Karchmer, 2006).

Vision

United States general population statistics indicate approximately 20 million reported having trouble seeing even with glasses or contact lenses, or being blind (Blackwell et al., 2014). Prevalence rates indicate no difference between men and women (Dillon, Gu, Hoffman, & Ko, 2010). At least one study reports that older persons with visual impairment were more likely to have hearing loss (Chia et al., 2006). People with combined vision and hearing loss represent a heterogeneous population of children and adults who may have minimum combined vision and hearing loss either congenital or acquired or, in the most extreme cases, complete Deaf-Blindness. The National Center on DeafBlindness believes that there are over 10,000 children, youth, and young adults from birth to age 22 who have been classified as DeafBlind, meaning that the combination of hearing and vision issues are such that their educational needs cannot be managed in programs solely for deaf or vision-limited children (Miles, 2008). It is estimated that there are approximately up to 40,000 adults who have been classified as DeafBlind (Watson & Taff-Watson, 1993). According to the Gallaudet Research Institute (2013), approximately 6 percent of the deaf and hard-of-hearing student population have vision conditions, including low vision, legal blindness,[3] and DeafBlind. In addition, approximately 36 percent of this population has one or more additional conditions (not including vision conditions). The fastest growing segment of the population to be affected by combined vision and hearing loss are the elderly. It is estimated that within this group, between 8 and 10 percent have combined vision and hearing loss (www.visionaware.org).

Cochlear Implants

As of December 2012, approximately 324,200 people worldwide have received cochlear implants, and in the United States, roughly 58,000 adults and 38,000 children have received them (National Institute on Deafness and Communication Disorders, 2014b).

The Deaf Community: Frames of Reference

Despite the fact that demographics indicate that the deaf and hard-of-hearing population is indeed diverse, there have been attempts to provide relatively homogenous descriptions of this population. The terminology used by the medical and deaf communities to label deaf Americans reflect different perspectives, with implications for how deaf people are treated by professionals and society in general. In the popular media, much has been written on how divergent the medical/disability and the cultural/linguistic models of explaining social perspectives of deaf people are. However, textbooks typically do not write about how each model affects deaf Americans in their daily lives. We now explore these two perspectives.

Medical and Functional Frames

The role of medicine in identifying, preventing, or curing medical conditions; treating symptoms; and improving or maintaining physical functioning has become the backdrop for treating hearing differences as something to be ameliorated, remedied, or cured through medical treatment (Gonsoulin, 2001), including surgery, particularly for middle ear issues or cochlear implants. Without surgery, the focus becomes that of enabling access to sound through auditory technology (hearing aids and other assistive listening devices), accompanied by intensive auditory and speech training to facilitate the use of spoken language as a means of approximating the hearing ideal such that the deaf person can function like a hearing person. This intensive auditory and speech training is also indicated for children and adults going through cochlear implantation. Overall, this process gives rise to the implied message that to hear differently is to be disabled and therefore this condition is unacceptable.

Overtly or covertly, society often equates disability with powerlessness, incompetence, burdensomeness, abnormality, forced dependency, or a condition to be overcome by sheer motivation. Therefore, the deaf person may strive to be as "hearing" as possible, thereby denigrating the condition of being deaf and increasing the comfort of hearing individuals around them. Some professionals encourage parents to place their deaf children in public schools with hearing children in the interest of "helping" deaf children "overcome their disability" and fit into mainstream society. Users of ASL use a sign of a box, made outside the ear, to illustrate what they see as a focus on the ear. This sign, with its English translation of "pathological model," encompasses their feeling that the medical/disability view imposes restrictions on them by overly focusing on their access to communication through sound via the ear instead of through vision.

Professionals who subscribe to the medical model will tend to use terms such as *auditory handicap, disabled, hearing-impaired, congenitally deaf, hearing-challenged, hearing-disabled,* or *having hearing loss* because these terms focus on a biological deficiency and not on how deaf people function. Such medically tinged terms imply a condition in need of "correction" or repair, which can be viewed as stigmatizing for those individuals who do not think of themselves as needing to have their ears "fixed" or "cured," because they can rely primarily on vision as an alternative approach to communication. Rather, they prefer to view themselves as a distinct linguistic and cultural group seeking equal access to communication, education, and employment opportunities, just like other diverse Americans (DeLuca, Leigh, Lindgren, & Napoli, 2008; Holcomb, 2013) (see the following for further discussion).

The term *hearing impaired* is the generic term most often used by professionals, who tend to use the term *deaf* only for children or adults who have a profound hearing loss of 91 decibels (dB) or greater. The terms *deaf and dumb* and *deaf-mute* were used in times past, leading deaf children to be placed in asylums such as the American Asylum for Deaf-Mutes (www.ct museumquest.com/?page_id=7789). But deaf people are not mute—they can communicate and speak, and the term *asylum* connotes a caretaking facility for persons with intellectual disabilities or mental health issues, not a school where children are educated.

Physicians, audiologists, and other professionals do not see the medical/disability view as limiting. They see it more broadly in the context of the health of the entire human body, since many auditory disorders have medical correlates (e.g., vascular, renal, and heart problems; nervous and immune-system disorders; vestibular dysfunction, syphilis; tumors; fungal, bacterial, and viral infections of the cochlear; and ototoxity) that require medical treatment and management. Not all auditory disorders, of course, have medical correlates. Many deaf Americans enjoy good health and can be perceived as healthy, hearing difference notwithstanding. Many do go to physicians for issues related to their auditory systems, such as earwax buildup, ear infections, earaches, and tumors, or for cochlear implant surgery. Deaf Americans will use audiological diagnostic services at certain junctures of their lives to attain eligibility for educational services, vocational rehabilitation, disability benefits, auditory and visual assistive devices, interpreting services, and otherwise to obtain all the protections and services provided by the Americans with Disabilities Act and other legislation.

Those deaf individuals who reflect the perspective of the medical model are typically termed *oral deaf* (Reisler, 2002) or *spoken language users*. They are comfortable in hearing society, and often the majority of their social interactions are with hearing people. Although spoken language users may not necessarily use American Sign Language fluently or join Deaf culture organizations, they do utilize the technology that the deaf community can take advantage of as needed—*visual* technologies such as visual alerting devices, vibro-tactile devices, captioned telephones, close-captioned TV, real-time captioning, speech recognition software, and so on, as well as *auditory* devices such as hearing aids, cochlear implants, and assistive listening devices such as audio loops. They will tend to view interpreters who mouth words, captioned TV, video or captioning relay systems, hearing aids, and so on simply as tools for accessing auditory information, just as, for example, hearing persons use microphones, amplifiers, and telephones to access auditory information. Clearly, both spoken and sign language users recognize common needs and have worked together, as part of the deaf community, on joint projects such as captioned television, captioned streamed videos, captioning in movie theaters, and universal newborn hearing screening procedures.

While some professionals view deaf persons as unable to function independently in society without significant help from others, such as an interpreter, in contrast, deaf persons view the use of an interpreter as allowing them to function very independently in the hearing world. For example, with an interpreter, a deaf lawyer can fully participate in the trial of his or her client, a deaf Ph.D. researcher can easily participate in a group discussion about theoretical linguistics or any other scholarly discipline, and a deaf person can use an interpreter when dealing with doctors, lawyers, realtors, and others, so that he or she does not have to depend on friends or family members. Such are the different views.

Although the medical/disability model is important for its concern with overall health, it focuses primarily on medical and audiological intervention, with secondary attention being paid to early cognitive, linguistic, and socialization issues, particularly for those whose ability to decipher linguistic information is not sufficiently developed. It is important to note that the literature is replete with research studies on how children raised using spoken language are functioning cognitively, linguistically, and socially and illustrate for the most part the strength of this approach, particularly in cochlear implant users. In the view of culturally Deaf Americans, the model does not adequately take into account their early cognitive and linguistic needs and social-identity issues (see Chapters 4, 5, and 6 for further discussion). These individuals would like physicians, audiologists, and speech-language pathologists to learn about their Deaf culture and to share this information with parents and other professionals. Thomas Gonsoulin, M.D. (2001) asks his fellow otolaryngologists to think philosophically about these different perspectives and maintain dialogue with culturally Deaf members who would prefer to be viewed from a multifaceted sociolinguistic/cultural perspective.

The Sociolinguistic/Cultural Model

Within the framework of this model, medically toned considerations such as etiology, type and degree of hearing loss, and even age of onset make little difference to many culturally Deaf persons in terms of how they function as adults with their Deaf peers. Being a deaf person has more to do with one's identity as a "whole person." It involves their shared experiences, language, culture, attitudes, social obligations to each other, and quality-of-life issues and how they cope in daily life (Holcomb, 2013; Leigh, 2009). It involves comfort with who and what they are, a different way of being, not deficit based, and confers minority group status rather than disability status per se. It involves greater emphasis on visual orientation in comparison to reliance on audition.

> Being deaf is not a disease. It's not a sickness that needs to be healed or cured. Being deaf is a way of life. It's a culture with a language and members all over the world.
> (Megan Gleason, sister of a deaf young adult, 2014, p. 37)

As with other cultures, Deaf culture can be viewed anthropologically as an adaptive coping mechanism through which Deaf people have developed signed languages to accommodate their necessarily visual orientation. It reflects the phenomenon of "a conspicuous social group" exclusively for deaf people (Rée, 1999, p. 231), who coalesced in a shared sense of bonding as a response to a hearing society that afforded minimal opportunities for full immersion because of language and communication barriers. One of the strongest features of Deaf culture is an emphasis on social relationships with other deaf persons who share similar experiences.

Although American Sign Language (ASL) is of great value for those who identify with Deaf culture, it is more the shared experiences involved with being deaf that encourage diverse deaf persons, including spoken language users, to explore the community. Within the sociolinguistic/cultural model, signed languages are viewed as natural languages equal to spoken languages. Many deaf persons, however, will additionally use ASL signs in English word order to communicate with other deaf people or with hearing people. They may also use a signing system of English and/or written English and, if possible, spoken English, with hearing friends, family, and coworkers. Consequently, they are more often described as being bilingual,[4] or users of two languages, than monolingual in, for example, spoken English or ASL.

Deaf adults who use ASL are viewed as positive role models, and involvement with Deaf people as a group is seen as collaborating with them to promote access to the same civil rights, opportunities, and privileges other diverse Americans enjoy. In addition, Deaf adults may not perceive themselves as responsible for communication failure, misunderstanding, and language problems; rather, they attribute responsibility for inadequacy to the hearing person's inability to understand ASL or Deaf ways of being.

Generally, audiology, medical, educational, and hearing/speech professionals do not interact frequently with deaf people. Consequently, there is limited professional awareness about the daily lives of deaf people, including those who are well educated, although publicity in recent years has emphasized the full lives that culturally Deaf people lead. More often than not, professionals may be susceptible to describing Deaf culture members as lonely, isolated, and living in a limited world rather than as socially fulfilled through interactions with deaf peers. This is understandable, given the low incidence of deafness in the population. The fact that there is a book titled *Deaf Gain* (Bauman & Murray, 2014) indicates how much hearing society, including hearing professionals, need to learn about the advantages of being Deaf and how Deaf people maximize their quality of life.

Instead of viewing the deaf community as a haven for the unsuccessful or as an isolating, separatist lifestyle, Deaf Americans see their culture as providing positive opportunities to learn, grow, and expand their interests and hobbies; to serve as mentors for younger deaf people, particularly those with hearing parents and those in mainstream education programs; to develop friendships; to develop wider links to deaf communities at the local, national, and international levels through its networks of organizations and institutions as well as via the Internet; and to manage their own affairs (Holcomb, 2013). Worldwide, deaf people have formed national and international organizations that arrange regular events such as congresses, festivals of arts and crafts, theater presentations, and seminars (e.g., Ammons, 2009; Goodstein, 2006; Rosen, 2009). There were almost 10,000 participants from 121 countries officially registered at the 2002 international Deaf Way II conference (Goodstein, 2006). At this cultural event, there were presentations of Deaf theater, art, history and heritage, education, linguistics, and other issues relevant to the deaf community. Counteracting the separatist perspective, these organizational activities require working with hearing people in the larger society at varying levels.

Reading this, you can get a sense of the cultural capital that the deaf community can provide. Cultural capital incorporates the use of cultural knowledge, skills, abilities, and interactions to influence aspirations, socialization, language use, family patterns, and resistance to disadvantages (Yosso, 2005). Looking at the cultural capital wealth of Deaf culture, the use of visual language, visual learning, and the relationships with Deaf people who are fully engaged with life lends support to a protective factor for Deaf people who confront lower expectations projected by hearing people and work to counter these.

Hearing people unfamiliar with Deaf culture are usually puzzled by the split Deaf people make between *Hearing* and *Deaf* cultures. While Deaf people share many values with hearing Americans, they understand the concept of hearing culture and how hearing culture behaviors differ from Deaf culture behaviors. Hearing culture focuses on things people do because they hear; with their culture being based on sound, the ways they orient themselves, such as in getting the attention of others, differ from how Deaf people orient themselves (Holcomb, 2013). Deaf people are more like Native Americans, Asian Americans, or African Americans who live as a minority within a larger culture. In the case of Deaf culture, Deaf people see themselves as a minority culture that is vision based in contrast to the larger hearing culture. While Deaf Americans do not have their own style of clothing, food, or their own country, as is typical for other cultures, they do have unique features, most notably more lighting in their surroundings and the use of visual alerting devices such as flashing lights to signal sounds, such as doorbell systems, baby crier setups, and alarm clocks. Additionally, Deaf people use video relay services[5] while hearing people use the telephone. They also use hearing dogs, TV and movie captioning, computer-assisted note-taking, sign language interpreters and video interpreting services, the Internet, electronic mail, instant messaging via text and video, smartphones, and so on. Gallaudet University's Technology Access Program (TAP) researches accessibility issues using technology (www.tap.gallaudet.edu).

Professionals in audiology, rehabilitation, and medicine often refer to such technology as adaptive devices or auxiliary aids to compensate for a deaf person's inability to hear. In line with the cultural view, these are not compensatory but rather enhancement devices, referred to as visual alerts and electronic devices for communication and signaling. This view reflects many deaf people's emphasis on the importance of vision for communication and the centrality of vision in Deaf culture.

Deaf people use their eyes, their expressions, spatial relationships of signs, body movement, and touch far more than hearing persons do in everyday conversations. A high value is placed on how the hands are used, particularly with ASL, while hearing people use spoken language. Hearing people use their voices to get the attention of others while Deaf people may wave or tap shoulders. When persons are introduced, information such as the place of birth and the name of the school attended are often included (Padden & Humphries, 1988). The assigning of name signs is another custom unique to Deaf culture (Supalla, 1992).

Culturally Deaf people have their own folklore, including ABC story-poems, ASL stories and poetry, stories and narratives, puns, riddles, jokes, theater, and visual arts, which provide avenues for the expression of feelings about the Deaf experience (Baldwin, 1993; Bauman & Murray, 2014; Clark, 2009; Holcomb, 2013; Peters, 2000; more details provided later in this chapter). ASL storytelling is an art. Themes often center on success stories of deaf persons (Byrne, 2013; Padden & Humphries, 1988).

Differences also stem from how children acquire their culture and how this leads to differentiation between hearing and Deaf cultures. For hearing children, the home culture is transmitted through auditory experiences, including conversations, social rules and routines, songs, poems, radio, TV, and family stories. They learn from listening to their family members, teachers, and friends and from incidental conversations around them. Deaf children try to follow as well, but even with auditory aids, their auditory world is significantly different and less clear than the auditory world of hearing people, even with cochlear implants. Many of them will tend to perceive what is around them visually, and as they accumulate these visual experiences into a visual memory, this memory enhances their ability to think, communicate, problem solve, and generally relate to other people. Based on this experience, once exposed to Deaf culture, they will more readily adjust to the different cultural ways.

Because many professionals are less than optimally familiar with Deaf culture, the ability to inform parents about the many successful Deaf adults who use alternative visual communication strategies such as signing, with or without ancillary auditory strategies, suffers. Often, parents have to seek out this information about sign language and Deaf culture on their own (Christiansen & Leigh, 2002/2005). By the time parents learn about these facts, their children may be teenagers who are struggling due to inadequate mastery of English or because they think they are the only deaf persons in the world. However, evidence indicates that more parents are using sign language with their deaf children than previously thought (Christiansen & Leigh, 2002/2005). The supplement to the 2007 Joint Committee on Infant Hearing position statement (Yoshinaga-Itano, 2014) includes a section that recommends the availability of a system of highly qualified early intervention service providers for all families across the spectrum of communication choices, including not only listening and spoken language but also ASL.

It is when parents are *not* informed about the benefits of sign language and Deaf culture when told about different approaches that concerns many adult Deaf Americans. They view themselves as the "end product" of auditory rehabilitation plans, which traditionally have not optimally included visual components, such as the use of sign language or other visual enhancements to facilitate language acquisition. It is true that some Deaf people express frustration at having been denied sign language when growing up, having had to go through speech therapy and wear hearing aids with little benefit and find solace at "converting" into Deaf culture (Bechter, 2008; Holcomb, 2013). But there are also Deaf Americans who benefit from speech and audiology services, including hearing aids and cochlear implants (Leigh, 2009), who implant their deaf children (Mitchiner & Sass-Lehrer, 2011), and who are appreciative of the help. Today, more audiologists, speech therapists, and other early intervention specialists are incorporating signing in therapy plans based on empirical evidence that the use of sign language is not necessarily detrimental to the development of spoken language and is helpful in situations when auditory aids are not being used (see Walker & Tomblin, 2014, for a review).

There exists a diversity of opinion, depending on individual experiences and the extent to which deaf persons may or may not have had the hearing ability or training needed to benefit from some of these services. Deaf people do vary in their use of speech. Some consider it to be a restriction and denial of the need to communicate comfortably in their own language (ASL) (Padden & Humphries, 1988). Others use speech freely, and many will "mouth" English sounds silently while signing.

Many deaf Americans prefer to use descriptions based on a communication mode using designations such as these: strong-deaf, deaf, oral, strong-oral. These labels suggest the diversity of communication modes, such as ASL; English in a signed, spoken, or written mode; or a combination. These designations provide more information about communication than the term *hearing loss* but still provide an incomplete picture of the person's individuality, feelings, interests, strengths, special talents, and so forth (Corker, 1996).

Currently, psycholinguists consider language acquisition to be a dual-channel activity involving both auditory and visual processes. Neurocognitive scientists and linguists have reported that age of ASL acquisition is important. The earlier the deaf child is exposed to a signed language, the better it is for the child's cognitive and linguistic development, particularly if hearing aid or cochlear implant use is less than optimal and there is insufficient spoken language reinforcement (Walker & Tomblin, 2014). The language-learning capacity of the brain includes both auditory and visual capabilities. Focusing only on auditory stimulation will not consistently guarantee language acquisition for deaf children. Yes, unquestionably, there are children and adults who have successfully acquired spoken English based primarily on the use of auditory amplification (e.g., Blamey & Sarant, 2011; Leigh, 1999; Schwartz, 2007). But there are also deaf individuals who have struggled to acquire language through auditory-verbal approaches alone and survive in mainstream school systems (Oliva & Lytle, 2014).

Low reading levels have historically been ascribed to the use of sign language and attendance at state schools for deaf students. The fact is that while the median is at approximately the 4th-grade level (Qi & Mitchell, 2012), this is due to various psycholinguistic variables, including level of reading exposure, intelligence, socioeconomic status, etc., that create significant variability in English proficiency among deaf persons, whether in the mainstream or in specialized schools for the deaf, and low reading scores are *not* directly attributable to the use of ASL (e.g., Easterbrooks & Beal-Alvarez, 2012; Marschark, Sarchet, Rhoten, & Zupan, 2010; Trezek, Wang, & Paul, 2011). As an aside, it is interesting to note that at the very challenging national Academic Bowl competition among high school programs for deaf students (www.gallaudet.edu/ outreach-programs/youth-programs/academic-bowl.html) teams from both state schools for the deaf (predominantly ASL-based) and mainstream programs with deaf students (utilizing diverse communication modes) have demonstrated significant and advanced academic knowledge of diverse areas, including English literature, en route to top place finishes in this competition. www.gallaudet.edu/academic_bowl/history.html). Additionally, deaf children of culturally Deaf parents who are well educated typically have continuous exposure to sign language and tend to read better than or equal to deaf youth with less or no exposure to ASL.

But as in mainstream society, not all succeed. There are some Deaf Americans who are uneducated, underemployed, or unemployed who lead, in Deaf culture vernacular, a "no good" life (Buck, 2000). The most recent statistical estimates we have are based on Blanchfield and colleagues (2001), who used three nationally representative data sets to calculate that of the severely and profoundly deaf population over the age of 17, about 44 percent did not graduate from high school, compared to 19 percent of the general population. Further, only 46 percent of those who graduated from high school attended some college, compared to 60 percent of the general population. Only 5 percent of the deaf students graduated from college, compared to 13 percent of the general population. While underemployment is no longer a serious problem for deaf college graduates at entry levels (Schroedel & Geyer, 2000), both underemployment and unemployment continue to be serious problems for too many deaf individuals (Punch, Hyde, & Creed, 2004; Wilkens & Hehir, 2008). Unquestionably, the problems listed here are in large part related to society's failure to provide deaf people with equitable educational and employment opportunities or to the fact that the individuals concerned, for whatever reasons, fail to achieve their human potential.

With a better understanding of what consists Deaf culture, we now turn to an exploration of deaf community membership and how Deaf culture is transmitted.

Membership and Cultural Transmission

Deaf people have used and continue to use their language to pass down social norms, values, language, the arts, and technology to younger generations (Holcomb, 2013; Padden & Humphries, 1988; 2005; Van Cleve & Crouch, 1989). This deaf community phenomenon has been around for at least two centuries, perhaps more (e.g., Rée, 1999; Van Cleve & Crouch, 1989). Even though Deaf people are geographically dispersed in cities and rural areas, most live near large populations of other Deaf Americans, usually near a state school or university such as Gallaudet University in Washington, DC, the world's only liberal arts university for deaf people, or the Rochester Institute of Technology/National Technical Institute for the Deaf in Rochester, New York. Such proximity only serves to reinforce not only Deaf culture ways, but also bonds between deaf people with different backgrounds who can feel they are part of a larger deaf community. Not only that, the use of social media nationally and internationally via the Internet has created opportunities to participate in nonphysical deaf spaces and virtual Deaf communities, thus reinforcing the transmission of Deaf culture (Kurz & Cuculick, 2015; Valentine & Skelton, 2008).

Membership

Deaf Persons in Hearing Families

Most deaf persons are part of hearing families (over 90 percent, Mitchell & Karchmer, 2004) and learn about the deaf community and/or Deaf culture later in life when they meet Deaf adults at school; go to a summer camp with other Deaf youth; join a sports team of deaf players; attend a deaf club, religious event, or Deaf cultural festival; get information from the Internet; or find work with other deaf persons, even if they have been completely mainstreamed growing up. They may enter Gallaudet University or the Rochester Institute of Technology/National Technical Institute for the Deaf or a university/college/community college setting that enrolls deaf students and employs sign language interpreters. In these ways, they learn about Deaf culture. Many become comfortable in the culture, whereas others may stay on the fringe, and many will remain comfortably within their hearing communities.

Deaf in Deaf Families

Unlike most people who are born into their culture of origin, Deaf children who have culturally Deaf parents represent the minority in this culture. They most often grow up learning ASL; attend special schools for the deaf, deaf social gatherings; and, through everyday experiences, learn the values of Deaf culture (Holcomb, 2013; Padden & Humphries, 1988; 2005). These individuals enjoy a special status in Deaf culture and often become leaders in the community. For example, the four finalists for President of Gallaudet University in 2009 not only were Deaf and fluent signers; they also were all from Deaf families. And Roberta "Bobbi" Cordano, the first female President of Gallaudet University starting in January 2016, is also Deaf and from a Deaf family.

Hard of Hearing

From an audiological perspective, the term *hard of hearing* refers to individuals who fall into the moderate hearing loss category rather than the severely to profoundly deaf category (Leigh, 2009; Ross, 2001). However, this term has also tended to encompass individuals who mostly use speaking and listening, relying on their residual hearing supplemented by speechreading and auditory aids (Israelite, Ower, & Goldstein, 2002; Punch, Creed, & Hyde, 2006). Hard-of-hearing children with Deaf parents will often become part of Deaf culture. Hard-of-hearing children with hearing parents may also belong, depending on the extent of exposure to the deaf community, but many do not (Leigh, 2009). Most of these children are educated in public schools but experience difficulty with language development due to missed auditory cues (Ross, 2001). They may meet deaf peers in high school or college and get involved in Deaf teams or organizations, particularly if they have the ASL skills to transition between the hearing and Deaf worlds. They will often learn ASL and use it as a second language, although some will reject ASL because they do not wish to mingle with signing individuals (Vesey & Wilson, 2003).

Deaf Individuals with Cochlear Implants

When cochlear implants first emerged on the scene, many in the deaf community reacted negatively, fearing an assault on their beloved culture (Christiansen & Leigh, 2002/2005). Deaf adults who decided to try cochlear implants were regarded as traitors and betrayers of Deaf culture because of their desire to access the world of sound. As time passed, there was increasing recognition that deaf people with cochlear implants, including those who were culturally Deaf, were still using ASL and maintaining connections with their deaf communities. Currently, cochlear implants are not a deterrent to membership in the deaf community (Paludneviciene & Leigh, 2010), although there is still resistance on the part of some to pediatric cochlear implantation because of concerns regarding unrealistic expectations for spoken language development and potential aftereffects of surgery, among other things (Christiansen & Leigh, 2010).

Deaf Adoptees

A good number of deaf and hearing individuals are adopting and/or taking in foster deaf children from multiple countries worldwide. For a deaf child, it can be enormously beneficial to be adopted into a hearing or deaf signing family who understands the psychological, social-emotional, communicative, cultural, and educational ramifications connected with being deaf and can acclimatize the child into Deaf culture. In a study of 55 deaf parents of adopted children, a major finding was that deaf adoptive parents perceived much stronger social support from social networks within the deaf community than from formal service providers, primarily because of inaccessible communication and professional lack of awareness of the needs of deaf clients plus skepticism about the ability of deaf parents to parent (White, 1999). Deaf parents in the sample demonstrated an unconditional sense of entitlement to their deaf adopted children, including those with language delays who were older at the time of placement. The author explained this based on a "goodness of fit" paradigm for adoptive placements.

Like other transracial adoptions, deaf adoptees must grapple with physical differences compared to their adoptive families. Deaf adoptees may want to learn more about their biological families and home countries as they get older. Adoptive issues related to bonding and identity compounded by being deaf can become acute, especially during adolescent and early adulthood. White (1999) notes that more research is needed into the experiences of deaf adoptees and their families.

Late Deafened

Many individuals who acquire a hearing loss after age 18 due to disease, noise, trauma, or other causes will benefit from amplification or cochlear implants because of their memory for spoken language. They will generally retain speech skills, although distortions and tone variation can occur due to difficulty in monitoring vocal production and volume (www.alda.org/hearing-loss/). While late-deafened adults may rely on speechreading, many will find this fatiguing and inadequate and try to maximize their ability to use hearing aids or cochlear implants, although such devices will never approximate the hearing they used to have. Disruptions in career and family life are typical if communication adjustments are not made. There typically is a grieving process for the loss of sound communication and the ability to adjust varies. Late-deafened adults may learn ASL as a second language or use simultaneous communication (signs and speech). There is a lot of variation in how much speech and how many signs late-deafened people use. It is often dependent on their social networks and jobs. Some late-deafened persons will associate with deaf people to a greater extent because of the difficulty of speechreading and the ease of signing. Some will enter the deaf community and enjoy its networks of sports teams and organizations. Some choose not to, preferring to communicate with hearing persons. Most elderly people who experience hearing loss will fit into this latter category.

Hearing People

Can hearing people be members of the deaf community? What about hearing persons who marry deaf spouses, hearing children of deaf parents, siblings of deaf people, coworkers, and sign language interpreters? These hearing individuals with deaf family members often live in hearing-deaf cross-cultural environments, depending on the level of Deaf culture involvement of the deaf family members, similar to those who live in bilingual and bicultural families (Berkowitz & Jonas, 2014; Hoffmeister, 2008).

Growing up as a hearing child in deaf families can involve complex communication, socialization, and cultural issues within the home and within the extended family. As children, these hearing individuals might acquire ASL and internalize Deaf culture to varying degrees depending on family interest and background. They also learn English as a second language. For example, there have been studies of hearing toddlers of deaf parents in Puerto Rico who learned Puerto Rican Sign Language as their first language and Spanish as their second language (Rodriguez, 2001). Studies show they acquire both languages on the same timetable as other bilingual children do (Pettito, 2000).

Deaf parents, even if they rely primarily on signing, may also use speech in addition to signing with their hearing children (Mather & Andrews, 2008; Mather, Rodriguez-Fraticelli, Andrews, & Rodriguez, 2006). This is particularly true if these parents come from hearing families. Deaf parents will also expose their hearing children to hearing neighbors, relatives, TV, teachers, and peers in preschool for speech development. Those who grow up bilingually also internalize two identities, hearing and Deaf, and learn to navigate between them (Hoffmeister, 2008; Knight, 2013; Leigh, 2009). On the other hand, if deaf parents communicate with their hearing children using only speech, these children will more likely develop English as their primary language (Hoffmeister, 2008).

Often, the hearing family member becomes the "go-between" between the deaf family and the hearing society. This can be a burden, especially for a young child of deaf parents. In some cases, it is a source of conflict, as parents may depend on the child to be the family interpreter (Hoffmeister, 2008). However, because of recent developments such as video relay services (paralleling telephone discourse with sign language interpreters relaying messages), electronic mail, smartphones that provide video capacity for communication, and TV captioning, these burdens are less common (Knight, 2013). In adulthood, some of these children will leave their deaf heritage behind as they enter adulthood, never to return to the deaf community, whereas others stay, or leave and return.

A good number of hearing individuals who work with deaf people professionally may consider themselves to be part of the deaf community if they socialize comfortably with deaf people. The deaf community may welcome them depending on the degree of comfort in joint communication. If the communication remains awkward, acceptance into the deaf community is jeopardized.

The Role of Vision

The role of vision is crucial for membership in the deaf community, considering that communication is much more visual than audiological. DeafBlind persons cannot be considered "people of the eye" because their vision is limited or lacking. Their membership in the deaf community is facilitated by their use of sign language, either constrained within the individual's visual field or via tactile signing that involves feeling the hand movements. DeafBlind individuals have their own communication preferences (Bailey & Miner, 2010; Ingraham, 2015; Stoffel, 2012). Depending on the etiology and age of onset of hearing and vision loss, those individuals may use adaptive technologies, including amplification, cochlear implants, magnifying devices, and Braille, while others may use sign language, utilizing a tactile mode if needed. Special equipment includes computers with glare-reduced computer screens; Braille output devices; voice output devices; text enlargement programs; closed circuit televisions (CCTV); large-print or Braille watches; vibrating or flashing alert systems; Braille, amplified, or large button telephones; assistive listening devices; and computerized Braille note-taking devices, to name some. In a study of eight DeafBlind adults ages 47 to 91, Ingraham (2015) found they used a variety of adaptive and assistive technology, such as guide dogs, labeling kitchen appliances with tactile Braille dots, cochlear implants, speaker functions on telephones, Braille books, Braille readers on computers, FM systems, ASL, fingerspelling, large-screen televisions connected to text telephone, videophones, iPads with zoom text function, hearing aids, corrective lens for glasses, vibrating alarm clocks, Braille note-takers, talking computers, talking books, wireless microphones, adapted furniture such as lever door knobs, additional lighting, raised flooring, and handrails and grab bars throughout the home and Braille-adapted apps to keep track of food intake.

Those with Usher syndrome, a genetic condition that leads to blindness, may have been born deaf and brought up using sign language. On the other hand, an elderly person who gradually loses hearing and vision may use hearing aids and magnifying devices. The deaf community may subtly shun DeafBlind persons due to prejudices about tactile contact and fears of loss, given how deaf people depend on vision for communication, although many do make an effort to welcome them. DeafBlind Americans also have their own societies, organizations, and information networks but also interact with the larger deaf community (Bailey & Miner, 2010; Ingraham, 2015).

The Diversity Component

As indicated earlier in the demographic section, Deaf Americans have differences based on ethnic background and disabilities but also gender; alternative life styles (gay, lesbian, bisexual, and transgender); and religion, among others (Holcomb, 2013; Leigh, 2009). Recent autobiographies and biographies of minority-affiliated Deaf Americans have provided insight into what it means to grow up with a double or triple minority status. For example, Mary Herring Wright (1999), an African American woman deafened by age 10, writes about her experiences with racial segregation in the 1920s, particularly her recognition of painful injustices when observing how much better equipped and furnished White schools were compared to her African American school. And Andrés Torres (2009) describes his deaf Puerto Rican migrant parents and how they struggled to integrate into the streets of New York City. Raymond Luczak's (2007) edited book describes homophobic attitudes related to coming out as a deaf person who is gay or lesbian. A small quality-of-life study of Latino deaf and hard-of-hearing individuals focused on the importance of being able to participate in Mexican-related family cultural activities (Kushalnagar, Draganac-Hawk, & Patrick, 2015).

The cultural forces that draw deaf people together have also created institutional racism within the deaf community. Deaf people, like their hearing counterparts, may also discriminate against other deaf people who differ across dimensions of skin color, sexual orientation, gender, disability, or age (Gutman & Zangas, 2010; Leigh, 2012; Luczak, 2007). This is in part due to inadequate education and limited access to information and in part due to having been socialized toward "being normal" and therefore mirroring the intolerances of group differences exhibited in the larger society. However, recent years have revealed increasing rapprochement and acceptance of diversity within the American deaf community.

Hearing and Deaf Communities

In some communities, hearing persons have learned sign language in order to incorporate deaf citizens into the economic, religious, and social milieu of their communities. There are historical accounts of large numbers of deaf and hearing people in the eighteenth century who all used sign language with each other, living in communities such as Martha's Vineyard, Massachusetts; Heinneker, New Hampshire; and Sandy River Valley, Maine (Lane, Pillard, & French, 2000). Within an international context, such bilingual societies of hearing and deaf persons have also been reported and documented in, for example, the Bedouin community of Al-Sayyid (Kisch, 2004; Sandler, Aronoff, Padden, & Meir, 2014); Nohya in Central Yucatan, Mexico (Johnson, 1994); Adamorobe in Ghana (Kusters, 2015); and Desa Kolok in Indonesia (Marsaja, 2008).

Transmission of Deaf Culture

Unless the family is Deaf, Deaf culture is transmitted horizontally mostly through peer socialization rather than vertically from parents or caregivers to child (Leigh, 2009; Holcomb, 2013; Padden & Humphries, 1988; 2005). Many become part of Deaf culture through exposure, either during their school years if they interact with significant groups of deaf peers or later as they join Deaf organizations or meet Deaf people and become exposed to Deaf ways of being, with the Internet increasingly a factor. Exposure occurs in state schools where Deaf culture is introduced informally through Deaf peer and adult interaction as well as through direct teaching of Deaf culture; this can also occur in mainstream settings. Transmission can occur via Deaf art, theater, hobby, and sport groups; religious settings; Deaf festivals; Internet sites focusing on Deaf issues; state Deaf associations across the 50 states; and Deaf advocacy organizations such as, for examples, the National Association of the Deaf (NAD), Telecommunications for the Deaf (TDI), and the American Sign Language Teachers Association (ASLTA). Parents can be exposed to Deaf culture through the American Society for Deaf Children (ASDC) and Hands and Voices.

Accounts of the transmission of Deaf culture can be found in written histories of deaf people forming their own communities to minimize isolation, establish a system embodying their own values and beliefs, preserve sign language, chronicle their achievements, and transmit Deaf culture. Such accounts, including their wider historical context, are often available in historical descriptions of the founding of schools for the deaf as well as in the controversies surrounding the question of spoken versus signed languages (Van Cleve, 1993; Van Cleve & Crouch, 1989). For example, the repression of sign language during the early 1900s can be understood within the context of Darwinism and evolutionary theories that fostered the perception that sign languages were "primitive" and inferior to spoken languages

(Baynton, 1993). Since 1991, there have been regularly scheduled international conferences on Deaf history that examine such issues.

Professionals providing services to deaf children and adults have a role in the transmission of Deaf culture. Medical personnel and audiologists are often the first to identify the presence of hearing issues; they often are not familiar with the deaf community or Deaf culture aspects (Andrews & Dionne, 2008). If they were, they could discuss Deaf culture as a welcoming culture in addition to providing resources as needed. Ethically, professionals in early intervention programs should follow the supplement to the 2007 Joint Committee on Infant Hearing that recommends informing parents of newly identified deaf children about all language and communication opportunities, including the use of American Sign Language (Yoshinaga-Itano, 2014). Follow-up on this includes information about Deaf culture. Educators in the mainstream also have a responsibility to help deaf students learn about Deaf culture, so that these students know there is a community they can identify with if they so wish. The presence of professionals who themselves are deaf can provide a welcoming avenue to Deaf culture for people just learning about the culture. There are deaf audiologists and deaf early interventionists who can facilitate this process.

The scholarly field of Deaf Studies is yet another venue for the transmission of Deaf culture. This field incorporates Deaf history and heritage, politics, ASL literature, art, and theater. The focus is on encouraging students to look at the *whole person* rather than focus on the hearing loss. Students can develop new theories and views to explain the rich diversity of the characteristics of the deaf community and broadcast it wherever they go. Deaf Studies courses can be found in other curricula and disciplines, such as education, interpreter training, vocational rehabilitation, psychology, social work nursing, and special education. Most sign language classes will also incorporate Deaf Studies components. Academic programs in Deaf Studies have been established at Boston University, California State University at Northridge, Gallaudet University, McDaniel College, and Ohlone College among others.

The literature of Deaf Americans can also transmit Deaf culture through poetry, stories, plays, storytelling, films, TV shows, YouTube videos, and the like (Byrne, 2013). Many ASL stories have been passed down through the years as folklore or "Deaf lore." Deaf literature can also be stories and poems written in English, such as the works of Robert Panara and others (Harmon & Nelson, 2012; Peters, 2000), through adaptations of plays or poems into sign language, or through original sign language versions such as Clayton Valli's (1995) DVD of his ASL poetry. ASL poetry incorporates complex poetic forms using the linguistic parameters of ASL in playful and meaningful ways.

Early deaf drama groups in America consisted of weekend skits, mime shows, and signed songs and poems at local deaf clubs. The National Theater of the Deaf (NTD) was started in 1965, having evolved from the collaboration of hearing and deaf people in writing grants for funding. It has become a versatile touring company that performs nationally and internationally. Other deaf acting companies include Deaf West Theatre and New York Deaf Theatre among others. These theater groups provide public access to actors who use ASL to convey dialogue and provide unique cultural experiences for the lay public. The SignStage theater group, originally the Fairmont Theater of the Deaf in Cleveland, Ohio, focuses its efforts on presenting interactive educational programs in local schools using performing arts, ASL, and Deaf issues, in order to create a greater sensitivity to deaf people and other diversity issues (www.chsc.org/Main/SignStage.aspx).

In addition to these specialized theater groups, Deaf actors have also performed in plays; on TV; and in soap operas, movies, and commercials. This is a welcome change from the 1950s and 1960s, when hearing actors were typically used to portray deaf people. Deaf characters were portrayed as "mute dummies" or "mute imposters" or perfect "lipreaders." After deaf actors protested of discrimination in using hearing performers in deaf roles, casting and script writing changed. By the 1980s, television programs began to explore the complexity of deaf persons (Schuchman, 1988) and teach more about Deaf culture through soap operas, children's shows such as *Sesame Street*, and TV serials such as the popular *Switched at Birth*, which portrays actors communicating in ASL. Deaf actors have now distinguished themselves, one prime example being film and TV actress Marlee Matlin, who won an Academy Award/Oscar for her portrayal of Sarah in the film, *Children of a Lesser God*. A recent Broadway production of *Spring Awakening* produced by Deaf West Theater, which uses both Deaf and hearing actors, has received rave reviews. Television and radio celebrities such as Nanette Fabray and Rush Limbaugh have used entertainment media to openly discuss their deafness, all of which has contributed to the public's sensitivity and understanding of hearing issues.

Art enlightens deaf and hearing viewers by presenting visually rendered experiences seen through deaf eyes. Deaf artists have developed a specific genre called Deaf View/Image Art (De'VIA); the focus is on the use of art to express cultural aspects of the deaf experience, including sign language and difficulties with hearing aids or speech training. These artists incorporate formal elements such as contrasting colors, intense colors, and textures, as well as facial features such as eyes, mouths, and ears (www.deafart.org/Deaf_Art_/deaf_art_.html). There have been traveling art shows that showcase the work of deaf artists, including paintings, sculpture, woodcuts, photography, and drawings, most often at the Deaf Expo, university museums, and other venues (Andrews & Lokensgard, 2010). Sonnenstrahl (2002) has written a comprehensive history of deaf artists and their work from colonial to contemporary times.

Conclusions

Whatever their race, color, ethnicity, religion, gender, socioeconomic background, lifestyle, cultural orientation, mode of communication and language use, hearing status, education background, and use of communication technologies, deaf Americans function in both hearing and Deaf worlds. Many deaf Americans utilize a diversity of communication and languages depending on their family background, education experiences, and with whom they are communicating. They may gravitate between being "included" and being "excluded" in hearing environments if they have no interpreter or captioning or cannot understand what is being said. Inclusion happens when they do have appropriate auditory and visual access to communication through technology and sign language interpreting with hearing family members or with colleagues in the workplace. By the same token, if they understand their deaf peers, whether using speech or signs, they are included instead of excluded. Daily, deaf people negotiate these differences and tensions by using different communication modes: speech or sign; different signed, spoken, or written languages; technology aids such as speech recognition tools; or a combination of these, similar to the hearing bilingual/multilingual, multicultural, and multimodal person who codeswitches between two or more languages, cultures, and modalities (Grosjean, 2010).

Suggested Readings

Bahan, B., & Supalla, S. *ASL literature series*. San Diego, CA: DawnSign Press. (One 60-minute videotape of two classic stories based on the Deaf experience.)
   Bahan's fable, "Bird of a Different Feather," explores the differences of a bird within a family of eagles. Rather than accepting the bird's differences, the eagle family tries to apply a pathological approach to raising the unusual bird, an odyssey familiar to many deaf people. Supalla's "For a Decent Living" portrays a boy who is searching for his deaf identity by escaping from his hearing family and going on a journey to prove himself to his family and the deaf community (www.dawnsign.com).

The books listed here represent a brief selection of biographies and autobiographies covering how Deaf people live their lives:

Cyrus, B., Katz, E., Cheyney, C., & Parsons, F. (2005). *Deaf women's lives: Three self-portraits*. Washington, DC: Gallaudet University Press.

Lang, H., & Meath-Lang, B. (1995). *Deaf persons in the arts and sciences*. Westport, CT: Greenwood Press.

Luczak, R. (Ed.). (2007). *Eyes of desire 2: A deaf GLBT reader*. Minneapolis, MN: Handtype Press.

McDonald, D. (2014). *The art of being deaf*. Washington, DC: Gallaudet University Press.

Stoffel, S. (Ed.). (2012). *Deaf-blind reality*. Washington, DC: Gallaudet University Press.

Torres, A. (2009). *Signing in Puerto Rican*. Washington, DC: Gallaudet University Press.

Wright, M. H. (1999). *Sounds like home: Growing up black and deaf in the South*. Washington, DC: Gallaudet University Press.

Notes

1   dB is the standard abbreviation for decibel, which refers to the unit of measurement of sound intensity or loudness.

2   It is important to keep in mind that the data reported by the Gallaudet Research Institute covers only participating public schools that were recruited from a variety of sources, including a registry of programs that continue to participate, with or without interruptions, volunteers and referrals, lists provided by many but not all state departments of education, the *American Annals of the Deaf* directory of programs, and random selection from the registry of public schools in the Common Core of Data of the National Center for Education Statistics. Therefore the information most likely underrepresents actual numbers since data reporting is voluntary and may not catch many missing students (www.gallaudet.edu/rsia/research_support/demographics.html).

3   Legal blindness is defined as having 20/200 or worse vision in the better eye.

4   *Bilingual* is defined as having the functional use of two languages but not necessarily having native proficiency in both languages (Grosjean, 1998; 2010).

5   Video relay services enable deaf people to use a sign language interpreter as an intermediary via the Internet while making phone calls to hearing users.

3 How It All Begins

An audiologist will wind up her audiological assessment with a written evaluation that is sure to label the patient with "mild," "moderate," "severe," or "profound" losses across frequencies taken both singly and then as a whole. And even though textbooks and living audiologists alike will advise us all to be wary of such labels, they persist.

Brueggemann (1999, p. 133)

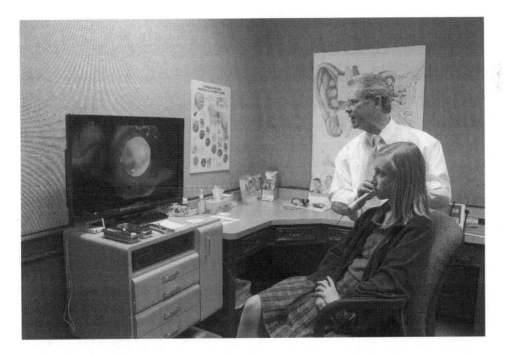

Figure 3.1 Photo of audiology session
Source: Used with permission.

For most people, "deaf" begins at the moment of identification, when hearing differences are reported. The reactions to this process carry the baggage of typical cultural perceptions of what it means to be deaf. Essentially, these perceptions involve the concept that "beyond sound are no human relationships, no government, no equality of existence, no inkling of knowledge" (Brueggemann, 1999, p. 106). In the eyes of those who rarely encounter deaf people, sound is life, and the lack of sound is the death of human connection. For this reason, many parents grieve when they realize their child has been identified as deaf and adults who used to be able to hear grieve as they experience the diminishing of their ability to hear. There is a full life after the identification of hearing differences, but it takes time for parents and others to realize this.

Chapter Objectives

This chapter explains why etiology is important and outlines the major causes of deafness. We discuss the importance of genetic information and the implications of genetic counseling for deaf and hearing people. Readers will become aware of the psychodynamics surrounding the identification process with particular focus on the reactions of both hearing and deaf parents. Having sensitive professionals who can appropriately provide services to parents during the period after identification—a difficult phase during which these parents are confronting the critical decisions they will need to make about audiological, communication, and educational interventions, including whether to proceed with cochlear implantation—is emphasized as important. We review psychological and ethical issues related to the identification process and follow-up intervention procedures.

Etiology: The Causes of Hearing Differences

The Significance of Etiology

If a person cannot hear, it means that the ear, auditory nerve, or brain is not doing the job of deciphering and interpreting sounds that these were designed to do. Multiple causes differentially affect hearing abilities, and the patterns of onset have implications for the psychological development and functioning of deaf children and adults. For example, if a child was born hearing and 2 years later contracted spinal meningitis that resulted in hearing, vision, and balance changes, this child's psychological experiences will differ from those of a child who is born deaf to deaf parents. Each etiology has its own sequelae; some cause only hearing loss or lack of hearing, while others may result not only in hearing issues but also changes or injuries in other sensory or neurological systems. Many deaf people are, to some extent, molded psychologically, not only by the functional effects of their hearing level, but also by physiological or neurological involvement depending on their specific etiology.

Recognizing the various ways in which each etiology and its potential consequences may interact with the environment and affect child development will therefore contribute to constructive audiological, linguistic, and educational approaches that can enhance psychological adjustment and educational progress. For this reason, differential diagnosis is of critical importance. It is facilitated by a good medical history that includes information about the hearing issues as well as the age of onset and other related factors. In the end, whatever the etiology, habilitative and educational needs for the deaf child often are complex and extensive and require long-term commitment (Marschark, 2007).

In our discussion of deaf people, we are basically looking at individuals with *sensorineural hearing loss*, defined as a hearing loss most commonly situated in the inner ear or, less frequently, in the auditory nerve, or both, and is the most common type of permanent hearing loss (www.asha.org/public/hearing/sensorineural-hearing-loss/). Sensorineural deafness can be congenital (dating from birth) or can occur at any time after birth. There may be delays in identifying deaf children with delayed onset if they are identified as hearing during universal newborn hearing screening (see later). Sometimes there are several possible causal conditions, such as deafness in the family and maternal exposure to diseases causing hearing difficulties.

Often the cause is unknown, but recent evidence indicates the importance of genetic factors (Morton & Nance, 2006). In contrast, there is conductive hearing loss, which happens when there is dysfunctional conduction of sound through the outer ear canal to the eardrum and the tiny bones (ossicles) of the middle ear (www.asha.org/public/hearing/Conductive-Hearing-Loss/). This condition is usually corrected with medical or surgical treatment.

Medical factors influence prevalence figures. For example, the rubella epidemic in the mid-1960s resulted in a temporary dramatic increase in the deaf population. Vaccines and medical advances not only have reduced incidences of hearing differences due to certain conditions, such as complications of Rh factor and rubella, but they have also increased incidences of hearing issues due to improved survival rates for infants, especially those born prematurely (e.g., Hille, van Straaten, & Verkerk, 2007; Marschark, 2007). For example, antibiotics help people survive meningitis, but the individuals often end up with changes in hearing ability (Worsøe, Cayé-Thomasen, Brandt, Thomsen, & Østergaard, 2010).

Here, we briefly present various leading causes of deafness to illustrate the complexity of etiological factors that will have implications for the developing child's psychological and educational pathways.

Major Nongenetic Causes of Deafness

Infections

The potential for particular infections, such as meningitis and those within the TORCH, group to contribute to hearing loss continues. TORCH infections are congenitally acquired infections, including cytomegalovirus (CMV), the herpes simplex virus, syphilis, rubella (German measles), congenital toxoplasmosis, and HIV among others, which can cause significant health and developmental issues in babies (Pediatrics Clerkship, 2013). Infections within the TORCH group occur when mothers pass infections through the placenta or during birth.

While viral meningitis may affect hearing, bacterial meningitis has been implicated as the most common infectious cause for sensorineural hearing loss and cochlear ossification (bone growth in the cochlea) (Du, Wu, & Li, 2006). Considering that meningitis is an infection of the membranes surrounding the brain, there is significant potential for neuropsychological sequelae (Brouwer, McIntyre, Prasad, & van de Beek, 2013), including, for example, aphasia, behavioral problems, emotional issues, impulse control, and distractibility in addition to vision, balance, and biochemistry changes. Since older children can verbalize symptoms, such as headache or stiff neck, earlier diagnosis and vaccination can occur before significant damage, including hearing loss, takes place (Weinberg, 2006). With infants and young children, diagnosis is easily delayed, with 15 to 25 percent developing sequelae such as deafness and neurological issues while up to 30 percent have mild residual issues including learning difficulties and mild hearing loss (Weinberg, 2006). Cochlear implants (see the Audiology Appendix for details) may be of benefit if inserted before extensive cochlear ossification sets in (Roukema et al., 2011). Roukema and colleagues additionally advise that language and speech outcomes will vary even in technically successful implantation.

Cytomegalovirus (CMV), a member of the herpes group of viruses, is typically a common infection with mostly mild symptoms, with 60 to 90 percent of adults being infected at some time (Pringle, 2014). However, congenital CMV has been identified as a major contributor to neurological and sensory impairment in children, including visual impairment, hearing loss, and intellectual disabilities (Dollard, Grosse, & Ross, 2007; Pringle, 2014). Out of 1,000 live births, the infection will be transmitted during pregnancy to less than 1 percent of infants, of whom 1–2 (0.1 percent) will exhibit permanent consequences (www.cdc.gov/cmv/trends-stats.html).

Infected children may not initially exhibit symptoms but experience progressive hearing loss (Dollard, Grosse, & Ross, 2007). Consequently, universal screening of hearing in newborns born with CMV infection can miss a significant number of cases. Ongoing hearing evaluations are critical for these cases. Emotional problems may be progressive or appear later. The extent of CMV in developing countries is likely high due to limitations in treatment availability.

Rubella, popularly known as German measles, is usually harmless except when the rubella virus infects a pregnant woman, particularly during the first trimester. Rubella has been significantly controlled by an effective immunization program in the United States, which was instituted after the last major rubella epidemic of 1964–1965, during which 50 percent to 90 percent of those affected ended up with some form of congenital rubella syndrome (www. historyofvaccines.org/content/articles/rubella). In this syndrome, while many exhibit only hearing loss, others may have visual and learning difficulties as well as intellectual disability, cardiac issues, and neurological problems (Caserta, 2013a; www.historyofvaccines.org/content/articles/rubella). Rubella is mentioned because of the 1964–1965 epidemic, during which at least 11,000 were identified as deaf. Adults may cite rubella as etiology, some of whom may also have other manifestations, such as behavior difficulties, language processing, and autism, that impact their quality of life (Vernon & Andrews, 1990). Globally, cases with rubella etiology continue to be reported. The varied, almost idiosyncratic way in which the rubella virus affects the auditory mechanism makes it difficult to predict potential benefit from residual hearing (e.g., Goldberg & Flexer, 1993; Vernon & Andrews, 1990).

Sudden sensorineural hearing loss has been associated with the herpes simplex virus, (Rubinstein, Jerry, Saraf-Lavi, Sklar, & Bradley, 2001), but this is relatively rare. This virus can cause nearly the same effects as CMV for infants born to infected mothers (Dahle & McCollister, 1988, as cited in Chase & colleagues, 1996). Twenty percent of the cases reviewed by Prasad, Bhojwani, Shenoy, and Prasad (2006) had otological issues, most commonly chronic otitis media (middle ear infections). A National Institutes of Health study reveals that 9 to 15 percent of children exposed to HIV during the mother's pregnancy are at greater risk for hearing loss (www.nih.gov/news/health/jun2012/nichd-20.htm). These children are also at risk for language, balance, and swallowing issues (Swanepoel & Louw, 2010) among other issues. Adults with HIV also have higher rates of hearing loss (Torre et al., 2015).

Infants affected due to congenital toxoplasmosis have up to a 26 percent chance for delayed onset hearing loss, therefore necessitating audiological follow-up (Brown, Chau, Atashband, Westerberg, & Kozak, 2009), and also are at risk for intellectual disability, seizures, or other neurological manifestations (Caserta, 2013b). Differential diagnosis can be difficult because of overlap of sequelae in various perinatal diseases, especially those caused by CMV, but early diagnosis will facilitate treatment.

Ototoxic Drugs

Drugs in the ototoxic category potentially may cause symptoms of hearing loss, tinnitus, imbalance, or vertigo. Particular care must be taken with aminoglycosides, a specific group of antibiotics including streptomycin, gentamycin, and neomycin among others (Rizzi & Hirose, 2007). These drugs tend to be prescribed in life-threatening situations. However, it is not always clear whether it is the disease or the treatment drug that causes hearing loss. Interestingly, it has been noted that some of those who lose their hearing subsequent to administration of aminoglycosides may have a genetic vulnerability for hearing loss (Bitner-Glindzicz & Rahman, 2007).

Abuse of some pharmacological and recreational drugs has also been implicated in sensorineural hearing loss, although this is not common (Lopez, Ishiyama, & Ishiyama, 2012).

Alcohol is also a culprit, with fetal alcohol syndrome creating the potential, not only for cognitive impairment, learning disabilities, facial anomalies, and behavior disorders, but also for hearing loss (Cone-Wesson, 2005).

Prematurity

This can result in permanent hearing loss, with approximately 10 percent of extremely premature infants (with gestation up to 28 weeks) affected (Robertson, Howarth, Bork, & Dinu, 2009). For premature as well as full-term babies, anoxia and trauma during delivery can affect not only hearing but also vision as well as cognitive and neuromotor development. Although medical advances have raised the survival rate for prematurely born infants, the risk of multiple disabilities is present.

Noise-Induced Hearing Loss and Hearing Loss Due to Traumatic Brain Injury

Noise-induced hearing loss (NIHL) is a significant problem, with approximately 500 million worldwide losing their hearing over time after exposure to entertainment or occupational noise (Alberti, 1998). In their review of statistics on NIHL, Griest, Folmer, and Martin (2007) report on estimates revealing that about 10 percent of Americans between the ages of 20 and 66 have permanent damage to their hearing and approximately 12.5 percent of school-aged children may have NIHL, possibly due to excessive exposure to noisy machinery such as lawn mowers, motorcycles, and loud music. Athletes who participate in high-contact sports such as soccer and football and who end up with concussions are at risk for brain injury that is often accompanied by balance problems and hearing loss (Omalu et al., 2005). For example, it is well known that I. King Jordan, a past president of Gallaudet University, lost his hearing at age 21 when he was thrown from a motorcycle and suffered a concussion.

Genetic Causes of Deafness[1]

It is helpful for professionals who work with deaf persons and their families to be aware of the complexity of various genetic manifestations of deafness and the effect they can have on the social, psychological, educational, and medical functioning of deaf individuals and how these may impact family members (siblings and offspring). Therefore, we provide some basic information to facilitate this awareness. See also Smith, Shearer, Hildebrand, and Van Camp (2014) for a brief overview.

It is highly likely that many individuals who attribute their deafness to unknown causes may have a genetic etiology. It is estimated that at least 10 percent of all genes are involved in determining the structure and functioning of the hearing mechanism. Increasing knowledge about the function of these genes has aided in understanding how mutations (changes) in a single gene can lead to hearing issues. Not only that, such mutations can also lead to syndromes with a variety of physical manifestations in different parts of the body. Since genes can also express themselves at different times prior to and after birth, the effects of specific mutations will vary such that, for example, the onset of hearing loss can occur at any time during one's life and possibly also be influenced by environmental events. Adding to the complexity, it has also been shown that some types of deafness may possibly be caused by the interaction of specific genetic and environmental factors (Usami, Abe, & Shinkawa, 1998).

At present, it appears that genetic factors are responsible for 50 to 60 percent of children identified with sensorineural hearing loss (Morton & Nance, 2006; Smith et al., 2014). Deciphering the specific type of genetic deafness is complex. Roughly 30 percent of all genetic deafness is syndromic (characterized by hearing loss in combination with other medical or physical characteristics), and approximately 70 percent is nonsyndromic (with only hearing loss) (Smith et al., 2014). In other words, most individuals with genetic deafness inherit only the trait of deafness. A complicating factor is that very often the child with an inherited hearing loss is the only such person in the family, therefore making it difficult to identify the cause of hearing loss.

The process of identifying genes is based on genetic mapping. This refers to the localization of a region on a particular chromosome. Each chromosome is composed of thousands of genes, which provide the biochemical instructions that "program" body development. The hundreds of genes that determine the structure and function of the ear are spread across all the chromosomes. One change in a single gene in the pathway controlling the development of the hearing organ, or other parts of the body, can result in a variety of physical manifestations, including hearing loss in isolation or with other characteristics.

Genetic deafness is inherited in specific patterns that vary such that the deafness may be congenital or occur any time after birth, even years later. Audiological characteristics of the hearing loss (type, degree, or progression); vestibular characteristics (balance problems); mode of inheritance; or the presence or absence of other medical or physical characteristics are additional variables that can distinguish between the more than 400 types of hereditary deafness that have been identified (Toriello & Smith, 2013).

There are four monogenetic inheritance patterns: autosomal dominant, autosomal recessive, X-linked recessive, and mitochondrial inheritance.

Autosomal Dominant Inheritance

This occurs when only a single copy of the gene is required for the trait to express itself. Dominantly inherited traits are usually, but not always, inherited from one of the parents, and account for approximately 20 percent of hereditary types of deafness (Marazita et al., 1993). The person with dominantly inherited deafness usually has one copy of the deaf gene and one copy of the hearing gene. Consequently, as shown in Figure 3.2, for each pregnancy there is a 50 percent chance of passing the deaf gene to each child. If both parents have a dominant gene for deafness, there is a 75 percent chance that each offspring will be deaf. In some families,

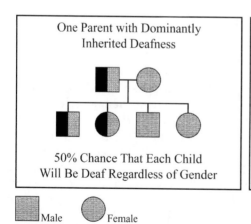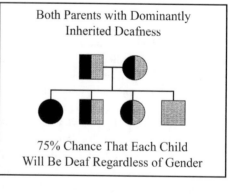

Figure 3.2 Autosomal Dominant Conditions of Deafness

Source: Used with permission.

even if all family members have the same gene for deafness, the hearing loss itself can range from mild to profound and vary in age of onset (variable expression). Rarely, the hearing loss may appear to skip generations (reduced penetrance). Variable expression and reduced penetrance can appear in both syndromic and nonsyndromic types of dominantly inherited deafness. In syndromic types, the associated physical and medical characteristics can even vary from one family member to another.

Autosomal Recessive Inheritance

The inheritance pattern for genetic deafness is autosomal recessive in 75 to 80 percent of identified cases of hereditary deafness (Marazita et al., 1993). To be deaf, a person must receive two copies of the altered gene, one from each parent. As shown in Figure 3.3, when both parents are hearing and are carriers of one gene for deafness, each pregnancy carries a one in four possibility, or 25 percent, that the offspring will be deaf. The child may have another deaf sibling or be the only deaf person in the family. Relatives can be carriers. Although one in eight individuals will be a carrier of a recessive gene for deafness, the parents must carry the exact same gene for the 25 percent chance of having a deaf child to apply. If one parent is deaf from recessive genes and the other parent is a carrier of the same gene, there is a 50 percent chance to have a deaf child. If the other parent is not a carrier, each child will be a hearing carrier. Since most types of recessive hearing loss are nonsyndromic, identification is often difficult when there is only one deaf child in the family.

Approximately 1 in 33 Americans is a carrier of the most common autosomal recessive gene for nonsyndromic deafness, connexin 26 (GJB2) (Smith et al., 2014). Depending on its mutation, the onset and progression of the hearing loss varies. One common mutation accounts for about 70 percent of deafness related to this gene (Denoyelle et al., 1997). Following the recessive gene pattern for inheritance, when an offspring inherits a specific mutation in the connexin 26 gene from each parent, that person will be deaf. Mutations in the connexin 26 gene are the cause of deafness in at least one-third or more of individuals who have congenital, moderate to profound hearing loss (Arnos, 2002). These mutations are also estimated to be the cause of deafness in 50 to 80 percent of individuals with deaf siblings and hearing parents (Denoyelle et al., 1997). In families with deaf parents and all deaf children, it is likely that

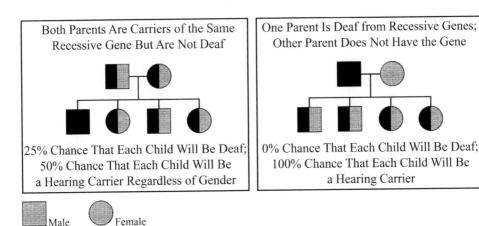

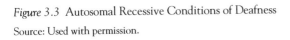

Figure 3.3 Autosomal Recessive Conditions of Deafness

Source: Used with permission.

the etiology can be attributed to connexin 26 (Nance, Liu, & Pandya, 2000). Another interesting attribute of this mutation is that it can foster faster healing of wounds by acting as a protective factor in that bacteria is less likely to invade skin wounds (www.researchgate.net/publication/236579598_Connexin_dynamics_in_the_privileged_wound_healing_of_the_buccal_mucosa). Due to the small size of this gene and the existence of a common mutation, testing for connexin 26 mutations is relatively easy and widely available in comparison to other, more complex genes.

X-linked Recessive Inheritance

This causes a small percentage of genetic deafness (Marazita et al., 1993). As shown in Figure 3.4, with a female who is a carrier for an X-linked recessive gene for deafness (Xx), each of her sons have a 50 percent chance to inherit this gene and be deaf (xY), and each of her daughters have a 50 percent chance to be a carrier (Xx). If the father is deaf from an X-linked recessive gene, his daughters will be hearing carriers while all the sons will be hearing noncarriers of this gene, since they inherit the Y chromosome from their father.

Mitochondrial Inheritance

Mitochondrial transmission involves mitochondria, which are tiny cytoplasmic cellular structures containing one circular DNA piece that produces energy for cellular activities. Mitochondria are transmitted solely from the mother through the egg cell; there is no transmission from the father. Several forms of syndromic and nonsyndromic deafness are caused by mutations in mitochondrial genes (http://hereditaryhearingloss.org/main.aspx?c=.HHH&n=86367).

Major Genetic Syndromes Involving Deafness

Several types of syndromes will be discussed here because of their relative frequency, because they represent conditions having psychological correlates, or because there are serious consequences. If identified and understood, appropriate treatment may be possible.

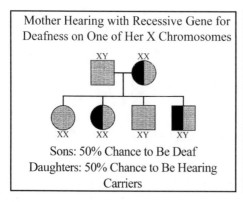 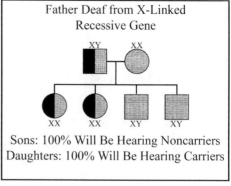

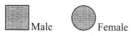

Figure 3.4 Sex-Linked Recessive Conditions of Deafness
Source: Used with permission.

Branchiootrenal Syndrome (BOR)

Prevalence is approximately 2 percent of the profoundly deaf category (Hoskins et al., 2007). Features include one or more of the following: malformed external ears; skin tags on the ear; ear pits (tiny holes) usually in front of the ear; tiny holes of the neck; kidney anomalies; and conductive, sensorineural, or mixed hearing loss. This is an example of variable expression of a dominant gene. Identifying those individuals is important because of the need to screen family members for potential kidney problems.

Jervell and Lange-Nielsen Syndrome

This syndrome, relatively rare, is inherited as an autosomal recessive trait, with profound sensorineural hearing loss. Fainting spells are caused by a defect in the conduction activity of the heart (Toriello & Smith, 2013), and sudden death is possible. For this reason, early identification is critical for treatment. Hearing carrier parents are also at risk for cardiac arrhythmia.

Neurofibromatosis Type 2 (NF2)

NF2 is inherited as an autosomal dominant trait that leads to bilateral acoustic neuroma or benign tumors of the eighth cranial nerve and other brain sites. These tumors arise from aberrant Schwann cells (a type of support cells, part of the peripheral nervous system) (Morrison et al., 2001). NF2 symptoms include progressive hearing loss, disturbances in balance and walking, dizziness, and tinnitus. These may emerge any time between childhood and early adulthood. NF2 acoustic tumors reaching large enough sizes or becoming malignant require surgery. In this process, the eighth cranial nerve is divided, thus precluding cochlear implantation. Auditory brain stem implants have resulted in varying degrees of understanding spoken language (Sanna, Di Lella, Guida, & Merkus, 2012).

Pendred Syndrome

Estimated to occur up to 10 percent of deaf children, Pendred syndrome is an autosomal recessive condition with a combination of sensorineural hearing loss, thyroid enlargement, and goiter, often with normal thyroid function (Arnos & Pandya, 2011). Some individuals will have a missing turn in the cochlea, usually characterized as Mondini aplasia and/or enlarged vestibular aqueduct (EVA) that can be diagnosed via MRI or CT scan. Cochlear implantation is possible for these individuals (Buchman, Copeland, Yu et al., 2004).

Stickler Syndrome (SS)

An autosomal dominant syndrome, this progressive arthro-opthalmopathy results in variable symptoms that can include flattening of the facial profile, cleft palate, vision problems such as myopia or retinal detachment, musculoskeletal and joint problems occurring over time, and hearing loss (Poulson et al., 2004). Mitral valve prolapse is possible; hence, a cardiology consultation is recommended. Due to symptom variability, SS is often underdiagnosed. Because of the multisystem impact, a multidisciplinary approach is critical to minimize the risk for associated problems.

Treacher-Collins Syndrome

This syndrome is a dominantly inherited condition that is associated with conductive hearing loss and malformations of the external ears, downward sloping eyes, flat cheekbones, a cleft palate, and other facial features (Vazquez, 2014). Since gene expression is so variable, diagnosis is difficult. Because of the physical appearance, severely affected individuals often require psychological support for psychosocial issues. Although facial surgical corrections are possible, these are complex and need to be tailored to the individual (Cobb, Green, & Gill et al., 2014).

Usher Syndrome

As a leading cause of DeafBlindness in more than half of all DeafBlind adults, its psychological and social effects can be devastating (Bailey & Miner, 2010). Three different forms each can result in blindness by adolescence or early to late adulthood. Individuals with Type 1 Usher syndrome have severe to profound congenital deafness, vestibular (balance) difficulties, and retinitis pigmentosa with onset before age 10. Retinitis pigmentosa is an eye disease that proceeds from night blindness to retina pigment changes, loss of peripheral vision, and eventually to blindness. Cochlear implants may provide additional sensory input to compensate for vision loss. People with relatively more common Type 2 have congenital, moderate sensorineural hearing loss, normal vestibular function, and later onset of retinitis pigmentosa in comparison to Type 1. Type 3 involves retinitis pigmentosa and progressive hearing loss. The progressive loss of vision necessitates ongoing readjustment in communication for those who have relied on vision activities of daily living become more difficult. Schools for the deaf, such as the Indiana School for the Deaf (www.deafhoosiers.com/apps/events/2015/1/15/20309 24/?id=2), have developed screening programs to facilitate early identification and modifications in the environment to lessen the impact of vision loss on educational and psychosocial development.

Waardenburg Syndrome (WS)

This common dominantly inherited condition consists of several features, including sensorineural hearing loss, vestibular dysfunction, wide-set eyes that can be bright blue or of different colors, white forelock of hair, a broad nose, and skin depigmentation (Toriello & Smith, 2013). Not all are necessarily present in any one case due to variable expression. Type 1 WS is characterized by the appearance of wide-spaced eyes; this does not occur for Type 2 WS, but both types have variable expression of features. About 25 percent of individuals with Type 1 have sensorineural deafness in contrast to about 50 percent for Type 2. Because of the dominant genetic transmission, it is typical to see WS in several generations of families, with many not knowing they have the gene because the features are so variable.

Genetic Testing and Counseling

A growing number of the estimated 400 genes for deafness have been characterized. The size and complexity of many of these genes currently preclude tests. However, genetic testing is now widely available for a few common forms of genetic deafness, most frequently for the nonsyndromic connexin 26 (GJB2) gene mentioned earlier. Clinical benefits of genetic testing (Alford et al., 2014) include elimination of the need for other invasive and expensive medical testing to identify syndromes that include complicating medical features such as thyroid and heart problems. The earlier the cause is identified, the more proactive parents and professionals can be in planning medical interventions if needed, accessible language programs, appropriate amplification, and educational interventions. There is a psychological benefit as well in that parental guilt can be alleviated, misinformation can be minimized, and parents have time to process acceptance of the information, particularly if it was unexpected.

Genetic counseling can assist families in getting accurate information about the causes of deafness, related medical or psychological complications, the chance for future children to have syndromic or nonsyndromic deafness, and reproductive options and consequently making choices that are appropriate for them (Arnos & Pandya, 2011). Even though an exact etiology cannot always be determined through genetic counseling or testing, parents can feel reassured about planning their future if they are informed that the possibility of additional medical complications is low or nonexistent. Also, families can be informed about new technologies in genetic testing and programs that offer testing for specific genes for deafness. Effective genetic counselors will assess the emotional state of the people seeking genetic counseling, work with them on grieving depending on the result, and help them with issues related to the results of genetic testing and making decisions that will impact the family.

Genetic counseling is often useful not only for hearing couples with deaf children but also for deaf adults. The etiology of deafness generally is not of major concern to people who have grown up deaf, since basically they adjust to life as deaf persons and do not dwell on why they are deaf. They often do not have other physical or medical conditions that warrant special attention. However, it is natural for deaf persons to wonder about the cause of their deafness and about the possibility of having deaf or hearing children as they approach reproductive age (Arnos & Pandya, 2004; Burton, Withrow, Arnos, Kalfoglou, & Pandya, 2006). A study of the relationship between genetic counselors' attitudes toward Deaf people and the genetic counseling session concluded that the more familiarity genetic counselors had about culturally Deaf people, the more comfortable they would be in offering genetic testing to culturally Deaf clients very comfortable with their Deaf way of life who may prefer to have a deaf child (Enns, Boudreault, & Palmer, 2010). This is easily understandable considering the fact that, on the other hand, hearing persons would be more comfortable having hearing children. Those deaf adults with health problems may want to know about the possibility of syndromes associated with deafness that may be impacting the ease of their lives.

The genetic counseling process generally involves an evaluation by a team of professionals, including a medical doctor specializing in clinical genetics, a Ph.D. medical geneticist, genetic counselors with master's degrees, social workers, and nurses (Arnos & Pandya, 2011). For the evaluation, information is obtained about family history, medical history, physical examination results, and medical testing as needed.

Family history provides details about family patterns of hearing levels or medical features of family members. Information about the health and hearing status of close and distant relatives is collected, as well as information about the blood relationship among relatives and the ethnic background of the family However, if there is nothing in the family history, this does not necessarily mean the etiology is not genetic, as some genes can be passed on with no one being affected for generations The medical history covers birth history, serious illnesses, or chronic health problems and also includes audiograms for the deaf person and other family members. This information can provide clues indicating the presence of a genetic syndrome or environmental cause. The physical examination, done by a board-certified M.D. clinical geneticist trained to recognize specific traits and features, as well as additional medical testing such as chromosome or metabolic testing, will contribute to a genetic diagnosis when combined with the family and medical history.

The final part of the genetic evaluation includes discussion of diagnosis, inheritance pattern, prognosis, and treatment options. This information must be provided to clients in a way that is sensitive to their emotional, cultural, and family needs, since there may be profound consequences for individual lives depending on the type of genetic conditions identified during the evaluation. The team can also make appropriate referrals as needed to educational programs, medical facilities, or organizations specializing in specific genetic conditions.

Ethical Issues

While there are health benefits to the identification and treatment of genetically transmitted disease, there are moral and ethical issues that have to be considered. The implications of genetic testing and genetic manipulation for altering human life are profound (www.who.int/genomics/elsi/en/).

The field of bioethics has emerged to deal with the application of ethics based on respect for human rights in the fields of medicine and health care (www.practicalbioethics.org/what-is-bioethics). As a response to the need to identify and address ethical issues connected with genetic findings and procedures that would affect individuals, families, and society, the Ethical, Legal, and Social Implications (ELSI) program was made an integral part of the Human Genome Project in 1990 (http://ghr.nlm.nih.gov/handbook/hgp/elsi). This program focuses on four main areas: 1) privacy (confidentiality) and fairness in the use of genetic information, especially in regard to the potential for genetic discrimination (see later discussion) and the need to respect cultural and religious beliefs; 2) integration of new genetic technologies and approaches into the clinical medicine process; 3) ethical issues related to genetic research, particularly informed consent; and 4) education of health care professionals, policymakers, students, and the public about genetics, access to genetic information, and its related emerging complex issues.

With comprehensive and inclusive informed consent, individuals who participate in genetic testing are fully informed of both benefits and risks involved in genetic testing. Risks include the possible psychological burden of the information, particularly if it is not what the parties involved expected, and potential negative effects on family dynamics, employment, and insurance coverage (where discrimination is possible). Participants might inadvertently learn potentially problematic information about their genetic makeup, possibly unrelated to their original request for genetic testing. If the potential implications for genetic testing are not made clear, individuals may have to make choices they are unprepared for. If genetic testing is focused on the purpose of prenatal diagnosis, choices regarding continuing the pregnancy or not depending on test results should be carefully presented by a genetic counselor who is trained to provide a clear overview of benefits and risks, including psychological risks, with respect for cultural, legal, and individual perceptions.

What are the ethical implications when considering hearing differences, deafness, or deaf people? Let us go back to the late 1880s, when eugenics became a hot topic focusing on selective breeding and/or the elimination of undesirable genes with the goal of increasing the "fitness" of the human race (Friedlander, 2002; Proctor, 2002; see also Branson & Miller, 2002; Burch, 2002, for brief reviews). Based on inadequate existing information about genetic transmission at that time, various state laws that permitted the sterilization of "potential carriers," including the insane, feebleminded, or criminal, to eliminate this "scourge" were passed in the United States during the early 1900s. These laws found support in two U.S. Supreme Court decisions, one in 1927 and the other in 1931 (Friedlander, 2002). Despite the fact that some deaf people were sterilized (e.g., Burch & Joyner, 2007), for the most part, deaf people were not subject to sterilization laws due to advocacy and educational efforts demonstrating the abilities of many deaf people to be good citizens.

The eugenics movement eventually culminated in the 1933 Nazi Germany doctrine of racial purity that condoned the sterilization and killing of victims who carried hereditary diseases, including deaf people (Biesold, 1999; Friedlander, 2002; Proctor, 2002). As a result of the Nazi policy, support for eugenics in the United States weakened, but this history does cast a long shadow over the field of genetics. There is a fear that eugenics is now cloaked in the guise of eliminating perceived genetic defects, including deafness, together with their associated and assumed negative quality of life. This adds to the urgency of extreme sensitivity in genetic decisions.

In the case of genetic deafness, the values attributed to a hearing child in comparison to a deaf child (depending on parent reactions) may differ and eventually affect reproductive decisions that can have repercussions for the future of Deaf culture and the Deaf community (Johnston, 2006). Hearing society and deaf people tend to have different perspectives on this issue, with culturally Deaf people seeing themselves as not having a medical problem while hearing people tend to frame "deaf" as a medical issue to be treated (Middleton, Emery, & Turner, 2010). For many deaf and hearing people, genetic screening may not be desired nor may it necessarily lead to termination of pregnancy. However, comparatively speaking, preliminary attitudinal research conducted by Middleton (2004) suggests that deaf people, particularly culturally Deaf people, were least interested in prenatal diagnosis for deafness, while hearing participants were comparatively more interested and would prefer to have hearing children. The fact that some genes, including connexin 26 mutations, can be screened in the embryo stage in preparation for in vitro fertilization has led to the approval of controversial procedures to remove the genes that would cause deafness. This was allowed in Australia because of perceptions that deafness is a medical condition that needs to be screened out (Noble, 2003). In Great Britain, fertility legislation enacted in 2008 stipulates that the use of embryos with genetic abnormalities with potential to create a serious physical or mental disability produced during in vitro fertilization procedures are not to be preferred to embryos without such genetic makeup (Emery, Middleton, & Turner, 2010). This sets the stage for classifying genes such as the connexin 26 mutation as falling into the category of a serious disability. Consequently, deaf individuals who wish to undergo in vitro fertilization would not be allowed to ensure that resulting embryos contain the connexin 26 gene to the exclusion of unaffected genes if they want to have deaf children. Those deaf individuals who opposed the bill in its original form saw themselves as leading perfectly normal lives; they resented being pathologized, having their lives seen as being of lesser value, and being left out of the debate regarding this legislation. Their protests led to minor modification, but the debate as to whether being deaf represents a serious medical condition continues (Emery et al., 2010).

In another example of genetic control and medicalization, a sperm bank informed a Deaf lesbian couple that potential donors were eliminated if congenital deafness was a possibility (Mundy, 2002). In this case, subsequently a deaf friend became the donor, and the baby was deaf. Public reactions ranged from support to overwhelmingly vitriolic opposition.

As they did in the Great Britain fertility legislation, members of the deaf community should continue to empower themselves through education about the genetics of deafness, form their own judgments about how emerging genetic technology may impact their own lives and the lives of deaf people, and share their perspectives with hearing society and legislative bodies. Ethically, it behooves society to respect the perspectives of culturally Deaf people.

Hearing Screening and Identification

Hearing Screening

Screening for hearing differences has emerged as an important aspect of neonatal care. Technical details of the screening process are described in the Audiology Appendix following this chapter. Early identification will enhance the child's opportunities to develop environmental awareness, language and communication, and academic and social skills (e.g., Calderon & Greenberg, 2011; St. John, Lytle, Nussbaum, & Shoup, 2016). In the United States, universal newborn hearing screening shortly after birth is now mandated in every state and territory (www.infanthearing.org/states_home/index.html). See www.infanthearing.org for further information on state implementation of Early Hearing Detection and Intervention (EHDI) systems. This screening has lowered the mean age of identification from the previous 30 to 36 months of age downward to 2 to 3 months of age for those infants who are followed up after the initial infant screening (Bradham, Caraway, Moog, Houston, & Rosenthal, 2015). However, this screening may miss children with, for example, progressive hearing loss, who may be identified later in the school setting (www.asha.org/Advocacy/state/School-Age-Hearing-Screening/). In addition, newborn hearing screening is far less available in developing countries, and there is an ethical issue as to whether to implement newborn hearing screening if appropriate follow-up programs are not available to assist family members with deaf infants (Leigh, Newall, & Newall, 2010).

For adults who lose their hearing, the process of confirming the hearing loss is done by otologists and audiologists through standard testing after individuals notice or recognize that something is wrong with their hearing. The Audiology Appendix following this chapter provides additional information on audiological aspects.

The Aftermath of Initial Identification

Hearing Parents

Once the initial screening identifies an infant in need of follow-up, the professional doing the hearing screening will then refer the family for a follow-up evaluation. If this evaluation confirms the finding of the initial screening, families are referred for more extensive evaluation. If the infant is identified as deaf, the next step is to recommend appropriate early intervention approaches (St. John et al., 2016). This can be an anxiety-producing process for parents (Khairi et al., 2011).

Some infants may appear to have typical hearing at first. Parents[2] may become concerned if they notice the infant not responding to sound and then consult with their pediatrician. The pediatrician may either tell the parents to be patient or may refer them to otologists and audiologists for hearing evaluations. The time lag from suspicion to final identification may be as long as six months (e.g., Denworth, 2014).

New parents may be dealing with unfamiliar and possibly confusing medical and audiological information, even more so if additional disabilities are involved. Some parents may experience relief that deafness is the only issue, but for many, this information may come as an emotional shock or as an intense disappointment, the full depth of which is not consistently sensed by professionals doing the evaluation unless they are well trained in sensitivity and understand the need to monitor the pace and process for sharing evaluation results and their implications (Meadow-Orlans, Mertens, & Sass-Lehrer, 2003; St. John et al., 2016). New parents often cannot immediately assimilate the irreversibility of sensorineural hearing loss and the implications of having a deaf child. They are dealing with the loss of the "normally hearing child" dream and substituting the vision of a child who cannot hear the parents' words of comfort or their spoken language.

For some, the emotional pain can be intense before subsiding into a dull ache, as parents acknowledge that their lives as parents will not be what they had expected. More information can be absorbed during follow-up visits, though parents may experience grief reactions of varying intensity and varying duration at different times (Young & Tattersall, 2007). During the grieving process, many feelings such as guilt, anger, and/or depression, either separately or simultaneously are expressed, as reviewed by various authors, including, for example, Elisabeth Kübler-Ross (e.g., 2000). Parents may wonder what they did to contribute to the child's deafness, particularly when there is no clear cause (e.g., Sass-Lehrer, Porter, & Wu, 2016). For example, the mother may re-enact each step of her pregnancy to ascertain what might have happened. For this mother, genetic counseling may help to deal with the guilt. Depending on the family's background, cultural explanations may predominate over Western medical inter-pretations. Eldredge (2010) presents several such examples for Native Americans, including one in which the mother, having seen an owl (an evil omen) during her pregnancy, believed that caused the baby's deafness. The deafness might be seen as a punishment for previous transgressions or as an act of God, both fatalistic attitudes that prevail in many Latino cultures (Hidalgo & Williams, 2010). Fatalism may also be a coping strategy in Chinese American culture (Wu & Grant, 2010).

Grief reactions are not necessarily pathological; rather, this is a normal process that allows the family to come to terms with the evaluation results and move ahead in exploring ways to cope with a deaf child in the family, with some families moving faster than others (St. John et al., 2016). The perceived burdens of having a deaf child may lead to anger if parents do not realize the possibility of joys that parents such as Lydia Denworth (2014) experience as they watch the child learn and grow. Some parents may run from doctor to doctor, searching in vain for a different result or cure. It takes energy to be angry—energy that can be channeled into constructive action when parents are able to acknowledge their fears and frustrations. Anger can also turn into depression if the parents feel that everything they do is futile. As a normal part of the grief reaction, bouts of depression may emerge. Depression is pathological if it becomes chronic and the parent cannot act in the interest of the child.

Grandparents, siblings, and other family members are also emotionally affected but can be excellent sources of support for parents as well (Meadow-Orlans et al., 2003; Sass-Lehrer et al., 2016). Some grandparents are able to provide warm support even when they are sad; others may be stuck in denial, offer well-meaning advice, or try to make the parents feel better by putting a positive spin on the situation. Siblings have to adjust to a new set of family circum-stances that may include changes in priorities as more attention is paid to the deaf child. For example, all of a sudden, the sibling has to go with mom and new baby to parent intervention programs instead of staying home and playing with neighborhood friends. Changes in how family members communicate may be perceived as another added burden.

When the emotional feelings surrounding the identification phase are cathartically expressed in a safe environment over time, parents can begin to psychologically let go of the "normal" child they had expected and internalize the fact that they have a deaf child who can still enrich their lives in different and equally satisfying ways. This helps them to accept and enact the necessary changes in the life situation of their family. They also feel supported and less alone when they meet with other parents who have been in similar situations (Krywko, 2015; Sass-Lehrer et al., 2016). It is also helpful to meet deaf and hard-of-hearing adults or deaf mentors who can help parents get some understanding of what is possible for their child (Pittman, Benedict, Olson, & Sass-Lehrer, 2016).

Deaf Parents

For deaf parents, the identification phase takes on different overtones. Many deaf parents will say that the most important thing will be to have healthy children, whatever the deaf or hear-ing status. They are more open to the possibility of having a deaf child, primarily because of their experience and comfort with being deaf (Meadow-Orlans et al., 2003). They also see the deaf child as a reflection of themselves, just as a hearing child is a reflection of hearing parents. Some culturally Deaf parents may experience temporary disappointment if their child is deaf, considering that the child may face many extra challenges in life, but this reaction usually does not last (Lane, Hoffmeister, & Bahan, 1996). Some deaf parents may prefer to rely on observa-tion rather than submit their infant to hearing screening (Stein, Barnett, & Padden, 2001).

However, the reality is that fewer than 5 percent of deaf students had at least one parent who was deaf (Mitchell & Karchmer, 2004). With their hearing children, deaf parents have to cope with a different set of realities related to social, communication, and educational needs. Other things such as socioeconomic and educational levels being equal, deaf parents are as capable of parenting children, deaf or hearing, as their hearing peers, and this is increasingly recognized in today's society. Various publications covering the hearing adult children of deaf parents indicate that their views about their childhood experiences are as diverse as those of other groups (Hoffmeister, 2008; Preston, 1994; Shultz Myers, Marcus, & Myers, 2010). Hearing children of deaf parents are generally not considered to be at risk for developmental problems. However, some deaf parents can benefit from support services to increase their level of comfort and efficacy in parenting hearing children. This is especially true if they have limited communicative experience with hearing family members while growing up. This is analogous to the problem that hearing parents of newly identified deaf children face in raising them.

Late-Deafened Individuals

While the focus has been on identifying youngsters who are deaf, we also need to direct the reader's attention to the significant population of late-deafened individuals. They have lived lives as hearing people. When they find out there is no way to restore hearing that is lost, they have to deal with a unique set of circumstances. Authors have described their reactions to hearing loss, depending on whether it was progressive or rapid (e.g., Aguayo & Coady, 2005; Meadow-Orlans, 1985). Grief and mourning for the hearing that has been lost is in the picture. Depression and withdrawal with resultant isolation are among the most prevalent psychological reactions. Individuals can also become nervous, anxious, fearful, fatigued, and irritable. On the other hand, there are individuals who respond with positive stamina and work to adapt to their hearing loss and thereby resolve their psychological issues (e.g., Maxwell-McCaw, 2001). Adjustment to hearing loss takes time as one goes through the grieving process and develops different ways of communicating with others, whether it is through hearing aid use, sign language, and/or speechreading. Learning American Sign Language and exploring the deaf community often represents a huge psychological hurdle since late-deafened individuals often prefer to maintain contact with their familiar hearing world (Harvey, 2003). Families are a critical component in providing social support as individuals transition through the process of accepting their loss.

Issues Related to Early Intervention

This period involves the recognition that there is a bewildering array of complex decisions that parents have to make about communication approaches, language choices, amplification (including hearing aids and cochlear implants), and type of education. Early intervention (see Chapter 7) is critical in helping parents develop effective approaches, particularly in communicating with their newly identified child. Providing support to families, whatever their needs, respecting cultural perspectives, and creating culturally inclusive environments for families provide opportunities for professionals to help families see the deaf child in a positive way (Cohrrsen, Church, & Tayler, 2009). Many studies focusing on family involvement support its importance in the academic achievement scores of deaf children (Carter, 2002, as cited in Sass-Lehrer et al., 2016). Rather than socioeconomic levels per se, high expectations, a home environment that encourages learning, and parent participation are critical factors in promoting achievement (Henderson & Berla, 1994, as cited in Sass-Lehrer et al., 2016). Comprehensive services that meet the needs of less educated and less affluent families will help in encouraging family involvement and optimal child development. This is an area that needs ongoing development (Meadow-Orlans et al., 2003; Sass-Lehrer et al., 2016).

Professionals need to recognize the resiliency of many families who can "rise to the occasion" in dealing with the aftermath of identification. However, stress is a factor to contend with. A review of studies covering parental stress levels reveals a pattern of mixed findings (Thomson, Kennedy, & Kuebli, 2011). Some studies indicate that hearing mothers may be dealing with more stress related to their difficulties in interacting with their deaf children than were mothers of hearing children; other studies indicate equivalent stress levels, and one study suggests that stress level is lower, possibly due to appropriate early intervention that enhances resiliency. However, this needs to be tempered by the fact that it can be stressful to raise a deaf child, with multiple issues such as decision-making about medical, communication, and educational options, attending frequent therapy appointments, learning and managing amplification devices, obtaining appropriate services, dealing with additional disabilities, relationships, and the child's communication abilities, in addition to dealing with socioeconomic issues (Zaidman-Zait, 2014).

Parents may experience feelings of inadequacy and confusion while learning how to raise a deaf child and considering the plethora of communication, language, amplification options, and educational approaches to choose from. In this situation, they may be overly willing to entrust hearing specialists, early intervention professionals, or other helping professionals with critical decisions about how to direct their child's life. Professionals need to avoid this trap and instead focus on teamwork with parents, using family-centered practice approaches to help parents increase their own feelings of self-confidence about their capacity to parent.

Language, Communication, and Educational Choices

Some of the decisions parents need to make involve language and communication choices, including ASL, signed English (following English word order), spoken English or spoken language in the home if not English (with focus on listening and speaking), and cued speech (a visual mode of communication that uses handshapes and placements in combination with the mouth movements of speech to indicate phonemes of spoken language (LaSasso, Crain, & Leybaert, 2010). Once the decision is made, parents need to learn how to maximize their child's ability to understand them. This means learning specific techniques, signs, or cued speech, all of which take time to master. If parents work, they may have to be resourceful in juggling time to cope with an avalanche of new requirements for helping their child. Educational programs have different communication and language approaches, and parents must select which program best meets their child's needs, depending on what is available in their area. As time goes on, parents face the need to consider whether to place their deaf child in a specialized school for deaf children or in a mainstream/inclusion setting. Parents are understandably fearful of making mistakes when facing this myriad of necessary decisions. They need reassurance that they are doing the best they can for their child and that any decision they make can be changed depending on their child's evolving communication and educational needs.

By selecting specific educational placements, parents are making choices about whether their child will interact with hearing or deaf peers, or both. This represents an additional factor to consider. Deaf children can be lonely or isolated if there are problems socializing with hearing peers, making this an important topic for research to identify factors that can improve this situation (Batten, Oakes, & Alexander, 2014). Parents who are relatively comfortable with having a deaf child will be more comfortable with their child having deaf friends. Exposure to the gamut of deaf adult role models, ranging from spoken language users to members of Deaf culture, can help increase parents' comfort level (Pittman et al., 2016). Parents rarely meet signing deaf adults. When they do, they may feel intimidated because of their limited signing skills (Christiansen & Leigh, 2002/2005). Professional can help facilitate this process of inter-action when parents are ready and willing (Pittman et al., 2016).

Deaf parents with deaf children are aware of language and communication opportunities, educational options, and amplification choices. Their decisions depend in large part on their own experiences growing up, what is available in their area, and what they perceive their children's needs to be (Mitchiner & Sass-Lehrer, 2011). Many will opt for special-ized schools for deaf children, which they see as providing full communicative accessibility and optimal socialization opportunities with deaf peers. Others are comfortable with main-stream settings.

Amplification Choices

Universal newborn hearing screening is likely to miss children with mild hearing loss who later on may demonstrate inconsistent responses to sound, miss softly spoken speech, and be at higher risk for speech-language, academic and social difficulties (McKay, Gravel, & Tharpe, 2008). Depending on individual needs, recommendations may include hearing aids and FM or sound-field systems for use in school. Hard-of-hearing children fall into the cat-egory of those with moderate to moderately severe hearing loss. They generally have the capacity to use hearing as the primary mode for understanding speech and acquiring lan-guage when appropriately fitted with hearing aids and use FM or remote microphone hear-ing assistance technology in background noise situations (McCreery, 2014). If needed, they can also supplement their listening with visual information, including speechreading and signing.

Parents of deaf children with severe and profound hearing levels tend to expose them to some level of spoken language from an early age regardless of the decisions made concern-ing communication method. Advances in digital hearing aids and cochlear implants have enhanced the usefulness of amplification, thus encouraging increasing numbers of families to initially focus on spoken language (Leigh, Morere, & Kobek Pezzarossi, 2014). Cochlear implants are typically recommended for those children whose hearing levels preclude sufficient benefit from hearing aids. Parents presented with this option have to decide whether to have their young child undergo the surgical procedure for a cochlear implant. For many of them, this can be an agonizing decision-making process (Archbold, Sach, Lutman, & Gregory, 2006; Christiansen & Leigh, 2002/2005; Hyde, Punch, & Komesaroff, 2010).

Cochlear Implants

As of 2000, the United States Food and Drug Administration (FDA) policy allows implanta-tion in children aged 12 months and older (National Institute on Deafness and Other Com-munication Disorders, 2014b). Some are implanted earlier, often in the case of meningitis as ossification of the cochlea may make it unfeasible to wait till 12 months. In retrospect, most parents see the implant as beneficial because of increased environmental awareness or com-municative competence. Most parents also focus on listening and spoken language, but some also value sign language (Christiansen & Leigh, 2002/2005).

A current issue has to do with how careful cochlear implant teams are in evaluating can-didates for cochlear implants. Hearsay has it that some parents will shop till they find a coch-lear implant site willing to implant their child. O'Brien et al. (2010) ask whether cochlear implantation is always the best choice, taking into account how well candidates meet criteria for implantation. They recommend the use of a cochlear implant team to carefully evaluate candidates and work with families after initial concerns are addressed.

Documentation of significant variability in speech and language outcomes for deaf children with cochlear implants (Pisoni, Conway, Kronenberger et al., 2008) means that there is no guarantee that deaf cochlear implant users will experience 100 percent auditory comprehension of spoken language. Current research focuses not only on how deaf children process information through spoken language, but also through vision alone or the combination of vision (e.g., speechreading) and sound, as hearing people do when processing spoken language (Morere, 2011). Regardless, it appears that cochlear implant use does not necessarily translate into reading achievement results that equal those of hearing peers (Geers, Tobey, Moog, & Brenner, 2008; Marschark, Sarchet, Rhoten, & Zupan, 2010). Essentially, academic achievement depends on multiple factors related to deaf and hard-of-hearing students themselves, their family environments, and their school experiences (Marschark, Shaver, Nagle, & Newman, 2015). Consequently, while there is evidence of improved access to auditory information, cochlear implants are not the miracle cure touted by the media. This is information that parents need before they make decisions for their children. This leads to the question of ethics, but first we review some history.

HISTORY

Starting in 1957, cochlear implants were developed by scientists whose goal was to provide sound for deaf individuals unable to benefit from hearing aids (Christiansen & Leigh, 2002/2005). It was their belief that access to sound meant a broadening of possibilities for these individuals. Interestingly, it was the scientific community that first raised concerns about the cochlear implant, primarily because they felt the structure of the ear did not permit it and the cochlea would be damaged. As time went by and research continued, scientists began to see the potential for cochlear implants. Early results indicated that adults who received cochlear implants could hear sounds at different frequencies, identify environmental sounds, and improve their speechreading. Because of these results, attention turned to children and the first pediatric cochlear implant took place in 1977.

While scientists began to feel comfortable about providing cochlear implants to deaf adults, pediatric implantation was not without controversy. Neurophysiologists were unsure if this procedure was appropriate for children. However, there was no stopping the momentum. In the 1980s, the focus was on clinical trials involving both children and adults in order to assess the effectiveness of cochlear implants. Nonetheless, during this period the number of adults and children receiving cochlear implants increased steadily despite limited research evidence considering risks versus benefits. Initially, implants were available only for older children for whom hearing aids did not work. As time went on, the age of implantation became younger, in order to take advantage of the critical period for learning language.

While the clinical trials indicated that children were doing reasonably well, the definition of reasonably well tends to be subjective. Does reasonably well include just recognizing environmental sounds, some speech sounds or words, sentence recognition, or some other criteria? Even with the improvement in technology, results continue to be quite variable, as mentioned earlier. Some children do not benefit, others demonstrate high recognition of spoken words and sentences, and then you have everything else in between.

DEAF COMMUNITY PERCEPTIONS

In the 1980s, significant opposition to cochlear implant development on the part of Deaf communities in different countries emerged (Christiansen & Leigh, 2002/2005). The opposition focused on the perception that cochlear implants implied deaf people needed to be able to hear and speak in order to lead productive lives because their lives were limited and lonely, which was not necessarily the case. There was a fear that Deaf culture would die out. Ongoing media portrayal of cochlear implants as a miracle cure and normalization for a condition that Deaf adults did not view as dire was a cause for concern. A May 4, 2003 advertisement published in the *New York Times Magazine* stated, "We turned a child who couldn't hear into a typical two year old who doesn't listen." A 2002 Michigan case illustrates how a Deaf couple had to fight in court to assert their parental rights not to implant their Deaf children in view of perceptions that cochlear implants are always in the best interest of the child and the parents were medically neglecting their children (Ouellette, 2011). The judge grudgingly ruled in favor of the parents on the grounds of parental rights and autonomy.

Some wondered why so much money was being spent on cochlear implants when other pressing needs were evident, including educational needs for deaf children. Deaf adults who opted for the implant were accused of choosing hearing and speaking over sign language, and therefore became traitors in the eyes of Deaf culture.

However, the increasing number of signing deaf adults with cochlear implants contributed to a tempering of the negative perceptions that were initially prevalent. Christiansen and Leigh (2011) compared results of two surveys distributed to deaf, hard-of-hearing, and hearing faculty, staff, and students at Gallaudet University, an institution much beloved by Deaf people. The first one was done in 2000 and the second in 2008. The researchers came to the conclusion that there was an overall increase in the percentage of respondents who agreed with the statement that it was possible for a person to use a cochlear implant and still have an identity as a Deaf person. Another survey of signing deaf adults conducted by Rashid, Kushalnagar, and Kushalnagar (2010) noted that less than half of the 47 respondents reported negative reactions that really were lukewarmly negative, primarily due to concerns about possible medical side effects rather than identity-related concerns.

In addition, an increasing number of Deaf parents are choosing to implant their deaf children as they see cochlear implants as providing more choices and opportunities to have access to both ASL and English (Mitchiner, 2015; Mitchiner & Sass-Lehrer, 2011), even in the face of some negative criticism by peers. A small study done in Belgium suggests that deaf parents debating between cochlear implants and hearing aids gave priority to Deaf identity, sign language, and ethical issues (Hardonk et al., 2011). The ethical issues that concerned both deaf and hearing parents included surgical risks and the loss of residual hearing capacities. Deaf parents felt there was insensitivity to culturally Deaf perceptions related to the importance of sign language as well as spoken language and the expectation that socialization would be better with the cochlear implant.

THE COCHLEAR IMPLANT DEBATE AND ETHICAL CONCERNS

As this brief history indicates, just as with genetics, there are ethical issues that constitute ongoing dilemmas. Benefits and risks have to be weighed very carefully. In the past, was it ethical to implant children with early versions of the technology before the establishment of a sufficient research database? Were parents fully informed of the potential risks as well as uncertain benefits? Was pressure to implant a factor? Do these issues continue?

Varied opinions on the effectiveness of this technology have contributed to the ongoing dilemma. The National Association of the Deaf's (NAD) initial 1991 position paper deplored the FDA decision to allow pediatric cochlear implantation on defenseless children due to the lack of scientific evidence for long-term physical, emotional, and social impact on children as well as concern that parents were poorly informed about alternate options and risks inherent in the surgical procedures (Christiansen & Leigh, 2002/2005). Fast forward to the 2000 NAD position paper, which indicated that quality of life can be good even without the implant, the diversity of deaf people is emphasized, as is the right of parents to make informed decisions for their deaf children, and cochlear implants are one of several tools that are available for these children (National Association of the Deaf, 2000).

Then we contrast these position papers with those of, for example, the American Academy of Audiology (1995) with its focus on the benefits of cochlear implants for speech production and auditory perception over those of hearing aids, though there is acknowledgment that reliable predictors of cochlear implant performance have not been identified. The Hearing Loss Association of America (HLAA) (2007) position statement states that current technology permits many, if not most, users to understand speech solely through hearing but qualifies this by explaining that the cochlear implant does not replace the ear but does improve functionality such that one can move from being functionally deaf to functionally hard-of-hearing. While caution is expressed regarding appropriate candidacy for young children, there is a strong recommendation for auditory-verbal training in order to maximize the potential benefit of the cochlear implant. Interestingly, in its position paper supporting the use of cochlear implants, the Alexander Graham Bell Association for the Deaf and Hard of Hearing (AGB) (n.d.) does not focus on auditory-verbal training. Rather, the focus is on ensuring that parents are fully informed of potential advantages and risks and that children learn to use auditory communication cues in speech together with attention to social, emotional, and cognitive development. There is support for implantation at a very young age for language learning. AGB (2008) has also posted a position statement on American Sign Language that indicates the importance of parents making informed decisions after being exposed to all language and communication options.

In examining these position statements, one cannot escape the issues that pertain to the ethical use of technology. The later position papers clearly acknowledge parental rights and the importance of being informed of not only risks and benefits but also information about varied language and communication opportunities. Notice is given that guarantees for optimal performance with cochlear implants cannot be made. It appears that the cochlear implant debates have interjected some caution into the process leading up to cochlear implant surgery and beyond. The ethical constructs of beneficence (extent of benefits), nonmaleficence (do no harm), autonomy (providing unbiased information to families), and justice (whether cochlear implants are available to all who can benefit) all must be considered by cochlear implant teams (Christiansen & Leigh, 2002/2005).

What is not clear is the extent to which cochlear implant users themselves participated in the development of the position papers. Bathard (2014) argues for their participation in debates about cochlear implants. They are the ones who deal with the impact of the cochlear implant on their lives, whether in terms of surgical/medical impact, technology reliability, language and communication, and interaction with others and can provide direct experience about the effectiveness and limitations of cochlear implants.

While professionals internationally agree that implantation is most effective at young ages for maximizing potential spoken language development, there is some disagreement about the sole focus on spoken language, particularly in view of the variability in results for both language and academics (e.g., Humphries et al., 2014c; Martin, Balanzategui, & Morgan, 2014; Pisoni et al., 2008). Due to concern about children with language delays, we need to ask how this harm can be circumvented. Researchers and educators have considered bilingual (spoken and signed languages) environments for children with cochlear implants based on the adage that whatever linguistic skills a child can master are all valuable, whether spoken or signed. Deaf parents are advocating for bilingual programs for their cochlear-implanted children (Mitchiner, 2015). They view having access to both languages as critical byways, not only to auditory stimuli and interactions with hearing peers, but also to connections with Deaf culture. For them, signing is not a failure but a pathway to mastery of a unique language. However, according to Knoors, Tang, and Marschark (2014), at present the academic advantage for bilingual programs for deaf children does not have a sufficient research base compared to results for monolingual spoken language programs.

Since an increasing number of deaf children with additional disabilities are receiving cochlear implants, there continues to be a question of benefit versus risk, considering the unique challenges in working with this population (Zaidman-Zait, Curle, Jamieson, Chia, & Kozak, 2015). Professionals must go beyond the usual course of candidacy evaluation and assess the potential for benefit, particularly in terms of communication access, education, and quality of life, and the ability to obtain services to meet individual challenges, no mean feat in an environment with limited services for children with additional disabilities. If services are limited, is it ethical to implant this population, or are the benefits sufficient to overcome this hurdle? Parents seem to feel the benefits are sufficient in terms of improved communication skills and well-being despite significant challenges (Zaidman-Zait et al., 2015).

Conclusions

If the "beginning" is handled in ways that facilitate parental adjustment to the presence of a deaf child in the family, the end result can be a deaf adult who functions effectively in society. When professionals help parents understand etiology and all the complex factors, including ethical issues, that need to be considered in making child-rearing decisions, parents are better enabled to do the best they can for their deaf child.

Suggested Readings

Paludneviciene, R., & Leigh, I. W. (2011). *Cochlear implants: Evolving perspectives.* Washington, DC: Gallaudet University Press.
   The chapters in this book indicate how the cochlear implant debate has changed and include information on both spoken and sign language users who use cochlear implants. Emphasis is placed on the value of both visual and aural pathways in the education of deaf children. The ethics of genetic engineering is also examined.

Schwartz, S. (2007). *Choices in deafness* (3rd ed.). Bethesda, MD: Woodbine House.
   This book provides user-friendly, nonjudgmental information about medical evaluation of hearing loss, audiological testing, and amplification options, including hearing aids and cochlear implants. Chapters present the various communication options for parents to consider together with vignettes describing deaf children and adults. There is a comprehensive list of national organizations serving individuals who are deaf and hard of hearing.

Smith, R., Shearer, E., Hildebrand, M., & Van Camp, G. (2014). *Deafness and hereditary hearing loss overview.* Retrieved from www.ncbi.nlm.nih.gov/books/NBK1434/
   This reference provides an excellent summary of the different types of hearing differences, hereditary forms of hearing loss, and syndromic/nonsyndromic constellations that include hearing differences. There is also a brief explanation of testing, genetic counseling, and management of different conditions.

Notes

1   Some of the information in this section has been extrapolated from Arnos, K., & Pandya, A. (2011). Advances in the genetics of deafness. In M. Marschark & P. Spencer (Eds.), *The Oxford handbook of deaf studies, language, and education* (pp. 412–424). New York, NY: Oxford.
2   In referring to parents, we recognize that they are part of many different family constellations, including single-parent families and families with nontraditional structures.

Audiology Appendix

The Basics of Audiology

Audiology covers the science of hearing. Audiology also includes the vestibular system and how information that is heard is managed by the central nervous system (Katz, 2009; Northern & Downs, 2014). Audiologists earn the Au.D. degree, which is a clinical doctorate in audiology. So exactly what does the audiologist do? With this qualification, the audiologist provides services related to the prevention; identification; assessment; and the habilitation or rehabilitation of hearing, auditory function, balance, and other related systems. As part of their services, they diagnose hearing loss; counsel families; select, fit, and dispense hearing aids and other hearing assistive devices; and also provide assessment and follow-up services for persons who use hearing aids or cochlear implants. Their functions also include hearing aid maintenance and repair, auditory therapy services, counseling, consultant services for noise reduction and ear protection in the workplace, the making of customized earplugs for swimming and noise protection, and other management strategies for hearing and balance issues (American Hearing-Language-Speech Association, 2004). Audiologists work in a variety of settings, including private practices; schools; offices with Ear, Nose, and Throat doctors (ENT); government agencies; university training programs; hospitals; and industry.

The Hearing Mechanism

Let's begin with the ear itself. How do people hear? What is described here is a very simplified explanation of the process, which starts at the outer ear (pinna or auricle) (Ervin, 2015; Lucker, 2002/2005). The pinna gently funnels sound waves into the ear canal (external auditory meatus) to the first part of the middle ear—specifically the eardrum (tympanic membrane) and causes it to vibrate. At that point, the sound wave's energy is transferred through three tiny bones (ossicles) called the *hammer (malleus)*, *anvil (incus)*, and *stirrup (stapes)*. The stapes is attached to the oval window, which separates the middle ear from the inner ear. As it vibrates, the sound energy is transmitted through the oval window to the inner ear. The inner ear holds the vestibular system (involved in balance) and the cochlea. The cochlea contains auditory receptor cells with hair-like structures called *cilia (hair cells)*. The fluid inside the cochlea transmits the sound energy along the hair cells, which convert the mechanical energy set up by the middle ear system to electrical energy. This energy then travels via the auditory nerve (eighth cranial nerve) to the auditory areas in the brain. The brain interprets the neural impulses into meaningful sound. See Northern and Downs (2014, pp. 7–49) for more in-depth information.

Four Types of Hearing Loss[1]

If the components of the outer and middle ear are operating inefficiently so that sound cannot get through, the related hearing loss is said to be *conductive* and is often temporary. Possible reasons include wax build-up in the ear, ear infection, or anatomical malformations. Conductive hearing loss can often be treated with medicine or surgery such as, for example, the draining of middle-ear fluid or reconstructing the middle ear bones. *Sensorineural hearing loss,* which tends to be permanent, is caused by problems in the way the hair cells of the inner ear transmit sound and the way that electrical impulses are carried to the hearing centers of the brain via the eighth auditory nerve. This happens when hair cells do not develop normally, are damaged, or have deteriorated secondary to aging or disease. Causes include environmental factors, such as noise, toxic medications, or head injury, and can also be genetic and progressive. Third, *mixed hearing loss* involves both conductive and sensorineural hearing losses. And lastly, there is *auditory neuropathy spectrum disorder,* which reflects hearing loss that occurs when transmission of sound from the inner ear to the brain is not organized in a way that the brain can understand due to damage in the inner ear or the auditory nerve. The individual may be able to hear sounds but cannot recognize spoken words (Northern & Downs, 2014).

The Measurement of Hearing

Traditional hearing tests use calibrated equipment to determine the type and degree of hearing level and assess speech discrimination. In the pure tone portion of the hearing test, the equipment generates pure tones within a restricted range of frequencies, usually in discrete intervals from 125 to 8,000 Hz, with Hz (hertz) representing cycles per second. The equipment can also vary the intensity level of each frequency. Pitch, a subjective term reflecting how high or low sounds are, is related to frequency. Specifically, pitch rises as frequency increases. Examples of low pitch would be men's voices, drums beating, doors closing, and vowels in words. High-pitch examples include women's voices, bird sounds, and consonants in words.

The technical term for loudness is expressed in dB (decibel), which represents the unit of measurement of sound intensity. The audiologist charts the loudness level (dB) where individuals just barely detect each pitch or frequency (Hz) presented. This represents the threshold level and is plotted on an audiogram. The audiogram is a graphic record that displays the results of the hearing test (see Figure A.1).

During the pure tone (PT) testing, sound is directed to the ears via earphones (air conduction) and via a vibrator held at either the forehead or mastoid part of the skull (bone conduction). Both air and bone conduction threshold responses are compared in order to get information about the type(s) and degree of hearing level that may be present.

Figure A.1 shows a sample form that audiologists fill out when conducting hearing evaluations. The audiogram on the form is designed to show both frequency and decibel information. The broken line at the 15-dB hearing level (HL) reflects the upper limit of typical hearing sensitivity. The degree of hearing level is often indicated by the average of the responses obtained at three different frequencies (500, 1,000, and 2,000 Hz). Hearing levels are classified into the following categories (Clark, 1981):

0–15 dB	Normal
16–25 dB	Slight or minimal
26–40 dB	Mild
41–55 dB	Moderate
56–70 dB	Moderately severe
71–90 dB	Severe
91+dB	Profound

Be aware, however, that even if two people both have a 70-dB hearing level, the audiogram may not necessarily look the same because the three PT tone-hearing threshold levels for each person may be at varying points, even if the end result is an average of 70 dB. People with a

GALLAUDET UNIVERSITY, HEARING AND SPEECH CENTER, Sorenson Language Communication Center (SLCC)
800 Florida Avenue, NE. Washington. DC 20002-3695 (202) 651-5328 (V/TTY) (202) 651-5324 (FAX) (202) 651-7328 (VP)

Name:_____ Date:_____ Age:___ ___ Sex:_____

DOB:_____ Referred by:_____

AUDIOMETER:_____ IMMITTANCE METER:_____

Audiologist:_____
Transducer: headphones insert
Response
Reliability: good   moderate   poor

AUDIOGRAM
FREQUENCY (PITCH) IN HERTZ (Hz)

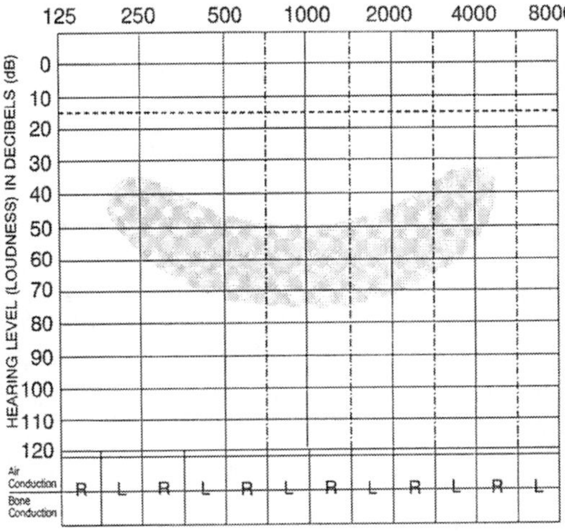

| | 125 | 250 | 500 | 1000 | 2000 | 4000 | 8000 |

HEARING LEVEL (LOUDNESS) IN DECIBELS (dB) — ANSI 1992
0, 10, 20, 30, 40, 50, 60, 70, 80, 90, 100, 110, 120

Air Conduction
Bone Conduction
R L R L R L R L R L R L

LEGE

		Right	Left
Air:	Unmasked	○	✳
	Masked		
Bone:—	Unmasked	<	>
	Masked		

No Response
Best Bone _____
Vibrotactile Response ✳
Unaided Sound Field   S
Narrow Band Noise
Warble Tone

PURE TONE AVERAGE (R:) (L:)

	Right	Left
AIR	dBHL	dBHL

TYMPANOMETRY (daPa)
1.75 / -.3
-300 -200 -100 0 +100 +200

daPa   Right Left
C₁=_____
SC=_____

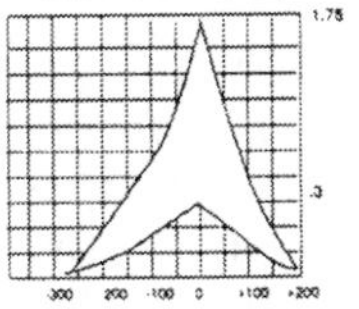

ABBREVIATIONS
C1 Canal Volume
CNA Could Not Average
CNE Could Not Establish
CNT Could Not Test
DNT Did Not Test
HL Hearing Level
MLV Monitored Live Voice
MTS Monosyllable, Troches, Spondees Test
MCL Most Comfortable Listening Level
NR No Response
PB% Word Recognition
SC Static Compliance
SDT Speech Detection Threshold
SRT Speech Recognition Threshold
S/N Signal To Noise Ratio
UCL Uncomfortable Listening Level

ACOUSTIC REFLEX MEASUREMENTS

Ear	Right				Left			
Stimulus	.5K	1K	2K	4K	.5K	1K	2K	4K
Contra (HL)								
Decay								
Ipsi (HL) (SPL)								

SPEECH AUDIOMETRY (dBHL)   MLV ☐   RECORDED ☐   LIST:_____

	SDT	SRT	MCL	UCL	PB% / HL	MASKING R L	PB% / HL	MASKING R L	PB% / HL	MASKING R L	MTS Categ%	HL Recog%
R		✳			/		/		/			/
L		✳			/		/		/			/
SF UNAIDED					/		/		/			/
AIDED					/		/		/			/

*Full ___ Select ___

TEST INTERPRETATION:

TYPE: R   L
☐ No Hearing Loss   ____   ____
☐ Conductive   ____   ____
☐ Mixed   ____   ____
☐ Sensorineural   ____   ____

DEGREE
R: _____
_____

L: _____
_____

RECOMMENDATION(S)
☐ Medical Referral
☐ Recheck Following Consultation
☐ Special Tests_____
☐ Hearing Aid Evaluation

☐ New earmold(s)
☐ Hearing Aid Check
☐ See Hearing Aid Worksheet
☐ Annual Reevaluation
☐ Other (Specify): _____

COMMENTS:_____
_____
_____
_____
_____
_____

_____   _____
Supervising Audiologist, CCC-A   Graduate Clinician

98-290M

Figure A.1 Typical Audiogram

Source: Used with permission from the Gallaudet University Department of Hearing, Speech, and Language Sciences.

70 dB hearing level do not necessarily hear things the same way, which is why they may prefer different types of hearing devices better suited to their individual audiometric configuration.

Figure A.2 provides some examples of where ordinary environmental sounds may fall on the audiogram when considering their decibel level and frequency range. Someone with a hearing level of 85 dB at 500 Hz will be unable to hear a dog barking, as indicated in Figure A.2.

In Figure A.1, there is a section on speech audiometry. This involves assessing the individual's ability to identify, recognize, and discriminate speech. Standardized tests are administered using the same calibrated equipment used for PT testing. Audiologists use different tests to assess speech capabilities. Results can often be very consistent with the type and degree of hearing level. Measurements are obtained in both unaided (no amplification) and aided listening conditions.

Additionally, Figure A.1 shows a tympanometry chart for an objective test that evaluates middle ear status, more specifically how well the eardrum moves. Specialized equipment measures eardrum movement with the introduction of a tone and various amounts of positive and negative pressure in the external ear canal. The individual remains quiet during the procedure. Abnormal readings can suggest conditions such as fluid in the middle ear space, Eustachian tube dysfunction, eardrum perforation, or disarticulation of the ossicles.

Other procedures have also been developed to predict the presence or absence of hearing sensitivity, particularly for infants, children, and difficult-to-test populations (Cone, 2011). Behavioral observation is one method that lacks reliability due to difficulties in separating responses from random behavior. More reliable and commonly used methods include auditory brainstem response (ABR) testing that uses electrodes (similar to EEG) on the back of the neck, forehead, and cheek or shoulder and measurement of otoacoustic emissions (OAE), which determines hair cell functions in the cochlea through cochlear emissions (waves) exiting the ear that are detected by a microphone in the ear, indicating that the infant's ear is responding to the sounds presented during the screening. Both procedures are noninvasive, although administering ABR sometimes requires sedation.

Hearing Aids and Cochlear Implants

Hearing aids are electroacoustic devices worn behind the ear, in the ear, and in the canal for the purpose of amplifying sound. Detailed information on hearing aids and their usefulness can be found in the following websites:

- www.asha.org/public/hearing/Hearing-Aids/
- www.audiology.org/publications-resources/document-library/pediatric-rehabilitation-hearing-aids

In contrast, cochlear implants are surgically implanted for the purpose of allowing the user to hear sound. The sound processer that fits behind the ear processes sound signals, which are then transmitted to the receiver implanted behind the ear. This receiver sends the signals to electrodes that have been inserted into the cochlea, which then transmits these signals to the auditory nerve and in turn to the brain for recognizing and interpreting these signals as sounds. These sounds differ from what hearing people hear. Training cochlear implant users to understand what the sounds mean is often required. Details can be found at www.nidcd.nih.gov/health/hearing/pages/coch.aspx. Those of you who are curious about what it sounds like to hear speech and music through a hearing aid and a cochlear implant can also check this website.

Note

1   Center for Disease Control (2015); Lucker (2002/2005).

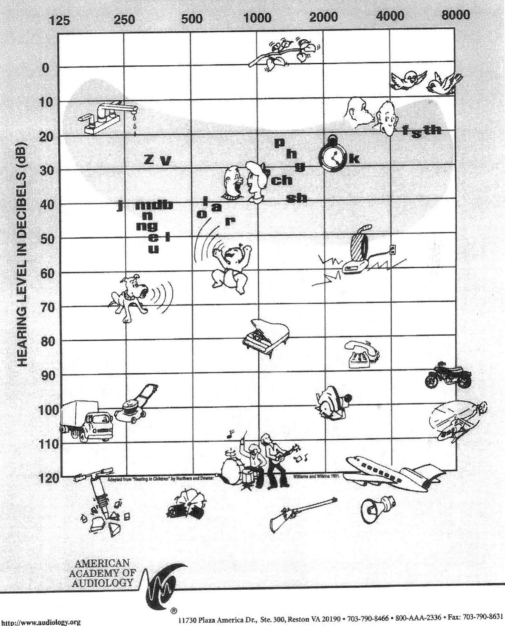

AUDIOGRAM OF FAMILIAR SOUNDS

Figure A.2 Audiogram of Speech Sounds

Source: Used with permission from the American Academy of Audiology.

4   Cognition, Language, and the Mind

We feel in one world, we think and name in another. Between the two we can set up a system of references, but we cannot fill the gap.

Marcel Proust (1871–1922)

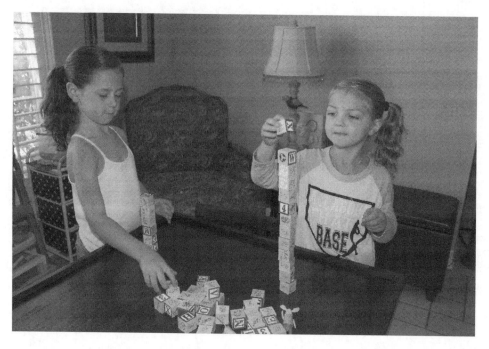

Figure 4.1 Two girls use their categorization skills as they stack blocks
Source: Used with permission.

Introduction

The psychological effects of being deaf are most obvious when the onset is early in life and when the degree of hearing loss is profound. If communication and language are not acquired early, there is a risk of cognitive and language delay. This, combined with poverty, can compound the deaf child's vulnerability for abuse, neglect, and maltreatment (Lomas & Johnson, 2012). Also, such delay can also significantly affect the child's educational, psychological, and social development, with repercussions for careers, marriages, friends, and overall quality of life. Ongoing findings in the areas of cognition, language, and neuroscience serve to create optimism for educational programs targeted to the needs of deaf children that can ameliorate the effects of earlier delays.

Chapter Objectives

Through a selective analysis of theoretical and empirical literature, we address how deaf individuals develop cognition, language, and thinking. We see how gesture and eye-gaze behaviors begin the development of both spoken and signed languages. A discussion about cochlear implants and their outcomes relative to cognition and language is presented. We conclude by raising the question of what research on thinking and language we can use to foster academic learning in the classroom.

Cognitive Abilities

Cognitive abilities include perception, attending, memory, problem solving, thinking, understanding, and language (Omstead & Kuhlmeier, 2015). From existing studies, we do know that deaf people use their vision, their sign language, their residual hearing, what spoken language capacity they have, their background and world knowledge, home and school experiences, communication modes, and learning styles (either visual, auditory, or both) to experience and interpret their environment (Andrews, Leigh, & Weiner, 2004). These cognitive processes may be similar but also different compared to those used by hearing persons (Marschark et al., 2015).

Intelligence Testing

Historically, intelligence has been linked to the ability to speak and read. Because many deaf individuals may have inadequate spoken and written language, they were believed to be inferior in intelligence to hearing people, as mentioned in Chapter 1. With the recognition of ASL and the understanding of cognitive abilities using sign language, the perspective of the intelligence of Deaf persons is better understood (Braden, 1994; Mayberry, 2002).

Expanding on what Chapter 1 states, prior to the 1950s, deaf people were given both verbal and nonverbal intelligence tests and were found to have lower combined IQ scores than hearing people in general. They were considered inferior in intelligence and abstract thinking (Braden, 1994). However, subsequent studies showed that when deaf adults and children were compared with hearing norms on measures of nonverbal abilities, they were found to have similar scores (Braden, 1994; Vernon, 1965/2005). The low performance on verbal and nonverbal IQ tests was often attributed to lack of language, test bias, not comprehending the test directions, or a combination of these factors (Vernon & Andrews, 1990).

Furth (1964) conducted some of the early empirical studies that examined deaf persons' performance on nonverbal cognitive tasks and found that deaf people perform similarly to hearing persons. He attributed deaf persons' poorer performance on some tasks to be related to their lack of experiences, with those differences decreasing as deaf persons became adults. Furth also determined that the so-called evidence for lower cognition in Deaf learners was not due to their performance entirely but was also due to inappropriate tests being used to assess their performance. This was a major breakthrough in our understanding of cognition as applied to deaf people during this time (see discussion of Furth's work in Martin, 2014).

In a meta-analysis of 285 studies that included 171,517 deaf children from 1900 to 1988, Braden (1994) found no significant difference in scores comparing nonverbal IQ scores that used norms for deaf children compared to studies that used norms developed for hearing children (Braden, 1994). Other studies showed that deaf children of deaf parents scored higher on nonverbal IQ tests than deaf children of hearing parents. This has been hypothesized to be due to nonsyndromic genetic etiologies (as opposed to etiologies caused by disease and genetic syndromes with neurological involvement) and early language experiences (Vernon & Andrews, 1990). Studies using verbal measures showed that if deaf children's early language interaction, whether in spoken or sign language, was of poor quality, their verbal IQ scores were lower than those scores of hearing children (Mayberry, 2002).

Thought and Language

Thought is connected to language, with language being the vehicle that conveys our thoughts to others. This requires symbols, either signs or words that we associate with objects, names of people, etc., that we store in our minds. The language of thought is called *mentalese*. This differs from *communicative language*, which makes use of symbols whose meanings we share (Corballis, 2002).

Although language and thought are not the same, they do influence each other. One theory called the *Whorfian hypothesis* or *linguistic determinism* proposed the notion that our language determines our thinking. While this theory has been debunked (Pinker, 1990), it is still accepted that language at some level affects thinking and may influence how individuals like deaf people will differ in their performance on a variety of perceptual and cognitive tasks (e.g., peripheral vision, face recognition).

Sign language may provide a path for deaf people to organize their thoughts, experiences, and perceptions of the world that may very well be different from nonsigners (Emmorey, 2002). Knowledge of sign language influences visual perception, visual-spatial perception, motion, and the use of facial expressions (Emmorey, 2002). So while language does not determine thought per se, our languages can direct us to pay attention to certain perceptual features and give us practice in performing some cognitive tasks (Traxler, 2012). Better understanding of these differences may assist us in developing more effective teaching strategies for deaf children.

All babies can think before they talk and have what Pinker (1990, p. 201) states is "a considerable amount of cognitive machinery in place before they start." And, by the age of 12 to 24 months, babies have developed nonverbal working memory (Hauser, Lukomski, & Hillman, 2008). As language is acquired, deaf children have a powerful cognitive tool to facilitate their ability to translate their thoughts into gestures, speech, signs, and written language. They can even form new thoughts without experiences with real objects and events. Hence, language expands the child's thinking skills.

Visual Attention Abilities

Language acquisition starts with visual attention skills. This is a cognitive process that can be categorized into the components of selective attention, sustained attention, and divided attention (Olmstead & Kuhlmeier, 2015). Due to limitations in how deaf people may use their residual hearing or assistive hearing devices, a common belief is that they compensate by having enhanced vision because they make use of it in place of hearing. Research suggests that the brain, as a multisensory processor, adapts to compensate for lack of auditory stimulation and this results in a cross-modal takeover of the auditory cortex region with visual stimuli (Dye & Bavelier, 2010). The compensatory plasticity hypothesis is a theory that explains how areas in the brain are programmed to respond to one sense that is taken over by another sense when sensory input is reduced (Olmstead & Kuhlmeier, 2015). But studies are far from conclusive for this theory. Indeed, other studies show that enhanced visual attention cannot be generalized to all deaf individuals because many have residual hearing and use audition for communication and learning (Marschark, Morrison, Lukomski, Borgna, & Convertino, 2013; Marschark et al., 2015).

What is known is that both deaf and hearing groups show the same visual processing when seeing shades of color and distinguishing between flashing items and visual motion. However, Deaf individuals who use ASL perform better than hearing signers and nonsigners on certain tasks such as being able to quickly change their visual attention, scan visual material, detect motion, and recognize faces (Dye & Bavelier, 2010). Further, when experiments using neuroimaging technology have compared two groups of early signers (deaf and hearing), researchers have found that native Deaf signers processed motion in the peripheral visual field faster than hearing signers. This peripheral processing advantage cannot be fully attributed to signing but rather to their lack of auditory stimulation (Bavelier et al., 2001).

Visual selective attention has a temporal component as well. For example, Dye and Bavelier (2010) found that young, native-signing deaf children below the age of 10 years are distracted when there is motion on either side of them. However, older deaf native signers are able to control their distractibility when movement occurs around them.

Visual Spatial Abilities

Studies have shown that native Deaf signing individuals who use sign language have advantages in visual spatial abilities, that is, the ability to perceive, analyze, and synthesize objects with visual patterns, compared to these same skills with hearing people (Emmorey, 2002). However, the effects on visual-spatial cognition of auditory deprivation and the use of sign language versus spoken language are complex. For example, Marschark and his colleagues (2015) examined language, visual-spatial, and nonverbal reasoning executive functioning (EF) abilities among deaf and hearing university students and found that the hearing students outperformed the deaf learners on selected visual-spatial tasks. They attribute this finding to the association of performance on visual-spatial tasks with differing cognitive abilities and suggest that different cognitive processes may be involved in visual-spatial processing for the deaf and hearing groups in their study.

Bimodal Processing

To remind the reader, hearing loss exists on a continuum from mild to profound, and there are many deaf and hard-of-hearing children and adults who process speech and language visually as well as through audition. This is called *bimodal processing*. For example, orally trained, nonsigning deaf people use both their vision to "read" language on the mouth (e.g., speechreading) or on the face (facial expressions) and on the body (e.g., body language) along with using their auditory processing through hearing aids or cochlear implants. They may also have developed an "inner language" based on the speech code, and this may help them in communicating, reading, and writing (Litchenstein, 1988).

Bimodal processing can also occur within models of reading for deaf children based on auditory phonological awareness, whether it is delivered via articulation, speechreading, residual hearing, through visual phonics or cued speech, or even through a signed English code delivered simultaneously with spoken language (LaSasso & Crain, 2015). See Chapter 6 for further details.

There are benefits to our understanding of bimodal processing for orally trained deaf persons, deaf persons who use cochlear implants and hard-of-hearing children. Deaf people who use spoken language look for ways to improve their auditory access in addition to depending on vision in their environment (Leigh, Morere, & Pezzarossi, 2014).

Memory, Learning, and Reasoning

Memory is a cognitive process that is important for thinking, language, and particularly reading (see Chapter 6). Studies show that signers and speakers use the same working memory

(WM) structures but with different subprocesses (Hall & Bavelier, 2010). For example, studies show that speakers use the phonological codes to a greater extent than signers who may use a combination of codes that include phonological, visuo-spatial, and also episodic processes (Hall & Bavelier, 2010). Differences in WM processes between deaf and hearing individuals are more indicative of auditory deprivation, language exposure, and language preferences rather than cognitive deficits (Hall & Bavelier, 2010).

Memory and cognitive development have been studied using Jean Piaget's (1896–1980) cognitive stage theory of development, which was applied to deaf children by Furth (1964). Following Piaget's model, during the sensorimotor stage (0 to 2 years), the first level of cognition focuses on motor reflexes. As deaf children move into the preoperational stage (2–6 years), there may be a delay for those who lacked communication and age-appropriate experiences with the environment. In the concrete operational stage (6–12 years), deaf children, if they lack language skills, will be limited in their understandings during interactions with adults to using only concrete examples. In the final stage of formal operations (12–15 years), they will need language to demonstrate abstract thinking in order to solve problems (Furth, 1964).

During each of these stages, deaf children's cognitive and linguistic functioning may have an impact on their ability to remember information. They may use visuospatial memory if they use sign language or verbal rehearsal strategies if they have more spoken language skills. They may have shorter spans of short-term memory for serial information and may have difficulty labeling their learning if they do not have language fluency in either spoken or sign language (see reviews of memory research in Marschark, 1993).

Lev Vygotsky (1896–1934) also studied memory and viewed language as a cognitive tool. Child social speech was developed through what Vygotsky (1978) called *inner-direct speech*. His theory underscored the importance of culture and social interactions with more knowledgeable others who scaffold or support deaf children's learning. Vygotsky makes the distinction between basic cognitive processes such as attention and memory and higher-order processes that are culturally shaped and socially mediated through language.

Short-term memory studies with deaf persons demonstrate conflicting results. For example, Conrad (1979) claims that, because of the linguistic demands of many of the experimental tasks used for studies, children were forced to guess and had to rely on their previous experiences or lexical knowledge. Therefore, deaf children with limited vocabulary were at a marked disadvantage. In many of these studies, the hearing subjects' performance on memory tasks was superior to deaf subjects' performance. However, on tasks such as memory for visual design, reversed recall, learning words matched with signs, discrimination of word pairs, recalling left to right digits presentation and forward recall of digits, and word recognition of fingerspelled words, the deaf subjects performed better than the hearing subjects who were tested. Many of the researchers noted that the deaf subjects were processing the information differently compared to their hearing peers, a finding that is consistent even today. (Again, see Marschark [1993] for further explanation.)

Long-term memory studies have focused on semantic bases for recall and have used nonverbal stimuli (drawings) to control for the language variable. Researchers have noted the importance of labeling in either spoken language or sign language so fluency in language was important in the ability to perform on these tasks. Also noted was the experience with stimuli. Deaf persons showed evidence of sign language coding in some memory tasks. In the main, hearing and deaf were found to use different strategies for remembering, as Marschark's (1993) review notes, and this has implications for teaching and learning.

Other studies show that native-deaf, signing children show better memory than hearing children on visuospatial tasks that do not require language. They use both visual imagery in place of verbal codes and spatial coding to remember information (e.g., furniture in the room) compared to hearing nonsigners (Marschark & Wauters, 2008). Deaf students can use signs to remember printed words, images, and sign phrases but need to be taught this strategy (Hamilton, 2011). Deaf children remember numbers and printed words less than hearing children do, but they remember better with tasks such as remembering unfamiliar faces and paths of lights arranged in space (Hamilton, 2011; Marschark & Wauters, 2008). In another study, researchers studied deaf children, deaf adults, and hearing adult fluent signers and found that they relied on top-down scaffolding in their working memory when remembering ASL sentences. In contrast, less fluent signers used a linear process of naming signs and imitating signs rather than remembering the meaning of the sentence. In other words, memory ability may be tied to mode of communication (Supalla, Hauser, & Bavelier, 2014).

Another cognitive ability, analytic reasoning, was also related to mode of communication. Deaf students, ages 9 to 10 years and 12 to 13 years from two different linguistic environments—deaf children of Deaf parents using sign language and deaf children of hearing parents using spoken language—were studied. Students were given three series of analogy tasks. Results indicated that early and consistent language and communication played an equivalent role in the development of verbal, numerical, and spatial reasoning similar to those of a comparison group of hearing children (Bandurski & Galkowski, 2004).

Metacognitive Abilities

Metacognition, or "thinking about thinking," is what students use to manage their cognitive processes, including aspects such as reasoning, comprehension, problem solving, and learning (Baker, 2002). While we do not need language to think, when we have language we can increase our thinking skills in tasks that involve play, Theory of Mind, and executive functioning as we interact with others. These are forms of social cognition and are important in the development of thinking skills and language skills.

Play

During play activities, children take on the roles of their toys such as dolls and stuffed animals, act out the routines of their lives, and engage in fantasy and pretend play. Studies show that deaf children with hearing mothers have similar play behaviors during the early stages of play, but when symbolic behavior or language becomes important, deaf children experience delays (Spencer, 2010). In a study of play with a 4-year-old deaf girl with deaf parents who was enrolled in a bilingual preschool, the researcher found that the girl's play behaviors were similar to those of 4-year-old hearing children as both had language skills to use during play activities (Musyoka, 2015). For further discussion on the role of play in early cognitive and psychosocial development, see Chapter 7.

Theory of Mind

Another metacognitive skill is Theory of Mind (ToM), which is another form of social cognition that covers how children begin to understand the feelings and perspectives of others. ToM is learned through observing and participating in conversations with others, particularly siblings and caregivers (Siegal, 2008). Two factors that were found to promote ToM are the mothers' sign language abilities and their proficiency in talking to their deaf child about feelings and beliefs (Moeller & Schick, 2006).

One study examined the behaviors of 176 deaf children who had Deaf parents and found that their ToM skills were equal to those of hearing children (Schick et al., 2007). Children who were late signers often did not have conversations at home where they could learn about other people's feelings, wants, and thoughts, and this impeded them from learning about the perspective of others. Even with factors such as syntax abilities, mental age in spatial ability, and executive functioning being factored in, late signers still had difficulty in understanding ToM tasks shown on pictures (Schick et al., 2007). While ToM often does not develop until the teen years for deaf individuals, most hearing children develop ToM as early as age 4 (Moeller & Schick, 2006; Schick et al., 2007).

Executive Function

Executive function (EF), another metacognitive skill, refers to a set of self-regulation skills that allow the individual to focus attention, remember instructions, organize, control one's impulses, have emotional understanding, and have the ability to problem solve, to plan and get things done. Similar to ToM, EF skills develop through early conversations with caregivers about everyday activities from childhood to adolescence to adult years (Center on the Developing Child, 2012).

One aspect of EF is problem solving. Marschark and Everhart (1999) found differences in deaf and hearing college students on their performance in problem-solving a 20-question task. In another study, Luckner and McNeill (1994) found differences in performance between deaf and hearing students on a Tower of Hanoi puzzle. In both studies, the groups of deaf students had difficulty in solving the problems.

Another approach to studying EF is to query teachers and parents and ask them to rate children on information related to their working memory, emotional control, and problem-solving capabilities using a questionnaire called the BRIEF (Behavior Rating Inventory of Executive Functioning), which has separate forms for parents and teachers (Hintermair, 2013). In its current form, BRIEF is an 86-item questionnaire that covers eight theoretically and empirically based clinical scales of behavior (www4.parinc.com/products/Product.aspx?ProductID=BRIEF). There are teacher and parent forms, as well as forms for children themselves. Hintermair (2013) had teachers assess 214 deaf and hard-of-hearing students using a German version of the BRIEF and found a significantly higher behavioral problem rate for EF compared to hearing norms. Hintermair (2013) also reviews EF studies indicating that, for example, there is a relationship between measures of social language ability and EF skills as measured by the BRIEF with young deaf children ages 6 to 14 (Rhine-Kalback, 2004, as cited in Hintermair, 2013). Hintermair concludes that the roles of EF and communicative competence are significant for behavior problems.

Another EF self-regulation skill noted by Hauser, Lukomski, and Hillman (2008) is the use of eye-gaze behaviors. Deaf children need to know when and where to look for linguistic information not only at home but when they enter school. Many deaf children who do not have early communication will enter school and not have the eye contact behaviors to follow conversations in the classroom, and this impedes their learning (Hauser et al., 2008).

Cognitive abilities, both lower-level perception and attention and higher-level cognitive abilities that include cognition and language during memory, reasoning, and metacognition tasks are interrelated. They continue to interact, build on each other, and co-evolve throughout the deaf child's mental development.

The psychological impact of processing language in primarily the visual modality has profound implications for how deaf children learn concepts, language, social skills, and academic subjects. This difference in processing has implications for how to set up early language learning programs as well as how to structure learning in schools (see Chapter 5 on educational aspects and Chapter 6 on bilingual approaches). In this next section, we see how language in the visual and auditory modalities is structured, how they are acquired, and how they develop.

ASL and English Languages

Structures

ASL is a fully developed visual-spatial language with a complex grammar and rules for sign formation. Both ASL and English have similar organizational principles with rule-governed features. Just as a person cannot make up a word with a set of random letters, likewise, a person cannot make up a sign with random handshapes, locations, and positions.[1] English sentences are linear in their expression of ideas whereas ASL uses simultaneous production of signs to show relationships among lexical items. ASL, like English, can be analyzed at the sign, word, sentence, and discourse levels as both have phonology, morphology, syntax, semantics, and discourse. While English uses intonation and other voice contours, ASL uses space, body shifts, eye gazes, and head shifts in conversations. The basic order for a sentence found in English, subject-verb-object, is not always found in ASL. With its flexible word order, ASL sentences can be expressed in a variety of ways such as the use of topicalization (Valli et al., 2011). For more in-depth discussions of ASL and English linguistic structures, see Andrews, Leigh, and Weiner (2004); Quirk, Greenbaum, Leech, and Svartivik (1972); and Valli, Lucas, Mulrooney, and Villanueva (2011).

Language Use and Environments

Deaf children of Deaf parents will learn ASL from birth. The majority of deaf children who have hearing parents will not learn ASL or an English-based sign system until they meet other deaf children or if their parents take sign language classes. Most deaf children, and even some with Deaf parents, will learn and use a spoken language. A limited number of Deaf parents send their children to schools that focus solely on spoken language.

Spoken language for all deaf children can be difficult to acquire even with a digital hearing aid or cochlear implant. Despite using the most up-to-date technology, the cochlear implant still produces a degraded signal that does not mimic what the hearing person hears. And when the child enters a noisy environment, the signal is even harder to hear. Sign communication is easier to acquire because of easy access to visual and gestural systems. Signing provides full and open access to language, particularly for deaf children of Deaf parents who follow the same developmental milestones for language that hearing children do, using the visual-gestural modality in signing rather than the auditory/oral modality in speaking (Newport & Meier, 1985). However, many hearing parents, siblings, and other extended family members do not learn to sign or do not learn to sign fluently so that the deaf child has limited access to signing in the home. Further, deaf children who are raised in spoken language as well as sign language learning environments are both at a disadvantage because they miss out on incidental learning around them when not everyone in their environment can sign. Even Deaf cochlear implant users and Deaf signing non-cochlear implant users who enter postsecondary programs will struggle with world knowledge that tends to be acquired through incidental learning despite learning to read and write proficiently (Convertino et al., 2014). The fact of being deaf is that language across all aspects such as phonology, semantics, morphology, syntax, and pragmatics will be delayed unless appropriate intervention is provided. Even with interventions, delays can still occur because of limited access to incidental learning and language, and this can be exacerbated if the child fails to learn to read and write (see Chapter 6).

The relationship between the environment, various etiologies that cause one to be deaf, and language learning has been studied with deaf as well as other exceptional learners. These cases provide "natural experiments" to examine the ways cognition and language develop even under unusual circumstances such as in deprived and abusive environments, in families where the parents are Deaf and the children are hearing, and in the cases of children who have cognitive abilities or issues or have Williams syndrome (WS, a genetic syndrome that includes striking verbal abilities in addition to other possible sequelae including cardiovascular disease, developmental delays, and learning disabilities (https://williams-syndrome.org/what-is-williams-syndrome).

The case of Victor (Lane, 1976) and Genie (Rymer, 1994) are examples of feral children who experienced severe environmental deprivation and who could only learn a few basic vocabulary words in later childhood when they were rescued. Another form of language deprivation occurs when preschool children arrive at school with limited or no language exposure (Vernon & Andrews, 1990). These children often invent their own language using a spatial syntax (Goldin-Meadow, 2003). The fact that many of these children will learn a sign language, though not as fluent as native signers, in late childhood and even early adulthood challenges the hypothesis that there is a sensitive period for learning language.

Children typically bring their thought processes to the language learning process. One group of children with Williams syndrome challenges this idea of the cognitive underpinnings of linguistic development. With WS, linguistic abilities are preserved, but there are mild-to-moderate intellectual disabilities or learning problems (Genetics Home Reference, 2016). These children tend to have outgoing personalities. When they speak, they show sophisticated use of language with a complex syntax and adult-like vocabulary and can learn by repetition (Genetics Home Reference, 2016). These children demonstrate that there are some parts of the brain that can process and acquire language in the absence of higher level cognitive skills previously thought necessary for language acquisition (Bellugi et al., 1994). In contrast to WS children, deaf children have normal cognitive abilities but struggle with mastering the words and grammar of English.

Language Origins and Theories

One anthropological view of language origins is that pointing and gestures were humans' earliest form of language. Speech development came afterwards, with grammar evolving through the use of gestures (Stokoe, 2001).

B. F. Skinner (1957) proposed a psycholinguistic view that claims children learn language when they imitate their adult caretaker's speech through stimulus-response conditioning. The Skinnerian view was debunked by the Chomsky (1965) linguistic revolution in the 1970s. Chomsky proposed the nativist or innate view that claims human brains are preprogrammed to learn language. He also claimed that every child in any culture will learn the language of their culture because of this mental device, called the Language Acquisition Device (LAD). Instead of the LAD, Pinker (1990) suggested that humans are born with a "language instinct."

A compromise perspective to the Skinner/Chomsky view is that of the interactionist perspective. Those who hold this view posit that both genetics and environmental input contribute to language acquisition (Chapman, 2000). Additionally, Chomsky's nativist approach has been challenged by another theory called the *probabilistic language learning approach*, which is supported by data showing that word categories and morphological knowledge can be learned through environmental exposure (Hsu, Chater, & Vitányi, 2011). Probabilistic language learning, also called statistical language learning, reflects implicit rather than explicit language learning, which relies on the ability of the infant to automatically pick up and learn from the statistical regularities that exist in the stream of sensory information processed by the brain. Statistical language learning is believed to be strongly influenced by both phonetic learning and early word learning (Kuhl, 2010; 2015). Thus, the role of the brain's computational skills combined with cognitive and social interaction is seen to foster infant language learning.

P. Kuhl (2007) proposes another psycholinguistic theory called the *Social Gating Hypothesis*. Her theory suggests that social interaction provides language learning by increasing attention, information provided by another, a sense of relationship using gaze following, and the activation of parts of the brain that link perception and action. All of these theories are most relevant for the young deaf child who needs early language intervention so that the brain can be exposed to these statistical regularities of language, whether these be phonemes in the speech stream (sounds of spoken language) or phonemes in the sign stream (visual phonology of sign language). And all of this must be done early if the deaf child is able to maximize cognitive and language development.

Language Acquisition

Hearing babies begin their psycholinguistic development even in the womb as they hear and feel the vibrations of their mother's talk. Babies learn about prosodic features of their native language in the third trimester before they are born and can tell the difference between speech sounds as early as 2 months of age (Kuhl, 2015).

From birth to 7 months, both deaf and hearing babies exhibit gestures primarily as part of their movement or motor development. From 7 to 12 months of age, they use gestures to show what they want. As they use these communication gestures in different situations, the gestures take on symbolic meaning. In hearing infants, gestures will emerge, be used in combination with speech (co-speech), and then dropped when speech becomes an easier means of communication (Volterra & Erting, 1998). For deaf babies with signing input from caregivers, these gestures will evolve into a formalized language of signs.

According to Kuhl (2010), babies are little scientists who learn about the world by conducting experiments, analyzing statistics, and forming theories to account for their observations. This is a consequence of having brains that are wired for learning and creativity. Brain imaging and behavioral studies show that when babies are exposed to sounds early and learn specific sounds in the second half of the first year, this establishes connections in their brain for the native tongue in the home but not for other languages unless a child is exposed to multiple languages (Kuhl, 2015). Specifically, at birth the infant brain can understand a large set of sounds or phonemes that can be combined to form words in every language in the world (Kuhl, 2015). A perceptual narrowing occurs where babies will only perceive the sounds of their native language. Neuroscientists talk about a "sensitive period" during which the baby's brain is ready to learn the basic rules of the home language. This sensitivity fades as the child gets older; however, a child can still pick up a second language later if innate ability is present and the language is accessible (Kuhl, 2015).

In the early stages, both hearing and deaf babies babble vocally reflexively. Deaf babies will stop vocally babbling at age 6 or 7 months if they do not hear sounds through auditory feedback. Deaf babies exposed to signing will develop finger babbling, along with vocal babbling in a systemic fashion, not by randomly fluttering their fingers (Petitto & Marentette, 1991). Both hearing and deaf babies produce sounds and handshapes in expected and regular sequences. Hearing babies will develop their babbling and then progress to the one-word stage using a sequence of sounds that resemble words (e.g., baby talk) while deaf babies make a sequence of handshapes that are close to looking like signs (baby signs) (Petitto & Marentette, 1991).

Parents and caregivers establish eye contact, smile, set up joint attention, and provide words or signs to label objects the baby wants (Acredolo & Goodwyn, 1994). For hearing children, these early gestures evolve into spoken words at approximately 1 year of age with constant support, scaffolding, and social interaction (Kuhl, 2015). Later the gestures decrease in number as the hearing baby begins to talk and speech becomes easier to use. But babies may still use gestures to support their spoken language (Volterra & Erting, 1998).

Just as hearing babies learn to communicate through gestures, deaf children who are exposed to signing use gestures; some vocalizations too; and names of objects and activities to build their language, thinking, and social skills. For children born deaf into a hearing family, the learning of signing can happen at different times from early to late childhood, or even not until their teen years or young adulthood (Mayberry, 2002). Typically, deaf children of hearing parents are exposed to a spoken language first and then learn a sign language later. This puts some children at risk for language deprivation. This deprivation does not have to happen, as witness the case of Deaf children of Deaf parents and hearing parents who learn sign language. This is not to say all deaf babies cannot develop spoken language. But the point is that, even with amplification and cochlear implantation, speech must be taught directly and the training can be intensive and laborious, and not every deaf child can master spoken language intelligibly. The learning of spoken language by the deaf child is radically different from the hearing child who effortlessly picks up the spoken language around the household. For deaf children, it's an instructional process and hard work.

Using baby talk, motherese, parentese, toddlerese, or child-directed speech, parents and caregivers talk with exaggerated inflections, slower speech, sing-song rhythms, and repetition in order to affectionately engage their babies. Unbeknownst to many parents, this special register serves other purposes. It teaches their babies the intonations and cadences of the baby's native language, and it creates a social-emotional bond (Kuhl, 2015). Using sign language, in a similar fashion, Deaf mothers repeat signs, exaggerate, and sign slower to make sure their babies are seeing and understanding them. The mothers make signs on their baby's body or on objects or near food items. Mothers and caregivers engage the baby in eye contact and use eye gazes to build joint attention as they set up *conversational triangles* using space, pointing to a book, toy, or food item while maintaining eye contact with their child (Mather, Rodriguez-Fraticelli, Andrews, & Rodriguez, 2006).

Both Deaf mothers and hearing mothers make extensive use of eye gaze, vision, and touch. The ability to regulate eye gaze is important for communication and language and is predictive for later vocabulary. Further, the eye-gaze behaviors scaffold later joint attention and set the stage for vocabulary learning and other aspects of language development (Clark et al., 2015). Table 4.1 shows eye-gaze patterns between mother and child.

Table 4.1 Eye-Gaze Behavior between Caregiver and Infant

Six Ways to Support and Develop Eye-Gaze or Visual Attention with Infants	
Caregiver Behaviors	Infant Behaviors
Waiting until the infant looks at caregiver, followed by **immediate** communication	Infant directs **eye-gaze** to caregiver
Pointing to an object **Gesturing** in the infant's visual direction and field of vision (waving arm or hand)	Infant directs eye gaze to the object Infant directs eye gaze to caregiver
Physical touch	
Stroking	Infant directs eye gaze to caregiver
Tapping	
Vibrating the floor or on an object	Infant directs eye gaze to caregiver
Vocalizing in the infant's general direction	Infant directs eye gaze to caregiver

Source: From Clark, M. D., Galloza-Carrero, A., Keith, C. L., Tibbitt, J. S., Wolsey, J.L.A., & Zimmerman, H. G. (2015). Eye-gaze development in infants: Learning to look and looking to learn. *Advance for Speech and Hearing*. Retrieved from http://speech-language-pathology-audiology.advanceweb.com/Features/Articles/Eye-Gaze-Development-in-Infants.aspx. Reprinted with permission from Advance for Speech and Hearing.

Motherese or parentese may very well help the infant in the segmenting of the sign or the speech stream. Using single word or sign utterances may help too. As in the theories mentioned earlier, the baby's brain is hardwired to look for statistical regularities or the repetition of syllables in either sign or spoken words; this promotes language acquisition (Kuhl, 2015; Petitto, Holowka, Sergio, & Ostry, 2001). For deaf children, whether the language input is spoken, signed, or both, the earlier the better for the deaf child's cognitive, linguistic, and social growth and development.

Language Development

Toddlers use tools to help them learn vocabulary. One tool is to use naming games with their caregivers during which they point to objects and name them (e.g., "Where is your nose?"), which leverage their object recognition skills (Traxler, 2012). Children can also learn new words by taking the perspective of others (ToM), and their child language can be humorous to adults. For instance, a 3-year-old boy in a swing watched as his grandfather, who was using ear protection, rode by on a noisy lawn mower. The young boy said, "Grandpa wears ear muffs to keep the grass out of his ears" (James Phelan, personal communication, December 1, 2015).

Signing children have been observed to produce signs as early as 8 months, which is earlier than when hearing children produce their first spoken words. This may be due to the fact that this research was conducted using parent questionnaires where deaf children were given more credit for having produced an earlier lexical item or because of the iconicity of early signs. Lexical comprehension and production was studied in eight second-generation, deaf-signing toddlers (meaning they had deaf parents) in Italy using picture-naming tasks (Rinaldi, Caselli, Di Renzo, Gulli, & Volterra, 2014). A control group of hearing toddlers was utilized. The results showed that both Italian deaf and hearing children had higher comprehension scores than production scores. The deaf toddlers had slightly lower lexical production, but both groups were similar on comprehension. The authors concluded that signing toddlers were able to acquire predicates easier than nominals compared to the hearing toddlers and attributed this difference to input modalities and language structures of Italian Sign Language.

For deaf and hearing toddlers, the first spoken words and signs are made alone, but then after the babies acquire about fifty words and signs, they start to string words into two-word sentences. These early sentences begin to expand as the toddlers acquire the grammar of their languages. From 2 to 3 years of age, vocabulary continues to increase and morphemes are incorporated into utterances, which expand into phrases, clauses, and sentences. The deaf toddler learns more grammar with signs, body movements, and facial expressions. By age 3, the deaf toddler uses topicalization, conditional sentences, and directional verbs and uses space to signify grammar. The hearing toddler also uses expanded sentences with morphemes, engages in dialogue, uses *wh-* questions, and overregularizes the verb system. For example, the toddler may add the past *-ed* on all verbs, regular and irregular (e.g., "I goed to school"). Talk is in simple sentences, using negatives, imperatives, questions, and pronouns. By ages 4 and 5, both the deaf child and hearing child have learned most of the grammar of their languages and have a vocabulary of about 8,000 signs and or spoken words and can understand thousands more. At this age, they begin preschool and may use complex sentence structures and continue to refine their grammar systems (see reviews of psycholinguistic studies in Andrews, Logan, & Phelan, 2008). Table 4.2 presents a summary of ASL, speech, and hearing milestones.

Table 4.2 ASL, Speech, and Hearing Developmental Milestones

ASL (Deaf Children of Deaf Parents)	Speech (Hearing Children of Hearing Parents)	Hearing (Hearing Children of Hearing Parents)
Birth to 3 Months	**Birth to 3 Months**	At 20 weeks' gestation, the hearing system begins processing sounds that filter through amniotic fluid.
Finger movements evolve into rule-governed fingerbabbling.	Vocal babbling.	At 6 months' gestation and beyond, the fetus processes linguistic sounds, qualities of the mother's voice, and the language she speaks and becomes sensitive to prosody.
At 3 months, fingerbabbling increases, and the baby attends to faces, movements, and signs.	At 1 month, the baby can discriminate among individual speech sounds.	During last 3 months in womb, the baby hears the mother's conversations.
	Reflexive cries, vegetative cries.	
	Makes pleasure sounds (cooing, gooing).	**Birth to 3 Months**
	Cries differently for different needs.	Eyes widen, blinks, startles to sounds.
	Smiles when sees a person.	Eye shifts, quieting, beginning head turns at 4 months.
3 to 6 Months	**3 to 6 Months**	
Fingerbabbling increases.	Can discriminate among sequences of sounds.	**3 to 6 Months**
Visual attention increases.	Variety of vocalizations significantly increase.	Head turns on lateral plane toward sound, listening, attitude.
Fingerspells to self.	Repeats the same sounds.	Responds to changes in tone of voice.
Makes facial expressions.	Transitional or marginal babbling single-syllable and consonant-like sounds.	Notices toys make sounds.
Fixates to face.	Babbling sounds more speech-like with many different sounds, including /p/, /b/, and /m/.	Pays attention to music.
Fingerbabbles back to conversations.	Vocalizes excitement and displeasure.	
	Makes gurgling sounds when left alone and when playing.	
	Uses sounds and gestures to indicate wants.	

6 to 12 months

Uses syllabic manual babbling and manual jargon to self and objects.
First sign reported at 8 months; first single signs "frozen" with no inflections.
Understands meaning of specific interpersonal communication.
Communicates with gestures, pointing, and pulling.
Responds to simple commands, questions, and statements.
Uses some "true signs" to satisfy needs or wants.

6 to 9 Months

Babbling has long and short groups of sounds, such as "ta-ta," "up-up," and "bibibi."
Reduplicated babbling ("bababa").
Uses speech or noncrying sounds to get and keep attention.

10 Months

First words emerge
Imitates different sounds.
Has one to three words (bye-bye, da-da, mama).
Understands "no" and "hot."
Responds to simple requests.
Understands and responds to own name.
Uses song-like intonation pattern when babbling.
Uses echolalia.
Variegated babbling ("dadu").
Jargon babbling (intonational changes added to syllable production).
Uses speech sounds rather than cries to get attention.
Uses nouns almost exclusively.

6 to 12 Months

Direct localization of sounds to side, directly below ear level, and indirectly above ear level.
Understands and responds to simple commands.
Direct localization of sounds to side, directly below ear level, and indirectly above ear level.
Enjoys games like peek-a boo and pat-a-cake.
Listens when spoken to.
Recognizes common words for items like "cup," "shoe," and "juice."
Begins to respond to requests like "Come here" and "Want more?"

(Continued)

Table 4.2 Continued

ASL (Deaf Children of Deaf Parents)	Speech (Hearing Children of Hearing Parents)	Hearing (Hearing Children of Hearing Parents)
12 to 24 Months	**12 to 18 to 24 Months**	**12 to 24 Months**
ASL sign babbling. Uses baby signs (which approximate adult signs). One-word signs include nonlinguistic pointing (pointing used gestural instead of part of syntax). Manual jargon babbling continues. First 10 signs produced. Passes 50-sign milestone. Follows simple commands and statements. Understands names of things in environment. Expands vocabulary from about five words to more than 250. Enters two-word stage with full range of semantic relations at two-sign stage. Sign order shows semantic relations (e.g., "doggie outside," "doggie run outside"). Overgeneralize the pronoun "you," using it to refer to self.	Uses words more frequently than jargon. Has receptive vocabulary of 50 to 100 or more words. Has receptive vocabulary of 300 or more words. Combines nouns and verbs. Begins to use pronouns. Answers, "What's that?" questions. Knows five body parts. Accurately names a few familiar objects.	Direct localization of sounds on side, above and below. Points to a few body parts when asked. Follows simple commands and understands simple questions like "Roll the ball," "Kiss the baby," and "Where's the shoe?" Enjoys listening to simple stories, songs, and rhymes. Points to pictures in a book when named.
2 to 3 Years	**2 to 3 Years**	**2 to 3 Years**
Single signs expand to two or three signs with facial expression and pointing. Morphology using movement begins after age 2 and continues until age 5. Begins to use classifiers to show objects and handshapes. Headshake or negative word "no" plus sign demonstrates negations. Can distinguish yes-or-no questions with raised eyebrows. Can make "wh" question with raised eyebrows and slight head tilts.	Uses two to three word sentences. Understands concepts of "one" and "all." Requests items by name. Points to pictures in books. Answers one-to-two word questions. Uses two to three word phrases. Speech is understood by familiar listeners most of the time. Name objects to direct person's actions. Begins to use appropriately irregular verbs. Beginning of morphemes, articles, pronouns, present progressive (-ing), plurals, past tense, contractions involving "is."	Direct localization of sounds on side, above, and below. Understands the differences in meaning of "go/stop," "in/on," and "up/down." Follows two requests (e.g., "get the book and put it on the table").

Acquisition of sign word order (SV, VO, SVO).
Begins fingerspelling.
Sporadically marks nouns and verbs with appropriate features but not systematically.
Begins to use verbs that require agreement but produces them in uninflected form ("I give you").
Uses words or signs more than motor activity to communicate ideas and desires.
Understands and carries out more complex commands.
Answers simple questions of who, why, where, how many.
Masters pronominal pointing.
Uses object classifiers (cup, baseball bat).

3 to 4 Years

Morphology increases, and morphological overgeneralizations are worked out.
Uses facial adverbs: pah, pow.
Uses simple handshapes, substitutes simple handshapes for more complex ones.
Combines three to four signs, including indexing and facial expressions.
Uses compound signs (friend-chum).
Acquires nominal establishment (establishes location with present object that is present).
Uses space for location.
Begins classifier predicates.
Begins discourse skills.
Seeks eye contact before initiating conversation.
Begins to use topicalization.
Increases sign language vocabulary to more than 1,000 signs (receptively and expressively).

Has receptive vocabulary of 500 to 500-plus words.
Has an expressive vocabulary of 50 to 250-plus words.
Shows multiple grammar errors.
Uses vowels correctly.
Consistently uses initial consonants.
Uses approximately 27 phonemes.

3 to 4 Years

Morphemes become consistent.
Irregular forms of verbs used (see/saw, eat/ate).
Simple sentences: negatives, imperatives, questions, relative pronouns.
Talks about activities at school and home.
Understands simple question words: who, what, where, why.
Follows two- and three-part commands.
Mean length of utterance (MLU) = 4.3 to 4.4 words.
Produces simple verbal analogies.
Comprehends 1,200 to 2,000 words.
Uses 800 to 1,500 words.
Sentence grammar improves, although some errors still persist.
Speech is 80 percent intelligible.
Uses some contractions, irregular plurals, future tense verbs, and conjunctions.
Consistently uses regular plurals, possessives, and simple past verbs.

---

3 to 4 Years

Hears when someone calls from another room.
Has TV or radio at same loudness level as other family members.
Understands simple questions asking who, what, where, why.

(Continued)

Table 4.2 Continued

ASL (Deaf Children of Deaf Parents)	Speech (Hearing Children of Hearing Parents)	Hearing (Hearing Children of Hearing Parents)
4 to 6 Years	**4 to 5 Years**	**4 to 5 Years**
Acquires more fingerspelling.	Continues to develop relative clauses, passives, other complex sentences, reflexive pronouns, comparatives, adverbial word endings, irregular comparisons, and grammar.	Pays attention to a short story and answers simple questions about it. Hears and understands most of what is said at home and in school.
Uses more complex handshapes ("3" bug, "V" see, "Y" play, "L" library).	Comprehends 2,500 to 2,800 words.	
Uses simple sentence types with complex sentence construction emerging, including topicalization, rhetorical questions.	Uses 1,500 to 2,000 words.	
	Uses "could" and "would."	
Complex sentences such as nominal references, classifier morphology, aspects of discourse.	Errors of noun/verb and adjective/noun agreement.	
	Mean length of utterance (MLU) = 4.6 to 5.7 words.	
Begins to use conditional clauses with "if" or "suppose."	Uses grammatically correct sentences.	
	Asks for word definitions.	
Complex verbs of motion continue.	Enjoys rhyme, rhythm, and nonsense syllables.	
Complex facial adverbs emerge (sta, cha).	Produces consonants with 90 percent accuracy.	
More complex ASL grammar emerges.	Significantly reduces number of persistent sound omissions and substitutions.	
Complex verbs of motion continue.	Talks about experiences at school and friends' homes.	
Sign vocabulary increases.	Relays a long story accurately.	
	Pays attention to story and answers simple questions about it.	
	Uses some irregular plurals, possessive pronouns, future tense, reflexive pronouns, and comparative morphemes in sentences.	
	Makes indirect requests.	
	Uses deictic terms (this, that, here, these).	
	6 to 7 Years	
	Continues to master complex grammar and new linguistic meanings during school years.	
	Uses all pronouns consistently.	
	Uses superlatives.	

Uses adverbial word endings (e.g., slowly)
Mean length of utterance (MLU) = 6.6 to 7.3 words.
Describes locations or movement with prepositions like through, away, toward, and over.
Comprehends 13,000 to 26,000 words
Understands "if" and "so" clauses
Develops perfect tense with "have" and "had"
Uses nominalization clauses.
Uses irregular plurals.
Refines syntax.

From Andrews, J., Logan, R., & Phelan, J. (2008). Milestones of Language Development. *ADVANCE for Speech-Language Pathologists and Audiologists, 18*(2), 16–20. *Advance for Speech and Hearing.* Retrieved from http://speech-language-pathology-audiology.advanceweb.com/Article/Milestones-of-Language-Development.aspx. Reprinted with permission from Advance for Speech and Hearing.

Deaf children who use sign and spoken languages will often naturally mix the two languages, just like hearing bilingual children who naturally mix their two languages. This provides them with an additional resource in learning language. With time and repeated exposure, they learn to separate the two languages. Some, however, will continue to mix the languages with hearing nonsigners using a bimodal bilingual strategy (explained in Chapters 5 and 6) (Waddy-Smith, 2012).

Because of limited language access, many deaf children enter preschool and kindergarten having to learn language and literacy at the same time. They often do not have the vocabulary and grammar to learn the concepts that teachers are covering in class. Some of the common language challenges include minimal vocabulary, English grammar, and difficulty with gram-matical markers such as *-ed*, *-ing*, and *-er*. Deaf children may also have difficulty in conversa-tional turn-taking, asking for clarification, or communicating to the teacher what they do not know (Marschark & Wauters, 2008).

Linguistic Creativity in ASL and in English

Still another cognitive and metacognitive ability is how children play with the formal features of languages, both ASL and English, through the use of puns, humor, jokes, metaphors, similes, and other poetic devices. There have been few, if any, studies on how deaf children use ASL literature, including ASL theater arts, to promote and measure ASL linguistic creativity. The recent burgeoning of research on ASL literature in the Deaf Studies discipline certainly bodes well for future empirical classroom and dormitory studies.

In his qualitative study of interviews with ASL scholars and storytellers, Byrne (2013, p. 49) defined ASL literature as the inclusion of

> not only stories in ASL but also ASL poetry, riddles, humor, and other genres of a "through the air" literary tradition. ASL literature is not English literature *translated* into ASL but is comprised of original compositions that have arisen from the thoughts, emotions, and experiences of culturally Deaf people, and have been passed on by "hand" (through ASL) from one generation to another.

Byrne's research also points out that ASL and its visual-spatial dimension provides Deaf chil-dren with opportunities to learn language, knowledge, values, morals, and experiences of the world around them. See Figure 4.2 for variety of ASL literature forms created by Dr. Andrew Byrne.

Deaf children can also use their ASL linguistic creativity through the dramatic arts. Kil-patrick (2007) studied six different children's theaters for the deaf established in the United States and noted how these performances provided theater arts education for thousands of deaf children.

Related to linguistic creativity with English, a review of studies shows that deaf children can be creative in their language production if the comprehension tasks are structured in ways that they can understand (Marschark & Clark, 1987). In a study of four deaf and four hearing 12- to 15-year-old students, participants were asked to generate stories using their sign language. The stories were videotaped and analyzed for use of creative devices. The researchers found that deaf students produced figurative constructions at a rate equal to their hearing peers and surpassed them in four other categories of nonliteral expressions. These findings contradict previous research that found deaf children to be rigid and literal in their language use (Mar-schark & West, 1985), at least for this sample.

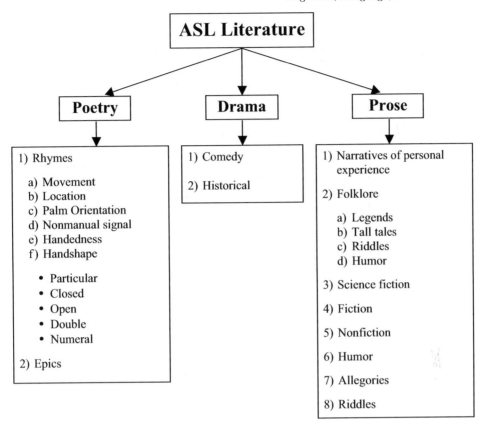

Figure 4.2 ASL Literature Forms

Source: ASL Literature Forms by Andrew Byrne (2013).

Cochlear Implant Outcomes

In any current discussion of deaf people, cognition, and language, one can easily see how cochlear implantation (see the Audiology Appendix for a brief explanation) has changed the landscape in deaf education (Archbold & Mayer, 2012). Since the 1970s, this prosthetic device has propelled a tsunami of research studies. Space allows us to only present a slice of cochlear implant research summaries pertaining to the domains of cognitive, speech, and language outcomes. We discuss cochlear implants and academic achievement in Chapter 5 and literacy in Chapter 6.

Cognitive Functioning and Deaf Cochlear Implant Users

Deaf children with cochlear implants provide researchers with the opportunity to study neuro-plasticity, reorganization, and neurocognitive learning when sound is introduced after a period of auditory deprivation. For example, in two research studies, Quittner, Smith, Osberger, Mitchell, and Katz (1994) investigated the relationship between audition and vision with a group of deaf, cochlear-implanted, school-age children and a group of deaf children without implants. The former group performed better on the visual attention tasks and had faster developmental rates than the latter group. Thus, auditory learning was seen as supporting visual attention task learning. This makes sense as auditory learning simply adds another cueing system that the child can tap into.

Pisoni and his colleagues (2010) examined the neurobiological mechanisms and neuro-cognitive processes related to executive functioning and organization-integration processes that contribute to the variability in speech and language outcomes following implantation. They propose that when early auditory experience is changed by electrical stimulation through the cochlear implant, the brain is reorganized with multiple interacting neurocognitive pro-cesses. Further, they propose that hearing impairment cannot be viewed as a simple sensory impairment but one that involves numerous neural and cognitive processes. They conclude that speech and language outcomes of cochlear implant use goes beyond conventional demo-graphic, medical/etiological, and educational factors and that neurocognitive assessments can assist those deaf children who are at high risk for poor outcomes following implantation (Pisoni et al., 2008; Pisoni, Conway, Kronenberger, Henning, & Anaya, 2010).

Conway and his colleagues (2011) assessed 24 deaf cochlear implanted children with age-matched hearing children on nonverbal cognitive measures of motor sequencing, tactile dis-crimination, response inhibition, visual-motor integration, and visual-spatial processing. The researchers reported that the children with implants showed deficiencies in motor sequencing and their scores were related to language scores as assessed on the Clinical Evaluation of Lan-guage Fundamentals (CELF-4). The researchers concluded that the period of auditory depriva-tion before cochlear implantation affects their motor sequencing skills, which in turn, causes language delays.

Another study examined ToM with implanted deaf children (Remmel & Peters, 2009). Thirty children at age 3 to 12 with cochlear implants and 30 children with typical hearing whose ages ranged from 4 to 6 years of age were assessed on ToM and language measures, including a syntax and semantics test and oral and written language tests. The deaf children with cochlear implants showed little to no delay on either ToM or spoken language. The researchers concluded that these deaf children had better language skills for their age than the deaf children of hearing parents without cochlear implants found in other studies (Remmel & Peters, 2009).

But another ToM study with deaf cochlear implant users found different results (Macaulay & Ford, 2006). In a study of 10 deaf children with cochlear implants ranging in age from 4 to 12 years, the relationship between language, age, and ToM in prelingually deaf children with hearing parents was studied. Three standard false-belief tests and the British Peabody Picture Vocabulary test were administered. All children used Total Communication. Compared to hearing peers, the deaf cochlear implant users were delayed in their ToM performance scores. The children's ToM performance was unrelated to the age they were implanted. In summary, the small sampling of neurocognitive studies mentioned here examine other domains of learn-ing rather than simply spoken language and illustrate the complex and sometimes contra-dictory research findings we note here. How professionals, including teachers, can use this information is a topic for future research.

Spoken Language and Deaf Cochlear Implant Users

Longitudinal studies of deaf students with cochlear implants followed over time from elemen-tary to high school have resulted in test scores indicating better speech production, speech reception, and language achievement for some deaf children who primarily use spoken lan-guage for communication (Geers & Sedey, 2011; Ruffin, Kronenberger, Colson, Henning, & Pisoni, 2013).

Geers and Sedey (2011) followed 112 deaf adolescents who had been using cochlear implants for more than 10 years. The teens were assessed twice, first between the ages of 8 and 9 and then between the ages of 15 and 18 years. Results from this study showed that deaf coch-lear implanted teens performed near their hearing same-age peers on single word vocabulary, isolated sentences comprehension, and factual information questions, but they still had difficulty with connected discourse and abstract reasoning tasks.

Ruffin and his colleagues (2013) studied 51 deaf cochlear implanted users who were prelingually deaf (prior to 3 years of age), received an implant before 7 years of age and had used the implant for at least 7 years. The majority of teens and young adults who had used their implants for 10 to 15 years had an average range or better performance in speech production, language, and academic achievement. The researchers reported factors that led to achievement, which included the following: earlier age of implantation, shorter length of time of preimplant auditory deprivation, more preimplant residual hearing, use of state of the art cochlear implant technology, use of spoken language, family income, and nonmenigitic etiologies.

Other cross-sectional and longitudinal studies show wide variability in deaf children's acquisition and rate of development of spoken language abilities (Geers, Brenner, & Tobey, 2011). Even those deaf children who acquire some speech skills continue to show delays compared to their hearing peers in general language structures (Niparko et al., 2010); acquiring vocabulary (Hayes, Geers, Treiman, & Moog, 2009); and developing spoken language grammar (Nikolopoulos et al., 2004). Some of the variability in outcomes have been linked to age of onset, the extent of the hearing loss and being implanted before age 2 (Connor, Hieber, Arts, & Zwolan, 2000; Nicholas & Geers, 2007), and communication mode in the family. Some researchers suggest that parents use auditory and listening skills only (Geers et al., 2011), while others suggest that parents use signs to support the learning of spoken language (Mitchener & Sass-Lehrer, 2015).

Because deaf children's mode of communication may change multiple times during their educational years and beyond, it is difficult to determine the impact of mode of communication and educational placement on language and academic achievement with deaf cochlear implanted students. Some may start with a spoken language mode, then switch to a Total Communication mode in junior high when the information load gets heavier and they use sign language interpreters, plus they may also develop friendships with signing deaf peers. Another reason why the findings of some cochlear implant studies are hard to interpret is because many of the children in these studies may use sign language and their sign language skills are seldom recognized as a variable that supports the development of their speech and language. For instance, in the Geers and Sedey (2011) study, a majority of the children used what the researchers phrased as "enhanced signing," which they report was not ASL. But without more linguistic descriptions of what "enhanced signing" looked like and how the children were using it to support their language development, it is hard to draw conclusions. All signing, even if it is English-based signing, comes from its mother-lode, ASL, at the very least in the majority of its lexicon. Where it differs is in the syntax. But even English-based signers will use a spatial grammar in their rendition of signing so it becomes more like contact signing. These issues could be added to future cochlear implant studies to provide information on the impact of signing on spoken language development.

The most direct way to studying the effect of signing on deaf cochlear implant users' language abilities is to study second-generation deaf students, that is, students with Deaf parents who use sign language.

Sign Language and Deaf Cochlear Implant Users

Studies of implanted Deaf children of Deaf parents have smaller sample sizes. However, results show that early sign language can be used to support the development of speech. In a case study, a deaf child who was implanted was taught Italian Sign Language at an early age and used sign language to support spoken language (Rinaldi & Caselli, 2014). In a language evaluation that included both Italian and Italian sign language, the child increased in vocabulary comparable to hearing age peers. The researchers concluded that bimodal bilingualism supported the child's use of spoken language.

In a retrospective study, seven Iranian deaf children of deaf parents and seven Iranian deaf children of hearing parents were matched on severity of hearing loss, age of onset, duration of deafness, age of cochlear implantation, gender, and cochlear implant model (Hassanzadeh, 2012). Assessments of auditory perception, speech perception, speech production, and language development were carried out with both groups of children; these showed growth in auditory and speech development. But the second-generation deaf children outperformed the deaf children of hearing parents in the language measures. No sign language assessments were carried out. The researchers concluded that deaf children can learn to communicate in sign language from an early age prior to implantation and that this can support their speech abilities.

In another study with five implanted Deaf children of Deaf parents, the researchers compared their language skills with those of 20 hearing ASL/English bilingual children with deaf parents (CODA children) (Davidson, Lillo-Martin, & Chen-Pichler, 2014). The children were administered a battery of tests that assessed ASL, nonverbal IQ, spoken English language measures, vocabulary, articulation, syntax, general language skills, and phonological awareness. The results showed that the five deaf, bimodal bilingual children had scores that were comparable with their hearing bimodal bilingual peers and with monolingual, hearing agemates using age norms.

Based on these selected studies, cochlear implants were found to support deaf children's visual as well as auditory learning (Quittner et al., 1994). Another study showed that language delays were related to deaf children's delays in motor sequencing (Conway et al., 2011). Findings related to ToM were conflicted with one study showing deaf children with cochlear implants had the same ToM performance as hearing children (Remmel & Peters, 2009) while the other study showed delayed ToM development among implanted deaf children (Macaulay & Ford, 2006). A consistent finding in several studies revealed that deaf children with implants increase their speech perception, speech production, and language abilities over time (Geers & Sedey, 2011; Ruffin, Kronenberger, Colson, Henning, & Pisoni, 2013). Further, children also show increases in vocabulary, isolated sentence recognition, and knowledge for factual information. However, implanted children studied longitudinally still have difficulty with connected discourse (Geers & Sedey, 2011). Other studies show contradictory evidence and report that even though deaf children's spoken language abilities increase (Geers, Brenner, & Tobey, 2011), deaf children with implants compared to children with typical hearing still show delays in general language structures (Niparko et al., 2010); acquiring vocabulary (Hayes, Geers, Treiman, & Moog, 2009); and spoken grammar skills (Nikolopoulos, Dyar, Archbold, & O'Donoghue, 2004). Factors in several studies that predict implant success included the following: early age of implantation, shorter length of time for preimplant auditory deprivation, residual hearing, use of state-of-the-art technology, use of spoken language at home, family income, and nonmenigitic etiologies (Geers et al., 2011; Ruffin et al., 2013). Furthermore, studies of implanted bilingual Deaf children of Deaf parents had scores in ASL and English that were comparable to their hearing bimodal bilingual peers, thus suggesting that early ASL can facilitate the development of speech as well as bilingual bimodalism (Rinaldi & Caselli, 2014). More studies are needed to substantiate this finding. It appears that researchers are beginning to recognize and document the use of signing even among deaf children who primarily use oral language. With the development of more ASL assessments for young deaf children (see Chapter 6), signing can be more accurately measured and examined as a variable that contributes to the development of spoken language. We also need to keep in mind that, as cochlear implant technology evolves and as children are implanted at younger ages, it is possible that future research results will portray a different picture.

The Brain, Language, and Neuroscience

Behavioral studies in laboratories and classrooms have provided much information about the cognitive and language learning processes of deaf individuals. Today, the field of neuroscience has added a new dimension to the study of cognition and language. With neuroimaging technology, scientists can scan the brain for neural activity to learn what happens when the brain is stimulated by cognitive and language tasks with the goal of providing fresh insights about how thinking and language develop. Patricia Kuhl's work with hearing infants and Laura-Ann Petitto's work with deaf infants are just two of the many examples of neuroscientific research that has provided fresh insights into the areas of cognition and language. Gallaudet University recently established a new Ph.D. program for neuroscientists and has enrolled Deaf graduate students who are preparing for careers in neuroscience. Undoubtedly the future contributions of Deaf neuroscientists will be significant.

Although we cannot see the inner workings of our thinking and language processing, we can look at the physical brain. The brain with all of its neural circuitry is the hub that controls the processes of our thinking, language, and learning (Sousa, 2007). Whenever we see, hear, sign, talk, think, touch, or learn something, this transfers to an electrical activity that takes place in our brain. Each time we stimulate our brains with learning experiences, we create new synapses that carry information within the brain.

Thanks to new neuroimaging technology, we are beginning to have a better picture of the functioning of different parts of the brain. For instance, the language center is located in the perisylvian region, which surrounds a fissure known as the Sylvian fissure that separates the temporal lobe from the parietal and frontal lobes. These parietal and frontal lobes are found in the left hemisphere where the understandings of speech sounds are found (Sousa, 2007). Spoken and sign languages both stimulate the language center of the brain. The brain is flexible for language acquisition and does not care if the information comes through the ear as a sound-based auditory/oral code or through a sign based visual/gestural code, or even as both. What the brain looks for is patterns (Kuhl, 2015). Carrying this further, Petitto (2012, p. 1) explains that the brain looks for patterns "pressed on the hands" or "pressed on the tongue."

Kuhl (2010) suggests that the social brain "gates" the computational mechanism that underlies the learning of language. She acknowledges that the social theories of language learning developed by Vygotsky (1978) and others are insufficient without the social interaction that is necessary to stimulate the learning of language; this begins at the phonetic level. It will help to remember that ASL also has a phonetic level that is called *visual phonology*. We provide more information on this in Chapter 6.

Kuhl and Rivera-Gaxiola (2008) describe four brain imaging techniques that are currently being used for speech and language processing in infants and young children: electroencephalography (EEG)/event-related potentials (ERPs), magnetoencephalography (MEG), functional magnetic resonance imaging (fMRI), and near-infrared spectroscopy (NIRS). These allow doctors and researchers to examine activity in the brain without invasive neurosurgery (see http://psychcentral.com/lib/types-of-brain-imaging-techniques/).

Today, these tools are used to advance the understanding of the infant's capacity for language and for diagnosing children with autism and reading difficulties among others (Sousa, 2007). Brain scanning also provides the opportunity to gain information on how two languages are acquired (Kuhl, 2010; Petitto & Dunbar, 2004). We provide more details on the deaf bilingual brain in Chapter 6.

Can Thinking Go to School?

Can teachers foster thinking skills with their students? Can students foster thinking skills with each other? The studies we present here indicate that yes, they can.

Teachers can harness the strengths that deaf learners have with visual attention, visual spatial, and peripheral vision by planning lessons where students can form pictures or visual image in their mind, remember pictures or objects in a room (visuospatial memory), and remember moving objects (Hamilton, 2011). Others have also suggested that teachers slow down their lectures to offset the disadvantage of divided attention between the teacher and sign language interpreter in mainstream classrooms by helping deaf students juxtapose their attention while speechreading the teacher and watching the interpreter (Marschark & Hauser, 2008). Setting up classrooms with semi-circled desks and chairs and restricting distraction activities in the periphery will assist deaf students in focusing on learning. However, even with visual learning, deaf students face challenges in learning academic subjects in the upper grades, including those of finding relationships between the cause and effect of events in social studies, math, and science as classroom experiments have found (Marschark & Wauters, 2008).

Studies conducted by Martin and his colleagues (Martin, 2014) over the past two decades in the United States, England, China, and South Africa have investigated metacognitive strategies in deaf and hard-of-hearing learners using the Feuerstein Instrumental Enrichment program (FIE) originally developed by Reuven Feuerstein (1980). The rationale for metacognitive activities in the classroom is to enable students (deaf or hearing) to become aware of their own mental processes, such that when they are on their own in life and face a problem, they will not be stuck—they will have a repertoire of cognitive strategies from which to choose (David Martin, personal communication, January 15, 2016).

Martin summarizes a number of empirical studies done since the late 1970s that show positive outcomes in deaf learners' cognitive skill acquisition. For example, the FIE program teaches thinking skills such as precision, comparison, analysis, systematic approaches to problem solving, and decoding. The students first use content-free paper and pencil exercises to learn about and practice the strategy, followed by a metacognitive discussion about the processes that were used, and then they practice a particular strategy matched to a particular content area in the regular curriculum. In his summary of the studies using FIE, Martin (2014) shows that deaf learners can acquire specific cognitive skills when teachers are trained with the appropriate methodology and the use of specially designed materials.

Direct instruction, specifically the use of explicit teaching instruction to teach specific skills, has been used as the anchor teaching strategy for deaf students and has never been challenged. Deaf children appear to need it because they miss so much with their language delays and decreased exposure to incidental learning. However, recent research with hearing children shows that direct instruction is not as effective as instruction that uses collaborative groups where students meet to discuss ideas and write about them. In a study of 764 fifth-graders from 36 classrooms in eight public schools who were primarily from African American and Hispanic homes, student learning through direct instruction was contrasted with learning within collaborative reasoning groups (Zhang et al., 2015). Students in the latter groups wrote essays that were significantly better than those of the students in the direct instruction classrooms on each of the three measures of decision-making that were evaluated. The direct instruction groups performed no better than the control students who did not receive instruction. Collaborative reasoning may be an innovative way to increase the learning of deaf children but would have to be delivered in a manner to accommodate their language levels.

Conclusions

To understand the psychological impact of being deaf on cognition, language, and the mind, it is important to understand the visual and auditory ways in which deaf persons' mental capabilities unfold, develop, and are organized. Visual paradigms of learning have been added to auditory paradigms in order to increase our understanding of the ways deaf people use their cognition, language, and minds to learn, think, problem solve, and be creative. In the next chapter, we review the educational aspects, special education laws, educational placements, academic achievement, curriculum, standards, and instructional practices with deaf individuals.

Suggested Readings

Bauman, H-D., Nelson, J., & Rose, H. (2006). *Signing the body poetic: Essays on American Sign Language literature*. Berkeley, CA: University of California Press.
   The linguistic creativity of ASL is an unexplored topic in deaf education classrooms because deaf children are seldom exposed to ASL literature from an early age. This book of essays with an accompanying DVD provides a stunning view of the rich literary, social, and performative aspects of American Sign Language, with scholars examining ASL poetry, narratives, and drama.

Pinker, S. (2013). *Language, cognition, and human nature*. Selected articles. New York, NY: Oxford.
   An eclectic collection of articles by Pinker and his colleagues explores the workings of language and its connections to cognition, perception, social relationships, child development, human evolution, and theories of human nature.

Wilson, F. (1998). *The hand: How its use shapes the brain, language, and human culture*. New York, NY: Pantheon Books.
   How the human hand has shaped our cognitive, emotional, linguistic, and psychological development is covered in this book within the context of research in anthropology, neuroscience, linguistics, and psycholinguistics. How our hands influence our learning is also discussed.

Note

1   The South African Deaf community was outraged when a man standing next to President Barack Obama faked the sign language interpretation of Nelson Mandela's memorial service in 2014 using movements and gestures that were not formal signs at all and were unintelligible to Deaf people watching (www.nbcnews.com/news/other/fake-sign-language-interpreter-nelson-mandela-memorial-provokes-anger-f2D11723934).

5 Educational Aspects of Deaf Education

We can—if given a chance. That chance has to begin with a good education.

Frank Bowe (1991, p. x)

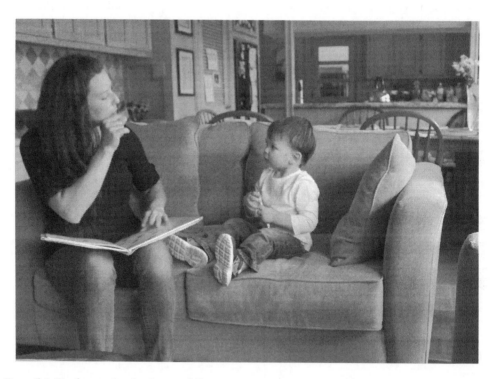

Figure 5.1 Teacher signing "cat" to a toddler
Source: Used with permission.

Introduction

Suppose, in a room sat a Deaf professional, a parent, a seasoned teacher, and a Ph.D. researcher. You ask each, "How do you educate a deaf child?" The Deaf professional says, "I can explain why a teaching method works or does not work. I can tell you how being deaf affects day-to-day living and working as well as the learning of English. My view is relevant." The parent says, "I have been communicating and guiding my deaf child since birth. I intuitively know what works and what does not work. And I care the most." And the veteran teacher says, "I have worked in the trenches (classroom) for decades, teaching all types of deaf children with different backgrounds, talents, and personalities. I have experience." And finally, the researcher says, "I can provide you with empirical support for best practices. I have the science."

Which viewpoint leads to a good education? A good education provides the deaf and hard-of-hearing child with linguistic and social capital[1] and makes available healing for the psychosocial traumas caused by frustrations due to lack of home communication (Chapter 7). All four viewpoints, which involve relevance, care, experience, and science, respectively, are involved in a good education. This chapter focuses on how these four perspectives intersect to create deaf education as we know it today.

Chapter Objectives

We summarize how deaf children learn given their cognitive and language abilities. We then provide theoretical frameworks that can inform our understanding of how they learn. We provide insight on how deaf children live and learn in Deaf and hearing home and school communities. We stress the importance of providing deaf children with a communication-driven program in the school environment that builds on their psychosocial development and is responsive in terms of enhancing their abilities to live and communicate in the Deaf and hearing worlds. The challenges of using state curriculum, standards, best practices, and technology are outlined.

How Deaf Children Learn and Theoretical Frameworks of Learning

How do deaf children learn given their cognitive and language abilities? In our selective review of studies in Chapter 4 and from comprehensive reviews of studies with practical teaching applications by Marschark and Hauser (2012), we can decipher that deaf children have the same cognitive potential as hearing children, but differences in their environment and experiences may affect their learning. What slows down deaf students' learning is not lack of intelligence, but lack of access to language. However, when given the opportunity, we know deaf children can regulate their eye-gaze behaviors and joint attention to learn language and academic content and use their memory and the study strategies provided by their teachers in the classroom.

With language access, deaf students can learn how to socialize with others; regulate their own behavior (e.g., impulse control, executive functioning); and maximize opportunities to master social cognition (e.g., Theory of Mind in terms of understanding the perspectives of others). But we also know that with less communication at home and, therefore, reduced opportunities for incidental learning of cognitive and social skills within family settings, these children arrive at school with learning challenges and socioemotional issues. For deaf children of hearing parents who cannot communicate with them effectively, the classroom is the major environment where learning for the deaf student occurs with the teacher functioning as a language role model (Singleton & Morgan, 2006). While in the classroom, research tells us that deaf individuals use their vision more and are more visually aware of their surroundings. And given their enhanced sensitivity to peripheral vision, the deaf child is more likely to become distracted in class with visual stimuli on either side, but as they grow older, they are able to better handle these visual distractions. Regarding other skills necessary for learning, what memory studies suggest is that deaf students may have difficulty remembering information they learn in school because of their strategies or because they cannot link new information with background experiences they have not had (Marschark & Hauser, 2012).

We also know that Deaf students have differences in world knowledge and how they organize that knowledge. This may affect their approaches to problem solving, metacognition, and social cognition. Given their learning issues, how can existing theoretical frameworks further inform us in maximizing learning opportunities for deaf students?

Moving away from Jean Piaget's (1952) model of individual learning, we gravitate towards theoretical frameworks that focus on cultural and group learning in the classroom and community (Rogoff, 2003; Vygotsky, 1978; Wenger, 1999) because these are the locations where learning takes place if there is limited access to language in the home.

In contrast to Piaget's developmental model that focuses on the individual's learning, Lev Vygotsky's (1978) cultural-historical theory focuses on the role of culture and social interactions from birth onward. Children develop through conversations with adults. Complex mental activities begin as social activities. Children learn best in the "zone of proximal development" that bridges the gap between what the child can do alone with what the child can do with the support or scaffolding provided by others.

Barbara Rogoff (2003) and Etienne Wenger (1999) make the case for learning as a cultural process with individuals developing within communities by interacting with others in shared endeavors or groups as well as building on the cultural practices of previous generations. Rather than looking at learning as the acquisition of certain forms of knowledge, they conceptualize learning as occurring in groups supported by social relationships. In this way, they pave the way towards widening the sphere of classroom learning to include groups of students with teachers engaging in "communities of practice" that also involves cultural practices.

Applied to deaf education, in order to learn, children need classroom communities that support their learning and provide multiple opportunities to use language to communicate, form relationships, build their dual identities within Deaf and hearing cultures, and learn academic content from both hearing and Deaf adults. For children who learn a sign language, it is in the classroom where they will learn this language, and it is their teachers who will become their language role models (Singleton & Morgan, 2006).

For learning to optimally occur, each deaf and hard-of-hearing child deserves a quality, communication-driven program that facilitates the development of age-level language skills, whether in spoken English, ASL, or some combination of both. Such a program should provide a critical mass of peers, teachers, and staff able to communicate directly with deaf and hard-of-hearing students, administrators who understand the unique needs of these students, deaf and hard-of-hearing role models, and access to extracurricular and other important school activities. The child's communication and psychosocial needs should be the prime determinant for his or her educational placement (Siegel, 2008).

The Role of Culturally Responsive Schools

Based on the learning models that incorporate the deaf students' cultures as discussed in the previous section, schools are challenged to develop a culturally responsive environment tailored to the support of deaf children's learning both individually as well as socially. We take a sociolinguistic view of deaf children who grow up using one or more languages, as they navigate two or more cultures—Deaf and hearing—to develop a healthy, bicultural identity (Holcomb, 1997; 2012; O'Brien, 2011). Rather than subscribing to a "deficit" view, which results in lowered expectations, overtesting of English, and a watered-down curriculum, we take an additive perspective that supports deaf children's deaf and racial/ethnic cultural identities and their sensory and cognitive strengths so that they can learn and grow in each of their communities: family, school, Deaf, and world communities. Our stance is not just for Deaf children from Deaf families; it also includes the 94 percent of Deaf children who live in hearing families and who belong to another variation of the deaf community that encompasses their visual ways of learning and their unique shared experiences of being deaf. In other words, they may be a "different kind of deaf" compared to the Deaf child from a Deaf family. Utilizing a bicultural perspective within the educational setting, we can widen their social spheres to include both Deaf and hearing conversational partners.

Setting up *culturally responsive* schools that align students' Deaf culture and home racial/ethnic background cultures with instructional practices may require a retooling of how teachers teach and how administrators lead. To measure cultural proficiency within K-12 schools, researchers have developed a cultural proficiency continuum as "a way of thinking about and creating cultural change in school leaders" (O'Brien, Kuntze, & Appanah, 2015, p. 298). As school leaders move along this continuum, they increasingly are able to learn about cultural differences and subsequently incorporate their awareness into actual practices, thereby creating biculturalism. A *culturally responsive* environment also includes the hiring of culturally relevant professionals, in this case, Deaf professionals; however, societal barriers often keep many out, as noted next (Andrews & Covell, 2006/2007).

Barriers Deaf Professionals Face

The barriers Deaf professionals face may take the form of low expectations, test bias, lack of accommodations, and discrimination in higher education (Smith & Andrews, 2015). The examples here are a poignant illustration of these barriers:

- *Low expectations*: Darlene S., a Deaf graduate student, prepared to sign fairy tales in ASL to her 5-year-old deaf students. Her supervising teacher said that the deaf children in the class did not have the language to understand fairy tales and that Darlene should, instead, focus on having the children identify colors and label objects.
- *Test bias*: Three Deaf teachers, who had master's degrees in deaf education, were denied teaching certifications because of their inability to pass a state teachers' competency test that consisted of questions requiring hearing and identifying sounds. All had graduated from different teachers' institutions with excellent reputations, had outstanding grades, and received exceptional student teaching evaluations. The case, *Deaf teachers v. the Texas Education Agency and the State Board of Education* never went to trial as a new law was passed—the Texas Education Code (TEC) 13.050, which exempted deaf persons from biased teacher proficiency tests (Smith & Andrews, 2015).
- *Lack of accommodations*: Walter Camenisch was denied sign language interpreters while studying for a master's degree in Educational Administration. In *Camenisch v. University of Texas*, a district court issued an injunction requiring the university to provide and pay for interpreters with the U.S. Court of Appeals for the Fifth Circuit, supporting this decision (National Association of the Deaf, 2015).
- *Discrimination*: The Dean of the College of Education expelled Nadelle Grantham from a teacher-education program during her last semester because she was deaf, as he believed she could not teach and supervise children in a student-teaching internship. Grantham filed a lawsuit under ADA and won the trial, and the U.S. Court of Appeals for the Fifth Circuit affirmed the jury's verdict (*Grantham v. Moffett*, 1998; National Association of the Deaf, 2015).
- *Lack of accommodations*: In a rural Appalachian classroom, when the fire alarm drill sounded, Mary T., a Deaf teacher and her deaf students were left behind because no one informed her of the drill (Andrews & Jaussi, 1993).
- *Discrimination*: Jack P., a Deaf teacher, had a doctorate in Deaf Education. His dissertation focused on reading, but he was passed over for a literacy coach job when a hearing woman with fewer credentials was selected. The rationale was that because the district adopted a phonics approach to reading instruction, it was felt a hearing teacher was needed to do the job.
- *Lack of support*: Hired to fill a tenured-faculty position, Dr. Michael Collier never had any contact with the department chair, was placed under the supervision of a nontenured professor, and was fired without any prior mentoring. A lawsuit was filed, *Michael L. Collier v. Texas Tech University*, and the jury awarded him a settlement (www.morelaw.com/verdicts/case.asp?n=&s=TX&d=48081).

Hearing teachers may have challenges in finding communities of Deaf people in order to learn how to be culturally responsive. Some may have learned ASL as second language in adulthood so their fluency in ASL likely will never approach that of a native user. Nonetheless, they are expected to be language role models as teachers (Schick, 2008). This also applies to educational interpreters. Some may join Deaf community organizations (e.g., NAD, state associations for the deaf, Deaf religious settings); attend events at state residential schools for the deaf; or meet Deaf senior citizens to learn about Deaf culture (Roberson & Shaw, 2015).

Aligning Teaching Workforce with Diverse Student Enrollment

Developing *culturally responsive* schools also means setting up deaf/hearing collaborative teams or working relationships (see further discussion in Chapter 11) and hiring Deaf and hearing teachers who represent the racial/ethnic background of their deaf students. This has been a challenge throughout the history of teaching in deaf education (Andrews, Leigh, & Weiner, 2004).

In the United States, historically, the teaching workforce in deaf education started with a deaf/hearing team—Laurent Clerc (Deaf) and Thomas Hopkins Gallaudet (hearing). Teachers in early America were primarily White men who taught children for a few years prior to entering the ministry, law, or politics, including, for example, Abraham Lincoln, and in modern times, Lyndon B. Johnson, both of whom eventually became President of the United States. Clerc represented one of many stellar Deaf students who graduated from a deaf school and who later returned to teach. When signing was banned from deaf schools in the 1880s, the number of deaf teachers decreased from 40 percent to less than 15 percent. There was also a decrease in male teachers, with men gravitating towards other professions. Subsequently, more women entered teaching and worked for less money, as their professional opportunities were limited (Baynton, Gannon, & Bergey, 2007).

Characteristics of Teachers

The deaf education workforce continues to be largely White, female, and hearing (Ausbrooks, Baker, & Daugaard, 2012; Simms, Rusher, Andrews, & Coryell, 2008). But by the year 2004, Deaf professionals, professionals of color, and male professionals were more frequently represented at residential schools. Further, there was a doubling of the representation of Deaf teachers in public schools from 7.3 percent to 15.4 percent. While this was a good sign in terms of addressing the need for language and cultural role models as the numbers of deaf children being placed in general education increased, the current representation continues to be a fraction of the need for Deaf teachers in the public school system.

Data on preservice teachers (students preparing to become teachers) show that, similar to inservice teachers (instructors employed in schools), the workforce is predominantly White, female, and hearing (Ausbrooks, Baker, & Daugaard, 2012). Both general education and deaf education have the same challenge—hiring more diverse teachers to mirror the current demographic picture of students from diverse backgrounds (Goldring, Gray, & Bitterman, 2013). The next section presents information on how the deaf student population has changed in terms of demographics.

Characteristics of Students

In the past four decades, White student enrollment has decreased from 76 percent in 1973/74 to 54 percent in 2012. The Black/African American child enrollment had been a steady 15 percent. On the other hand, the Latino/Hispanic enrollment has increased from 7.3 percent in the 1970s to 28.4 percent in 2012, as indicated in surveys done by the Gallaudet Research Institute (GRI, 2013). These figures are based on the GRI headcount of 23,731 deaf and hard-of-hearing students. It is important to note that this headcount is likely an underestimation of actual numbers since not all schools with deaf students, including state and public schools, report statistics to the GRI.

Deaf students also differ on degrees of hearing loss, age of onset, etiology, presence of additional disabilities, and parent hearing status. Children with profound hearing levels (90 dB and above) and severe hearing levels (66 to 90 dB) were typically taught in separate schools or schools for the deaf but now increasingly attend public schools in general education. Children with moderate hearing levels (41 to 61 dB) and mild (26 to 60 dB) hearing levels are taught in public schools. Public schools enroll about 85 percent deaf students either in day classes or with hearing students (Shaver, Marschark, Newman, & Marder, 2013). Many of these children will not form social networks with deaf people until a much later age, with potential repercussions for their psychosocial development and identity formation (Leigh, 2009), a concern that we address throughout this book.

Hard-of-hearing children comprise a special case, with many feeling they are in "cultural limbo" and unsure of their place in society (Grushkin, 2003, p. 34). They may develop a dual deaf/hearing identity similar to profoundly deaf children if they are exposed to this group. They also may have language delays, and similarly to children with profound losses, they are found to perform 2 or 3 years behind hearing students on academic tests (Ross, 1990). Hard-of-hearing children typically experience difficulty getting the accommodations they need such as special, acoustical, and teaching accommodations; classroom listening equipment; and sign language classes, basically because they are perceived to be able to hear, even if inadequately. Some will transfer to a school for the deaf in high school in order to improve their academics, and there they can learn ASL as a second language and develop friendships with deaf peers (Grushkin, 2003).

If the age of onset is at birth (congenital) or before the age of 2, many deaf children will access a spoken language program, an approach that does not include sign language (Northern & Downs, 2014). Alternatively, deaf children can be exposed to a bimodal bilingual approach that emphasizes the use of both a natural sign language and a spoken language (Emmorey & McCullough, 2009; Fish & Morford, 2012). A third approach is the ASL/English bilingual program that focuses on ASL and the teaching of English as second language (ESL). The ASL/English approach recognizes the importance of both ASL and English for deaf children's language development. In this approach, it is expected that deaf children will develop expressive and receptive language abilities in signing, attending to signs, reading, writing, listening, and speaking when it is appropriate for individual deaf students (Gárate, 2011; Fish & Morford, 2012; Nover & Andrews, 1998). Children who lose their hearing at age 5 or 6 may need speechreading instruction and auditory training to retain what language they have as well as ASL instruction for communication and academic purposes (Andrews et al., 2004).

A finding reported in the late 1960s (Vernon, 1969) and still robust today is that 40 percent of deaf students have additional disabilities that impact learning (Gallaudet Research Institute, 2013). These include visual impairments, intellectual disability, learning disabilities, emotional disturbance, attention deficit hyperactivity disorder, autism, developmental delay and other conditions. A specialized teacher-preparation program and curriculum are also required for this challenging population (Guardino & Cannon, 2015). Center schools will have special units where they employ teachers who are certified in special education as well as deaf education, such as at the Texas School for the Deaf. See the Suggested Readings section for additional information about special needs deaf children.

Table 5.1 Topic Areas for Teachers of Deaf Students in K-12 Settings

- History, trends, and issues
- Early intervention
- Itinerant teaching and collaboration with general education settings
- Bilingual instruction in residential and center-based settings
- Listening and spoken instruction in residential, center-based, and general education settings
- Parent and professional collaboration
- Evidence-based assessment and instruction with students who are deaf and hard of hearing and who are multiply disabled concerning
- Learning
- Audition
- Language
- Literacy
- Mathematics
- Science
- Social studies
- Behavior management
- Prevention, recognition, and reporting of maltreatment of students
- General education curricular benchmarks and mandated assessment protocols
- State and federal special and general education legislation, mandates, and educational trends
- Response to interventions and curriculum-based measurements
- Multicultural and multilingual families and children
- Assistive listening devices and cochlear implants
- Assistive and instructional technologies and strategies
- Early intervention and postsecondary transition
- Student learning and advocacy skills
- Receptive and expressive signing competency
- Appropriate practicum and student teaching experiences

Source: Johnson, H. A. (2013). Initial and ongoing teacher preparation and support: Current problems and possible solutions. *American Annals of the Deaf, 157*(5), 439–449. Permission by American Annals of the Deaf.

A Diverse and Well-Prepared Workforce

Given the diversity in race/ethnicity and other background factors, the development of a diverse and well-prepared workforce that employs both Deaf and hearing teachers is necessary to create a *culturally responsive* school-learning environment.

Deaf children of color often are underrepresented in special education and experience neglect, oppression, and discrimination (Simms et al., 2008). One way to address this issue is to prepare more teachers and leaders who are deaf and persons of color (Andrews & Covell, 2006/2007; Ausbrooks et al., 2012; Simms et al., 2008). Overall, well-prepared teachers need to have knowledge of content areas and competencies across different topics ranging from history, trends, and issues to appropriate practicum experiences (Johnson, 2013). See Table 5.1 for recommended topic areas.

Trends, Laws, and Placement Changes

Enrollment Shifts from Centers to Public Schools

In 1975, when one of the authors (Andrews) began her teaching career in middle school at the Maryland School for the Deaf in Frederick, an estimated 80 percent of deaf children were educated in center or special schools. But since 1975, there has been a migration from center or special schools to public schools, as mentioned earlier. According to a sample of 22,665 deaf students, 29.6 percent are enrolled in center or special schools, while the rest of the students attend public schools in regular education classes, either partially or fully (Gallaudet Research Institute, 2013).

One historical factor that contributed to the increase in deaf children being educated in the public school system was the rubella epidemic (1963–1965), which resulted in a large population of deaf children that center schools could not absorb, so new local programs were set up to accommodate the "bulge" of students.

Another historical factor for mainstreaming was the *Education for All Handicapped Children* (PL 94–142) enacted in 1975, which placed more deaf children in regular education. Spearheaded by parents who wanted their cognitively disabled children educated in general education classrooms rather than in segregated settings, this law affected deaf children too (Andrews et al., 2004).

A current factor influencing the current shift to public schools is the increase in the numbers of deaf children receiving cochlear implants. Approximately 38,000 children have received cochlear implants (www.nidcd.nih.gov/health/hearing/pages/coch.aspx). Although some deaf children with implants will attend a center school, the majority attend public schools. As discussed later, public schools have different options for placements ranging from full inclusion in regular education to self-contained classrooms and co-enrollment programs.

Special Education Laws

Following PL 94–142, called the *mainstream law*, the Individuals with Disabilities Act (IDEA, 1990) was passed. The *No Child Left Behind Act* (NCLB, 2001) followed. These laws created concerns in the Deaf community because of the lack of emphasis on the continuum of placements. Instead, the laws were interpreted to place all deaf children in classrooms with nondeaf children, with this setting being considered the least restrictive environment with limited or no consideration for how linguistically accessible this environment was for many deaf children, thus making it a more restrictive environment. Leaders felt that the language needs exhibited by many deaf children and the need for socialization with deaf peers and adult deaf role models were not being addressed. In response to their concerns, the Council of Educational Administrators for the Deaf (CEASD) and the National Association of the Deaf (NAD) set up the *Child First Campaign* (www.ceasd.org/child-first/child-first-campaign). This campaign advocates for providing parents with information about the continuum of services from center schools to public schools to meet the unique needs of individual deaf students. Leaders have also introduced legislation into Congress to this end—H.R. 3535—the Alice Cogswell and Anne Sullivan Macy Act (Tucker, 2010/2011).

Part C of IDEA specifically assists families with children from birth to age 3 with a mandate to develop the Individual Family Service Plan (IFSP). Both professionals and parents develop the IFSP based on the child's strengths and needs. Educational placements for these infants and toddlers include private clinics, home visits, and programs that are at center schools. Deaf mentors play a role in providing families with information about Deaf culture and ASL (Sass-Lehrer, 2016). There are also programs in center schools that provide Deaf teachers within their parent-infant and early childhood programs (Laurene Simms, personal communication, February 2, 2016).

Planning for provision of services for the deaf child from ages 3 to 21 is included under Part B of IDEA (2004). Placement opportunities for preschool and kindergarten through high school students include center schools, public schools, day schools, resource rooms, and self-contained classes. Parents and professionals together develop an IEP or Individualized Education Plan for the child that must be revisited each year. The IEP specifies the services the child will receive. These include speech therapy, counseling services, audiological services, tutoring, and sign language or oral interpreters. Part A of the IDEA (2004) requires that states provide a free and appropriate public education (FAPE) and placement in the least restrictive environment (LRE). Please note that we mention earlier how the least restrictive environment needs to be redefined for the deaf child. Part D of IDEA covers elements such as confidentiality of information, transition services, disciplining of students, and providing appropriate technology support (Raimondo, 2013).

Another law, the *No Child Left Behind Act* (NCLB, 2001) required states to set up a testing accountability system with the goal of having every child reading and performing in math on grade level by 2014. This law affected schools and programs for the deaf, and many had to develop alternative testing to account for adequate yearly progress (Cawthon, 2011). A largely unpopular law, the NCLB was recently replaced by the *Every Student Succeeds Act* (ESSA, 2015), which allows states to have more control. States can now develop their own testing accountability system, choose to use the Common Core Standards (CCS) or their own standards, determine teacher-preparation criteria, and reduce annual tests. ESSA also provides funding for early childhood, arts education, and homeless children (www.whitehouse.gov/the-press-office/2015/12/10/white-house-report-every-student-succeeds-act).

Placement Changes and Consequences

The deaf child's overall best interest should be considered in all placement decisions. This includes communication abilities, educational achievement, personality, social and emotional adjustment, and family support (Siegel, 2008). Parents have the right to ask any questions regarding whether the educational placement they are considering, or one their child is already in, provides an environment conducive to learning. Parents can be better advocates for their deaf child if they are familiar with the school's philosophy, administrative structure, instructional program, faculty/staff qualifications, support services available for child and parents, extracurricular activities, and interpreter quality if their child is placed in a center or public school, as well as know how their child will be evaluated (Andrews et al., 2004; Siegel, 2008).

Parents dissatisfied with final IEP recommendations have had to resort to litigation, not always with results in their favor (National Association of the Deaf, 2015). Litigation has focused on communication issues, the provision of support services, and the definition of LRE as applied to specific cases. The outcome of court cases tends to rest on how well school districts comply with IDEA procedures and how well they document their efforts. In one case, the court ruled in favor of the parent that a deaf student should be admitted to the state school because the school district did not provide a FAPE (*Barbour County Bd. of Educ. v. Parent,* 1999). Required services had not been given to the child, and there was no demonstrable educational progress.

In two more cases, the court ruled for the school district, which argued that the proposed IEP was reasonably calculated to provide an educational benefit to the student and therefore was appropriate under IDEA, even though the parent preferred a different educational methodology (*Board of Education v. Rowley,* 1982; *Brougham v. Town of Yarmouth,* 1993).

In a highly publicized case, in 1982, the United States Supreme Court ruled against Amy Rowley, a deaf 6-year-old whose family requested sign language interpretation in her public school classroom where she was fully integrated with hearing children. The court ruled that she was achieving on grade level and thus did not need a sign language interpreter (*Board of Education v. Rowley*). According to the court, a child has no right under IDEA to a particular program or methodology but rather to an appropriate education per se, which they determined Amy was receiving and therefore did not need this additional service.

In two other due processes hearings, the parents were not successful in gaining accommodations they felt their child needed. Joey, age 7 and profoundly deaf, was placed in a neighborhood public school classroom setting with hearing children and had an aide who could not sign. Thus, he had difficulty both in developing language and having access to the language around him (Siegel, 2008, p. 28). In another case, Debra, age 11, who functioned on grade level, was placed in a special class with deaf children ages 6 to 14 years who had different cognitive abilities. Her parents wanted to educate Debra in the neighborhood school that was closer to their home with her peers. The school district refused, citing its inability to afford a speech therapist for Debra (Siegel, 2008, pp. 44–46).

Siegel disagreed with the court's ruling in the Amy Rowley case, and the school districts' decisions regarding Joey and Debra. He argued that "Debra, Joey, and Amy Rowley have a fundamental right to access the 'flow of information' in their classrooms, whether through a qualified interpreter or through a language aide" (Siegel, 2008, p. 47).

Siegel provides a fresh interpretation of IDEA by connecting the communication rights of deaf children to the 1st Amendment and the 14th Amendment of the United States Constitution. Siegel believes that, when deaf children are denied an interpreter in the public school, they are denied access to school activities and the "flow of information," and they are denied appropriate interaction with their hearing peers—all of which are rights protected under the 1st Amendment. Further, he believes that deaf children are denied "equal protection" under the 14th Amendment, which states their education must be equal to that of hearing students.

There are procedural safeguards provided by IDEA to ensure that parents are able to fully participate in the decision-making process for an appropriate education for their deaf child. The NAD also provides information on how parents and school districts can prepare for the due process hearing, as well as how to appeal to the state education agency if a decision is not acceptable to parents and even to proceed to litigation (National Association of the Deaf, 2015).

Types of Placements

Newborn Infant Screening, Early Identification, and Early Intervention

With Universal Newborn Infant Screening (UNHS) required in every state, currently 98 to 99 percent of all children are screened for hearing loss by age 1 month (Yoshinago-Itano, 2013). In addition to the information presented in Chapter 3, we note the following: Diagnostic testing as follow-up to screenings that were not passed occurs for only about 52 percent of the children who fall into this category. This has been acknowledged as an area in need of significant improvement. About 65.1 percent of those children who get additional testing have hearing loss. As a reminder (see Chapter 3), a good number of children are not identified until later. In addition to those children lost to follow-up, children with mild-to-moderate hearing levels, progressive hearing losses, or conductive hearing losses may not be identified until early childhood or even later (Northern & Downs, 2014).

The Joint Commission on Infant Hearing (JCIH), a blue ribbon committee of professionals, recommends the 1–3–6 guidelines, which means that all children need to be screened for hearing loss by 1 month, identified by 3 months, and appropriately fitted with amplification by 6 months. Each state has its own guidelines on forming an eligibility service team made up of audiologists, deaf educators, speech-language pathologists, and early interventionists, all of whom assist in conducting the multidisciplinary assessment. They also develop the Individual Family Service Plan (IFSP), which includes recommendations for intervention strategies, communication opportunities such as ASL, sign codes, cued speech, and listening and spoken language, and technology options such as cochlear implants, hearing aids, and FM systems (Northern & Downs, 2014). Chapter 7 provides more details about the early intervention phase for deaf children.

Goals 3a, 10, and 11 of the Joint Committee for Infant Hearing Position Statement (JCIH), made in 2007 and updated in 2013, acknowledge the role of Deaf sign language teachers, mentors, and developers within the Early Hearing and Detection Intervention (EHDI) system at the federal, state, and local levels (Muse et al., 2013). This addresses the need for more participation by Deaf professionals in the early intervention phase, and as such has been enthusiastically supported by the Deaf community.

Deaf/hearing collaborative efforts in early childhood education is evident in the 2005 establishment of The National American Sign Language & English Bilingual Consortium as part of the Gallaudet Leadership Institute and Center on American Sign Language and English Bilingual Education and Research. This group formed an Early Childhood Advisory Focus Group to coordinate and collaborate on curriculum and resources to be used with home-based, school-based, and community-based programs. Their mission is "[t]o promote the development, management, and coordination of ASL/English bilingual early childhood education for children who are deaf and hard-of-hearing and their families, so that families are afforded the option of choosing ASL/English bilingual early childhood education for their child." (www.bilingualece.org./about/mission). To date, more than 20 center schools and public school programs have joined this consortium, which has held seven national 3-day summits annually for the purpose of exchanging ideas. About 20 early childhood Deaf teachers have joined this group. This consortium has created a website for parents and early childhood professionals that provides information on products and research articles. The year 2016 summit was slated to focus on Deaf, racial, and gender identity issues and the young deaf child (Laurene Simms, personal communication, February 2, 2016).

Residential or Center Schools for the Deaf

The history of deaf education in the United States began in 1817 with the establishment of the first state residential school for the deaf in Hartford, Connecticut. Today, almost every state has one residential school, with California and New York having two. Residential schools have rich histories and heritages with many having museums housing collections of books, uniforms, photographs, and memorabilia that preserve an era gone by. Nowadays, state schools are increasingly known as center schools that provide a variety of services, such as outreach to day programs and public schools that need expertise on deaf-related issues.

Center schools for the Deaf represent an exemplar of "communities of practice" (Wenger, 1999) where teachers or education experts scaffold or support Deaf children's language learning and cultural modeling (Rogoff, 2003; Vygotsky, 1978; Wenger, 1999). Deaf adults can model problem solving, metacognition, Theory of Mind (the perspective of others), as well as executive functioning skills (see Chapter 4) for deaf children across the ages in addition to teaching deaf children strategies for coping with the hearing world. Children also have a community of peers who are of the same age with whom to communicate.

Center schools provide comprehensive programming, with students engaged in academics, vocational training, sports, clubs, academic bowl competitions, student government, extracurricular activities, dormitory living, and, for the 18 to 21 age group, independent living skills. Staff work with state vocational rehabilitation agencies to plan for the students' transition to postsecondary education or to the working world. Yesterday's vocational training was shoe repair, printing, and culinary arts, while today's trades include graphic design, digital drawing and printing, and photography. Advantages of center school include those listed here as well as direct instruction without sign language interpreters. Support services include speech therapy and counseling among others. Center schools also have innovative programs such as summer camps to provide socialization and recreational activities for deaf children in the mainstream, classes on robotics, graphic design, and digital photography and the distribution of ASL storytelling throughout the state using videoconferencing technology (Claire Bugen, personal communication, January 27, 2016). To offset the disadvantage of children missing out on family life, center schools typically close on the weekends and provide transportation to children's homes to foster home-school connections. See Table 5.2 for innovative programs at the Texas School for the Deaf.

Public School Placements

Providing a *culturally responsive* curriculum in a public school is a challenge because there is neither a critical mass of deaf students or Deaf faculty. However, with increases in hiring Deaf teachers in public schools (Simms et al., 2008) and co-enrollment programs, administrators are finally beginning to recognize the importance of Deaf faculty as well as having groups of Deaf peers learning in classes together rather than having Deaf "solitaries" so changes may be in sight.

Deaf children can be partially or fully included in the public school classroom. In *mainstreaming* and *inclusion* placements, deaf students can be in regular education classes with an educational interpreter, can receive services individually, or be in small groups from specialized teachers available in a self-contained classroom or resource room. These teachers are trained to work with students who vary in age, hearing loss, presence of additional disabilities,

Table 5.2 Innovative Programs at the Texas School for the Deaf

---

Discovery Retreats for Solitaires* in the Mainstream

Brings together deaf and hard-of-hearing teens of *all* backgrounds and providing access to *all* modes of communication. The retreat's surface agenda is always focused around fun, engaging educational or career exploration activities while the deeper agenda is the opportunity for students to improve self-esteem as well as acceptance of self and others. To that end, deaf and hard-of-hearing adult role models/mentors abound as group leaders, instructors, and staff.

ASL Storytelling

Introduces gifted storytellers who are Deaf and have native ASL fluency to deaf and hard-of-hearing students across the state through interactive, videoconferencing. The storyteller makes constant connections between the ASL used to bring the story to life and the book's illustrations/English print projected in the background. For many students, ASL storytelling provides their only opportunity for interaction with a Deaf adult. The program is also building an online archive of stories told in ASL.

Online Classroom Resources

Allows teachers and students access to entire online units of instruction built around engaging videos that are accessible through sign, caption, and voiceover. Lesson plans include state standards for knowledge and skills as well as suggestions for expansion activities. Videos feature skilled communicators including hearing and deaf or hard-of-hearing adults and students.

Personalized, Interactive Instruction through Videoconferencing

Taking advantage of the ubiquity of personal devices, whether phone, notepads, or computers, parents are given the opportunity to learn sign language or get tutoring for reading to their children. By using devices as the classroom, flexibility, accessibility, and reach are built into the program. Parents have the opportunity to participate in personalized classes conducted at the time of their choice and in the location of their choice. For many, the latter is the comfort of their own home. It is also easier to staff the program when instructors can be anywhere in the state.

Young inventors build robots; their teams will participate in one or more of the regional and district events that measure the effectiveness of each robot, the power of collaboration, and the determination of students. Our current high school team has advanced to the finals.

---

* "Solitaires" refers to the isolation of the deaf child who is alone in the mainstream with other hearing classmates and without deaf classmates. It was coined by Gina A. Oliva in her book, *Alone in the Mainstream: A Deaf Woman Remembers Public School* (Washington, DC: Gallaudet University Press, 2004).

Source: Courtesy of Superintendent Claire Bugen, Texas School for the Deaf, Austin.

and academic achievement. Their services cover consultation and collaboration with teaching staff who may request assistance with specific students in need of general education classroom support (Andrews et al., 2004).

Itinerant teachers travel from school to school to serve mainstreamed students when there are insufficient students in any one school to justify a resource room teacher on site. Focusing on students' needs, they provide assessments in the academic, speech, audiological, and social needs and write goals, objectives, and necessary accommodations for the student's annual IEP and 3-year evaluations (Luckner & Ayantoye, 2013; Norman & Jamieson, 2015).

Day schools, found in larger metropolitan areas, tend to be similar to center schools, except for the lack of dormitories. In the past, in comparison to most mainstream and deaf/hearing integrated classrooms, day schools provided a more accessible communication environment in that teaching was directed specifically at students and there was a concentrated body of deaf peers with whom to socialize (Andrews et al., 2004). However, this is changing with more children being fully integrated into public schools. A different option is that of co-enrollment, which offers a promising possibility for deaf socialization.

In the co-enrollment model, one finds both hearing and deaf students in the same class. Two teachers work as a team, with one being a trained teacher of the deaf and the other a regular education teacher. There is a sufficient number of deaf students in these classrooms to provide socialization among themselves, plus opportunities to socialize with hearing classmates who are also being taught sign language. One outcome study focusing on co-enrollment shows that while deaf children have opportunities to develop deaf and hearing friends, their academic achievement still is not up to par with hearing classmates, showing where more work needs to be done (Antia & Metz, 2014).

Alternative Placements

Deaf children can also attend private schools, be home schooled, attend charter schools, or receive services in juvenile corrections units. Private schools can focus on specific areas such as religion (e.g., Catholic parochial school) or provide a monolingual listening and speaking curriculum. Home schooling of deaf children has increased to approximately 3.7 percent (GRI, 2013). In one study with 21 families, parents reported they chose home schooling because of lack of services in public schools (Parks, 2009). Others mentioned they wanted to provide religious instruction.

The charter school model operates under a "charter" contract with the local board of education. Some focus exclusively on listening and spoken language such as at the Ohio Valley Voices in Loveland, Ohio, and Child's Voice in Woodvale, Illinois. The goal of these schools is to educate deaf infants from birth to elementary school and, by age 8, to integrate them full-time in a public school. There are also charter ASL/English bilingual schools that aim to teach ASL as the instructional language and to teach English as a second language. Charter schools that use this approach are the Blossom Montessori School for the Deaf in Clearwater, Florida; the Jean Massieu School for the Deaf in Salt Lake City, Utah; the ASL Academy in Albuquerque, New Mexico; the Minnesota North Star Academy and the Metro Deaf School in Minnesota; the Rocky Mountain Deaf School in Denver, Colorado; the Sequoia School for the Deaf in Arizona; and the Las Vegas Charter School for the Deaf. These schools may also accept hearing siblings and hearing children with Deaf parents.

Academic Outcomes and Social Skills

Research is inconclusive on which educational placement provides better academic outcomes and social skills. Some children will move from one placement to another. Deaf children who are not succeeding may transfer to the center school in junior high or high school. Or they may change to a center school for more socialization or to join a sports team or after-school club.

Antia and Kreimeyer (2015) report that deaf and hard-of-hearing children in general education outperform their peers in self-contained classrooms, making a year's progress in a year's time. However, the authors recognize that deaf children in self-contained classrooms may differ on background characteristics such as levels of hearing loss and early access to language, may lack social skills, and may need more language support that a self-contained class may provide.

Other researchers found that it was instructional factors (e.g., the teacher) that contributed to the deaf students' academic achievement scores. For example, in a review of 20 years of research, Stinson and Kluwin (2011) found that only between 1 percent and 5 percent of the variances in deaf students' academic achievement was attributed to school placement, with 75 percent due to instructional factors, thus emphasizing the important role of the teacher.

Related to social competence skills, Antia and Kreimeyer (2015) summarized research that confirms the ability of deaf students to make friends with both hearing and deaf peers in public schools, thus widening their social circles. Just how deaf children in regular education can develop an early bicultural identity has not been investigated in depth. Case studies reveal that deaf and hard-of-hearing children may feel isolation and loneliness in the general education system (see Chapter 7). If they move to a center school in early adolescence for this reason or for academic needs, they may make deaf friends and learn ASL, thus becoming bilingual and bicultural (Grushkin, 2003). Further research is needed on ways to help administrators and teachers develop bicultural sensitivity for deaf students in general education.

Education Interpreting

In regular public school placements, educational interpreters provide communication access between deaf students and the teacher. They will utilize a communication modality used by the school that may incorporate the two languages—American Sign Language and English. These language and communication modalities may include American Sign Language, Total Communication, Sim-Com (Simultaneous Communication), Signed Exact English, Spoken Language (Oral), Cued Speech, PSE (Pidgin Signed English), or CASE (Conceptually Accurate Signed English) or combinations of these. Each of the languages and modalities are defined in Chapter 6. Interpreter duties may include interpreting classroom activities, field trips, club meetings, assemblies, counseling sessions, and athletic competitions. In some schools, the interpreter may also teach sign language and explain deaf-related issues to hearing school staff and children if qualified to do so.

Schick (2008) has conducted studies of educational interpreters and documented the challenges they face in providing quality services in K through 12 settings. Even though educational interpreters play an important role in providing access to the general education curriculum for deaf students, she reports that many interpreters do not have the knowledge of the content, translation skills, or professional training—all of which are needed to effectively translate the teacher's and student's communication. Many are not consistently able to interpret at the deaf student's level of understanding. Many interpreters are unable to pass state certification exams. This lack of training provides a disservice to young deaf students whose attention is tied up in sitting through or resolving communication breakdowns and errors caused by the interpreter rather than focusing on learning. To better understand these issues, Schick has proposed a model of student and interpreter factors that account for students' learning during the process of educational interpreting. Challenging issues also exist related to teachers' beliefs about the role of the interpreter. Some may feel uncomfortable having to slow the pace of their teaching to give time for the deaf students to follow lectures and participate in class discussions or even to use the interpreter as a teacher's aide (Marschark, Lang, & Albertini, 2002).

Academic Achievement and Assessment

Whether they are educated in the public schools or at center schools, we need evidence of how deaf students are achieving academically. An exemplar of Deaf youths' academic achievement is the Academic Bowl program sponsored by Gallaudet University (www.gallaudet.edu/out-reach-programs/youth-programs/academic-bowl/about-ab.html). Started in 1996 with teams from just six schools, in 2015, teams from 78 schools competed to answer challenging questions in various categories such as math, science, social studies, current events, literature, popular culture, and Deaf culture. If you view the videotape of the 2015 championship match, you will get a holistic view of Deaf youth using their cognitive and language skills, including visual attention, memory, executive functioning (e.g., planning and goal setting), thinking before answering, self-correction, critical and analytical skills (metacognition), and Theory of Mind (e.g., understanding the perspective of the other team and the announcer). In addition, the youth showed speed in recall of facts, communication, reading, writing, spelling, math calculation and word problem-solving skills, cooperative and collaborative learning, motivation, thinking under the stress of the stopwatch, and knowledge about the world, not to mention the hours of research and study skills they utilized before they came to the tournament. How did they do it? This is difficult to answer without knowing the background of the students and the roles their families and teachers played in their success. Observing and interviewing them to gain a better understanding of these academically achieving Deaf students' developmental histories and the strategies used in the competition would yield a goldmine of data that would help clarify the cognitive, neurocognitive, language, and motivational underpinnings of their learning.

Current data on school achievement based on standardized, norm-referenced tests indicate that deaf students tend to score lower compared to hearing children (Qi & Mitchell, 2012). Over a 30-year span, high school graduates were found to score at the median grade level between the 4th to the 7th grade levels compared to hearing peers. It is important to remember that the median indicates the presence of a range from high to low scores. While delays in English language development may be a significant factor, other reasons for low scores can include test-taking factors such as not receiving appropriate accommodations, including additional time or small group or individual administration, and not receiving the test directions in their primary language. And as these deaf students move through the grades and encounter more challenging academic material, this achievement gap widens (Cawthon & Leppo, 2013). Keep in mind, as we mentioned earlier, that standardized achievement scores are not necessarily related to school placement but rather to other instructional aspects (Stinson & Kluwin, 2011).

The mathematics scores for Deaf students are higher than their reading scores, leveling off to about a 7th-grade level in calculation abilities but with noted difficulties in addressing word problems. Pagliaro (2015) summarizes the mathematics skills of deaf students from preschool to school age by stating that deaf children and youths are behind in their understanding of concepts in various areas of numeracy, including numbers, geometry, measurement, fractions, and problem solving. She attributes some of these problems to the teachers who may subject deaf students to "rote and routine-based pedagogy" rather than higher-order thinking skills that align with cognitive strengths (Pagliaro, 2015, p. 186). See Chapter 4 on cognitive strengths.

Standards, Curriculum, and Teaching Strategies

Teachers of deaf students may find it challenging to use state standards to develop learning objectives for deaf students. Most states have K-12 standards that teachers are required to follow. Center and public school may adopt, differentiate or adapt those standards for deaf children. For example, at the Texas School for the Deaf, teachers use the Texas Essential Knowledge and Skills (TEKS) standards for English Language Arts, Math, Social Studies, and Science in grades K-12. They will adapt it depending on the students' background knowledge, learning styles, language, and modality needs (www.teksresourcesystem.net/module/profile/Account/LogOn). The Maryland School for the Deaf follows its state department of education curriculum just like the public schools do and also participates in the Maryland Assessment Program.

The Common Core Standards (CCS, 2012) is a set of standards that include expectations for student knowledge and skills starting at each grade level. The CCS, which have been adopted by 45 states (Dolman, 2013), place more emphasis on informational texts and require students to develop closer reading of texts to learn academic vocabulary. This represents a shift of emphasis for teachers of the deaf. Traditional deaf education class activities incorporated preteaching lessons during which the teacher built background knowledge pertaining to the topic prior to reading about it in a text (Dolman, 2013). Now the CCS focus is for students to get information directly from the texts with teachers adapting their lesson plans to follow this requirement. There is also an increased emphasis on research and analytical skills; English grammar, usage, and mechanics; parent involvement; and career readiness. The new assessments with CCS may also have "embedded universal accessibility systems" such as directions in ASL, closed captioning for English Language listening items, and a scribe for constructed response items (Pepnet 2, n.d.). States now have the option of accepting these standards or using their own due to changes in the legislation (ESSA, 2015).

Researchers have advised teachers to move toward using evidence-based practices (EBP) or instructional practices that have verifiable or emerging outcome data to support their use. Information on EBPs in science, mathematics, social studies, and literacy can be found in *Evidence-Based Practice in Educating Deaf and Hard of Hearing Students* (Spencer & Marschark, 2010); in *Educating Deaf Students: From Research to Practice* (Marschark, Lang, & Albertini, 2002); and in Easterbrooks and Beal-Alvarez's (2013) *Literacy Instruction for Students Who Are Deaf and Hard of Hearing*.

ASL and Deaf studies can be integrated into the curriculum and expanded beyond the limited focus inherent in events such as Deaf Awareness Week. Separate coursework in Deaf studies, Deaf culture, and ASL can be offered to Deaf children as well as hearing children in public schools as well as co-enrollment programs.

Transition

The current IDEA 2014 definition of transition entails a set of activities for the child with disabilities that focus on improving the academic and functioning of the child so that he or she can move from school to postschool activities, including postsecondary, vocational, and integrated employment as well as adult education, independent living, and community participation. The program should be based on the child's strengths and needs and take into account their preferences and interests. Transition services include instruction, related services, community experiences, the development of employment and other postschool adult living objectives, and daily living skills and functional vocational evaluation (Section 602(a) [20 U.S.C. 1401(a)]; Luft, 2014).

Many deaf students transition from high school to a college or university, go on to graduate degrees and become professionals in all walks of life (see Chapter 9). Those who do not go on to college may transition into the workforce or into vocational schools.

Vocational rehabilitation (VR) counselors will work with deaf clients to provide information about postsecondary education, administer assessments, and provide vocational training or work placements. In a survey of programs providing transition services to deaf and hard-of-hearing students, Luft (2014) found residential (center) schools offered significantly more transition services than large or small programs. She also found that programs focused on early and initial transition services rather than long-term needs and strategies. With new patterns of student placement in public schools, this has created challenges in providing deaf-specific transition services. Although deaf students may receive increased opportunity for instruction in the general curriculum, they often have fewer support services for their unique transition needs (Luft, 2014). The use of professionals with years of experience predicted more positive outcomes for transition goals (Cawthon et al., 2014).

Pepnet is a federally funded entity that provides transition resources for teachers, VR staff, special education professionals, and transition specialists who work with deaf and hard-of-hearing students and their parents. Pepnet provides training for professionals, newsletters, and listservs that address transition topics (www.pepnet.org).

Postsecondary Education and Accommodations

Today, approximately 30,000 students who are deaf or hard of hearing transition to colleges and universities. Gallaudet University, the Rochester Institute of Technology/National Technical Institute for the Deaf, California State University at Northridge, and Southwest Collegiate Institute for the Deaf are four postsecondary programs with multiple support services in place including ASL and oral interpreting, Communication Access Real-time Translation (CART), and note-taking. Only about 25 to 30 percent of deaf students graduate from 2- or 4-year programs, and it takes them longer to complete their programs compared to hearing students (Cawthon, Schoffstall, & Garberoglio, 2014; Luft, 2014). Individual factors such as strong academic preparation, self-efficacy, and problem-solving skills as well as postsecondary institutional factors such as adequate advising, quality of accommodations, and providing multiple learning formats that are accessible to students with a broad range of English literacy skills contribute to the success of deaf students who do graduate (Cawthon et al., 2014).

Accommodations for postsecondary students are protected under four laws: 1) the *Individuals with Disabilities Act* (IDEA), 2) *Section 504 of the Rehabilitation Act of 1973*, 3) *the American with Disabilities Act* (ADA), and 4) the *Twenty-First Century Communications and Video Accessibility Act* (CVVA, 2010; 2012; 2013). When postsecondary and graduate education are accessible through the use of interpreters, voice-to-text software, video relay services, real-time captioning, tutoring, and distance learning, many deaf adults succeed in their respective programs, whatever the discipline. Even though postsecondary programs are often well equipped to handle accommodation policy for Deaf students, they are often not prepared to meet the needs of Deaf students applying for faculty positions (Smith & Andrews, 2015).

Vocational Programs

Deaf students who do not attend an academic postsecondary program will transition to vocational programs for additional training or go directly into the workforce. As each state provides vocational rehabilitation services, these students may be assigned to a vocational rehabilitation counselor. VR counselors can be community-based or connected to a school for the deaf.

The Texas School for the Deaf has a Career and Technical Education department that provides work-based training for high school and transitional students (ages 18 to 21) with equipment and software training so students can develop marketable skills. Other technical skills include auto repair, cabinet making, culinary arts, fine arts, welding, digital interactive media, and child development. The Texas School for the Deaf also provides a variety of programs to assist families with transition planning, including career assessments and counseling, academic advising, early college start/dual credits, career education, computer lab to explore careers, college information and planning, parent training, employer partnerships, annual transition fair, and coordination with the onsite vocational rehabilitation counselor from the Texas Department of Assistive and Rehabilitative Services (www.tsd.state.tx.us/apps/pages/index. jsp?type=d&uREC_ID=169968&pREC_ID=350020).

Employment Data

For those deaf and hard-of-hearing persons who enter the workforce, their employment rate grew up to 44.2 percent after 2 years of leaving high school (Luft, 2014). But compared to their hearing peers, deaf adults are underemployed and underpaid. They are, however, employed at a higher rate than their peers with other disabilities (Newman et al., 2011). Other data provided by Pepnet shows that, in 2011, 47.9 percent of deaf adults were employed and that on average they made $4,000 less than the general population with Deaf men earning more than Deaf women, a disparity that was also parallel to the general population (www.pepnet.org/sites/ default/files/employmentbrief_v5.pdf). See Chapter 9 for an extensive discussion of transition and employment issues for this population.

There are also specialized training programs for deaf students with special needs such as the Helen Keller National Center for DeafBlind Youths and Adults. This center helps DeafBlind individuals transitioning to more limited vision. There are numerous kinds of technologies available for DeafBlind adults related to Braille readers on computers, print enlargers, print to voice software, and so on (Ingraham, 2015).

Bill of Rights for Deaf and Hard-of-Hearing Children

Fourteen states have passed a Deaf Children's Bill of Rights (DCBR) to address the unique needs of deaf and hard-of-hearing students (NAD, 2015). Each state's DCBR differs in content but have similar fundamentals. For example, each of these focuses on communication as a basic human right for every child. The availability of qualified and certified personnel who can communicate directly with deaf students is another essential requirement. The availability of same language mode peers who are of the same age and ability level, ample opportunities to interact with deaf and hard-of-hearing adult role models, equal opportunity to benefit from all services and programs at their schools, and appropriate assessments all are additional components of DCBR. Other rights, such as the addition of provisions supporting the need for early and consistent communication access from birth to 3 years, are also included. Professionals are prohibited from denying the family and child information about communication options and the possibility of considering center schools as a least restrictive environment option. Explicit directions are given for some states to involve Deaf and hard-of-hearing adults and other experienced deaf educators in the IEP process. Other states provide outreach programs to assist families (National Association of the Deaf, 2015).

Technology

The twenty-first-century classroom looks very different from the classroom of old that used chalk, blackboards, filmstrips, mimeograph machines, pencils, and paper. Today's computer age classroom has problem-based learning, universal design for learning, blended learning, and online instruction through the use of podcasting or screencasting, (Bennett et al., 2013). New models such as the flipped learning model allow teachers to shift from teacher-driver instruction to student-centered learning (Hamdan, McKnight, McKnight, & Arfstrom, 2013). The flipped learning model provides resources for the student to work on at home such as videos, podcasts, readings, and lecture notes so that they can come to class better prepared and thus enable the teacher to focus on helping them integrate and apply their knowledge in student-centered activities with their classmates.

In general education, there are sign language interpreters, C-Print, real-time captioning, and note-takers. Students and teachers have at their disposal smartphones, iPhones, iPads, e-books and other electronic tablets and books. Students are motivated to learn with ASL/English bilingual books, audiobooks, laptops, and wearable devices such as Apple Watches, Fitbits, and Google Glasses. In the classroom, there are laptops, videoconferencing software, visual paging systems, v-logs, signing avatars, multimedia materials, and text intercoms. Smartboards, white boards, and LCD projectors allow English text and signing to be presented side by side. There are multimedia encyclopedias and sign language dictionaries, games, and gaming devices. Teachers can purchase subscriptions to download digital tools that make it possible to create sign to print instructional materials (www.idrt.com). Children can view ASL storytelling on YouTube videos from their home or at school. Parents can also subscribe to ASL classes online. Translation software can be used by teachers, parents, and students to bridge signing and English. Mobile augmented reality (MAR) and Auras are increasingly coming into use as innovative technology. The MAR technology uses cell phones with computer tablets to scan a Quick Response (QR) code, which calls up a video to describe some object, and ASL videos can be added. The cell phone can also use Auras, a mechanism that triggers it to go to a server and pull down a video for information. QR codes and Auras provide equal access for deaf people for museums and tourist areas in place of audio recordings (Parton, 2014; 2015). Undoubtedly, these innovative uses of technology will be subjected to empirical testing in controlled studies of educational approaches for evidence-based practice purposes.

Conclusions

Just as there are many ways to be deaf—oral deaf, culturally Deaf, late deafened, hard of hearing, and DeafBlind (Leigh, 2009), as a corollary, there are many ways to educate deaf children within school environments that are *culturally responsive* to their Deaf and racial/ethnic hearing cultures. To enhance cultural responsiveness, deaf/hearing collaborative teams should be included at all levels. Input is needed from all four stakeholders: Deaf adults, parents, teachers, and scientists—each of whom brings relevance, care, experience, and science to deaf education. Early access to spoken language, bimodal, or bilingual languages or a combination of these will allow deaf children to form a healthy, bicultural identity and to learn language and academic content. Barriers, however, still persist in deaf education, and these need to be addressed. In the next chapter, we discuss the theories, outcomes, and practical applications of the monolingual, bimodal, and bilingual language learning and language teaching approaches and literacy.

Suggested Readings

Knoors, H., & Marschark, M. (2015). *Educating deaf learners: Creating a global evidence base.* New York, NY: Oxford University Press.

Taking an international perspective, these authors deliver a comprehensive synthesis of up-to-date scholarship in deaf education in the areas of language, literacy, numeracy, cognition, technology, and learning environments.

Lang, H., & Meath-Lang, B. (1995). *Deaf persons in the arts and science: A biographical dictionary.* Westport, CT: Greenwood Press.

The authors present a detailed biographical dictionary of 150 deaf individuals who have distinguished themselves in the arts and sciences, including deaf individuals known for their leadership in education. A must read for social studies, science, and literacy teachers.

Rogoff, M. (2003). *The cultural nature of human development*. New York, NY: Oxford.
   Human development and learning is viewed as a cultural process during which persons engage with others and build on the cultural practices of previous generations.

Santiago, D. A., Galdeano, E. C., & Taylor, M. (2015). *The condition of Latinos in education: 2015 Factbook*. Washington, DC: In Education. Retrieved from www.edexcelencia.org/research/2015-factbook
   This publication looks at the educational pipeline and the context of learning for Latino students. Current information is provided about Latino student achievement, practices, and policies as well as partnerships to serve Latino students.

Wright, C., Standen, P., & Patel, T. (2010). *Black youth matters: Transitions from school to success*. New York, NY: Routledge.
   Based on ethnographic research of Black youth excluded from school, this book examines their resourcefulness and resilience as they overcome school failure and create positive futures for themselves.

Note

1   According to Yosso's Cultural Wealth Model, linguistic and linguistic capital are two of his six types of cultural wealth. Linguistic capital includes intellectual and social skills that are developed through communication experiences with more than one language.

    Social capital refers to networks of people and community resources with their peers and other social contacts providing emotional support for learning (Yosso, 2005, pp. 78–79).

6 Language Learning and Language Teaching Approaches

A language-in-education approach—be it monolingual or bilingual—that does not acknowledge and build upon the hybrid language practices in bilingual communities is more concerned with controlling language behavior than in educating.

Ofelia Garcia & Jo Ann Kleifgen (2010, p. 43)

The speech classes helped me understand the syntax, semantics, and phonetics when writing sentences in the correct order.

Chatman Sieben (2014, p. 112)

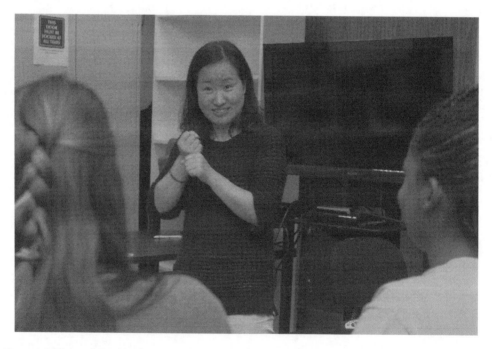

Figure 6.1 Photo of Deaf professor teaching at college

Source: Used with permission.

Introduction

The teaching of language for deaf children and instructional decisions do not operate in isolation. Rather, they are influenced by language debates, parental decisions, professional advice, and the perspectives of the larger Deaf community. For the last decade, deaf education has transitioned from students attending specialized schools to inclusive settings, including deaf/ hearing co-enrollment classrooms. In one respect, this constitutes a dismantling of the historic deaf education communities with roots in these specialized schools that for centuries have supported deaf students' cultural and linguistic development. Today, this responsibility has been somewhat relegated to public schools, which more often than not have limited knowledge sources and reduced resources.

In light of these trends, our major task as educators is to keep the needs of the deaf child paramount and consider what is in his or her best interest—in the long term. Today, we are privy to a wealth of new research related to earlier identification and intervention, neurocognitive and behavioral findings on the underpinnings of how deaf students learn, language and literacy practices, and cochlear implant technology (Knoors & Marschark, 2015). As a community of educators, how should we respond? Does deaf education need to be reformed? Increasing the number of culturally responsive language environments in inclusive or public school systems would be a major step (see Chapter 5). This includes not only a strong base in evidence-based language, literacy, and academic practices but also ongoing monitoring of progress and the hiring of Deaf faculty and staff in these inclusive settings because they bring with them a wealth of experience and knowledge relevant to the education of deaf children. It also means forging stronger alliances and sharing resources with center schools for the deaf, which have specialized faculty and expertise in providing for the psychosocial, language, and education needs of diverse deaf school-age populations. In this chapter, we explore traditional and innovative language learning and language teaching approaches.

Chapter Objectives

Using a sociocultural framework, we describe bilingual, bimodal, and monolingual approaches. We discuss the history, theoretical base, pedagogical techniques, language planning considerations, teaching strategies, materials, and outcomes for each approach. We also discuss the biological advantages of having early access to dual languages that reap future language and literacy learning benefits.

Diversity of Language Use by Deaf Individuals across the Lifespan

Over the past 40 years, Deaf college students have shared their language and literacy histories with one of the authors (Andrews). These stories seldom focus on "one method." Rather, these stories reveal a variety of practices including spoken language, speechreading, gestures, ASL, contact signing, fingerspelling, initialized signs, bimodal communication, reading, and writing that were used from childhood to adulthood. Some students remark that they are more comfortable separating the two languages, while others prefer to integrate, blend, and mix their two languages cross-modally.

We take into consideration these insights as we believe that a long-range view of the communication and language behaviors of Deaf adults across the life span will lead to a better understanding of the language strengths and needs of young deaf children. Adult language needs are seldom considered because many medical, audiological, and even professionals in deaf education have never interacted with Deaf adults. That is why, throughout this book, we underscore the importance of Deaf/hearing collaborative teams being involved in the deaf education process from the EDHI process forward to the creation of the IFSP and the IEP, the teaching process itself, and eventually to transition planning, postsecondary schooling, and the work environment (see Chapters 5 and 9). Our long-term goal is to help deaf children integrate into and become bicultural in both Deaf and hearing environments. The classroom is a good place to start this process.

Across Deaf communities in the United States, we see diversity in dual language and multilingual practices, which include spoken and sign languages. For example, deaf individuals may learn some spoken English, Navaho, Spanish, Chinese, or Taiwanese depending on the family heritage. They may learn a sign language such as ASL or Mexican Sign Language, a Taiwanese or Chinese Sign Language, or any other sign language from their home country. They may use a contact sign language along with the written language of their society or combine, mix, or change (codeswitch) languages depending on their communication partners as well as become biscriptal in alphabetic and logographic scripts, as in the case of Asian Deaf adults (Wang, Andrews, Liu, & Liu, 2016).

Early dual language or bilingual learning is not always available for every deaf child. For the 96 percent of deaf children from hearing-speaking homes, the language of the home tends to be a spoken language, whether English, Spanish (as 28.4 percent of deaf children are from Spanish-speaking homes), or some other spoken language. In total, to further challenge access issues, up to 35 percent of deaf children come from non-English speaking homes (Cannon & Guardino, 2016). Depending on their contact with professionals or peers, ASL, contact signing, or an English sign system will be introduced at different times from early childhood to high school or even in early adulthood.

In light of changing language demographics and other evidence, today's early childhood professionals and deaf educators are recommending that deaf children be exposed to a visual language from birth in order to take advantage of the sensitive period for language acquisition (see reviews in Humphries et al., 2014a; 2014b) as well as to support later reading and school achievement (Hrastinski & Wilbur, 2016; see also Chapter 4).

Language Conflicts

Throughout history, both approaches—signed and spoken languages—have been used in schools for the deaf (Moores, 2010; Nover, 2000). The two approaches were framed as the oral-only approach supported by Alexander Graham Bell and the Combined Approach led by Edward Miner Gallaudet (Winefield, 1987). Several historical events such as the Milan Conference of 1880 (during which it was determined that spoken language took precedence over sign language) and meetings of the Conference of Educational Administrators of Schools and Programs for the Deaf, popularly known as CEASD, resulted in a severe reduction of the use of sign language and the hiring of deaf teachers in schools by the year 1926 (Nover, 2000). During the early twentieth century, more oral schools were established, and spoken language was the focus of many programs for deaf children. Even among schools for the deaf, administrators set up separate oral and sign classrooms under one roof (Winefield, 1987).

In the early 1960s, the research of William C. Stokoe, an English professor at Gallaudet University who described the linguistic structure of ASL, encouraged national and global interest in studying the sign languages of Deaf people worldwide (Brentari, 2010). In the United States, both ASL and English were taught in the schools in various ways, either maintaining ASL grammar in ASL/English bilingualism, maintaining the two languages in bimodal bilingualism, or providing access to one complete language—English—using Total Communication (TC), Simultaneous Communication (SC) or Signed Supported Speech (SSS) within comprehensive language approaches (Andrews et al., 2004; Nover & Andrews, 1998).

Of interest is the fact that language conflicts have existed in the United States as far back as during the Civil War, when slaves were punished for not speaking English, when Americans Indians were forced to drop their tribal languages and go to boarding schools to learn to talk like White Americans, and when German Americans were prohibited from speaking the

German language in public during World War I (Lake, 2002). And internationally, a language war erupted when the former Soviet Union tried to force a single national language to replace the regional languages already in place (Calvet, 1998).

Hearing people often do not understand the feelings Deaf individuals may harbor when ASL is suppressed and oppressed. Such prohibitions strike at the heart of how Deaf persons may feel about their language, culture, and identity.

Viewed in this context, one can see why many Deaf adults want dual language programming that includes both ASL and English to be included in the education of deaf children. They have personally experienced ASL's identity connections, their cherishing of ASL, but also its utilitarian use in the learning of English. For hearing educators, this idea makes sense for the small population of Deaf children of Deaf parents who acquire ASL from birth onward, deaf students with additional disabilities, or deaf students from multilingual backgrounds whose acquisition of first and second languages can be challenging. In contrast, hearing educators are inclined to encourage the support of spoken language and minimize the importance of sign language for those deaf children with hearing parents in the mainstream (Smith & Wolfe, 2016). For hearing parents, spoken language methods are more commonly the preferred mode of communication to start with. As a result, deaf children of hearing parents typically acquire ASL later and this learning occurs horizontally, from peer-to-peer in childhood or adulthood, but not vertically from parent to child. Further, many parents find it difficult to learn ASL. Despite this difficulty, many families do learn to sign. But for many deaf children, the classroom is their only opportunity to learn and be immersed in ASL if they are enrolled in a program with other signing deaf peers and Deaf adults (Geslin, 2007; Myers, 2011; Nover & Andrews, 1998).

The oral-manual controversy has resurfaced in the two decades with the use of the cochlear implant and the tendency of hearing health professionals, including physicians to discourage parents from using sign language (Smith & Wolfe, 2016). This is a disservice to those children who may have difficulty accessing spoken language despite cochlear implantation. To address this challenge, two organizations with contrasting perspectives—the Conference of Educational Administrators of Schools and Programs for the Deaf (CEASD), which advocates for the increased use of sign language, and Options Schools, Inc., which emphasizes listening and spoken language have joined together. They have co-wrote and published a manifesto, called *Common Ground* (2015), that details shared understandings in order to identify areas for collaboration (www.ceasd.org/child-first/common-ground-project).

Communication and Language Learning Approaches

Before looking at language programming approaches, we review the languages that are being learned. For background information on milestones for ASL and speech, see Chapter 4.

ASL and Fingerspelling

ASL is easier to acquire for all deaf children because its grammar and lexicon are visually accessible. Deaf parents tend to teach their child English as a second language either simultaneously with ASL or sequentially in the home. Shared book reading is a common English teaching practice during which the parents use books to translate stories by pointing out the sign to print connections and matching fingerspelling to print (Herbold, 2008). For deaf children born into hearing families, the language learning journey of both ASL and English is more challenging because of the lack of ASL adult and peer models in the home.

Deaf children acquire fingerspelling relatively early. Typically, their first fingerspelled word is their name. The child first learns to fingerspell words as whole units. Then later, they "relearn" fingerspelling when they learn to read and spell words by matching the fingerspelled handshape to the English letter (Padden, 2006). Fingerspelling is part of adult Deaf discourse so children in contact with them can pick up fingerspelling from them. When speech is combined with fingerspelling, this is called the *Rochester method*, which was popular in schools for the deaf in the 1970s but has fallen into disuse (Andrews et al., 2004). See Figure 6.2 for a sample finger-spelling chart.

English

Deaf children are exposed to and directly taught English through multiple methods, including spoken language, fingerspelling, signs combined with speech, manual codes of English, and reading and writing. How these forms of English are taught and allocated in the home and school is what constitutes language planning in educational programming (Knoors & Marschark, 2012; Nover, 2000). We look at each form of English in this section; however, in actual practice, signs and spoken words are mixed, blended, and combined. Some deaf children learn ASL as the first or dominant language and English as a second language. With other deaf children, English is learned as a first language, and ASL as a second language.

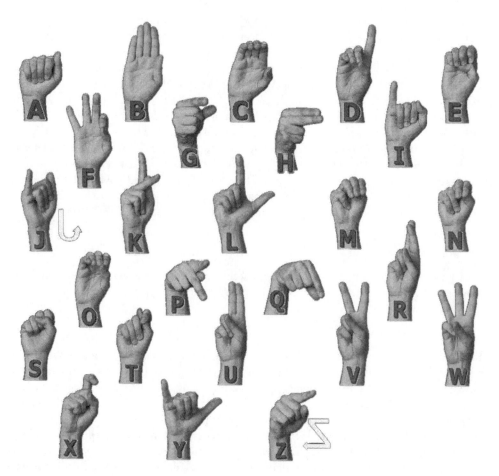

Figure 6.2 Manual Alphabet

Spoken Language, Speechreading, or Lipreading

Hearing children learn the articulation, phonation, and respiration of spoken language effort-lessly while deaf children must be taught through direct instruction using repetition and practice. Even if every deaf child is given the opportunity to learn to speak, not all deaf children are successful. The results of increased speech production and language abilities of deaf children with cochlear implants have given parents and professionals reasons for optimism. However, it is important to keep in mind, as we covered in Chapter 4, that there is significant variability in success rates, with much depending on factors such as age of implantation, auditory memory, neurocognitive correlates, family support, and intensive speech therapy (Marschark & Hauser, 2008). Further, the reading and language achievement gains acquired by young children are not always maintained when they become older (Convertino, Borgna, Marschark, & Durkin, 2014).

Other avenues of English learning are speechreading or lipreading. But these can be limiting in the learning of language as deaf individuals vary significantly in their ability to speechread, ranging from zero comprehension to almost full understanding of what is spoken (www.lipread ingtranslation.com/faq.htm). Many of the sounds are ambiguous, appearing the same on the lips, and lighting and the fatigue factor further decreases comprehension (Vernon & Andrews, 1990). Before speechreading can assist in deaf children's overall communicative and language ability, these children first must have an established language base. Deaf adults with cochlear implants do report benefits to lipreading as visual speechreading helps with the identification of sounds (Peterson, Pisoni, & Miyamoto, 2010). Deaf graduates students, too, most of whom were ASL signers, often asked one of the authors (Andrews) to mouth her lectures silently so they could use speechreading to decipher academic vocabulary.

Total Communication, Simultaneous Communication, Sign Supported Speech, Manual Codes of English, and Cued Speech

In traditional deaf education, English and sign have been combined for instructional purposes. The focus is on one language—English, with signing as a support. Total Communication (TC), Simultaneous Communication (SC), and Sign Supported Speech (SSS) have been devised to teach English using the hands. These are pedagogical tools to teach vocabulary and structures of English such as morphemes and grammar. This approach uses ASL lexical signs for the vocabulary component (see reviews in Andrews et al., 2004).

The Deaf adult community seldom uses these codes for communication among themselves, and with hearing people, they tend to use what is typically called *contact signing*. However, hearing teachers and parents may use these codes to communicate with their deaf children (Mayberry, 2002).

Total Communication (TC) is a philosophy (not a methodology) of communication that incorporates ASL, gestures, spoken language, lipreading, fingerspelling, body language, reading, writing, and manual codes of English depending on the needs of the child. Ray Holcomb, a deaf administrator who supervised a large day school program in California in the early 1970s, developed TC, which continues to be widely used. From the late 1960s to the 1980s, numerous studies showed that deaf children who were in signing/TC programs outperformed children in programs focused on spoken language (see reviews in Andrews et al., 2004; Vernon & Andrews, 1990). These studies were conducted before the cochlear implant.

Simultaneous Communication (SC) is a methodology rather than a philosophy like TC. SC focuses on the use of signs and spoken language at the same time. It is also referred to as Sign Supported Speech (SSS). Additional types of English-based signing that combine speech and signs are systems collectively termed Manually Coded English (MCE). These can include

Signed English (SE; Bornstein, 1982), Signing Essential English (SEE 1; Anthony, 1971), Signing Exact English (SEE 2; Gustason, Pfetzing, & Zawolkow, 1978), Linguistics of Visual English (LOVE; Wampler, 1971), and other forms such as Conceptually Accurate Signed English (CASE) (Vernon & Andrews, 1990). SEE 2 is most commonly used in schools today. You can find definitions and examples of these sign codes on the Internet and YouTube.

TC, SC, SSS, and MCE systems have been criticized based on difficulties in signing and speaking at the same time. When ASL, a visual-spatial grammar, is combined with English, an auditory-vocal-linear sequential language, speech can be slurred and slowed. The quality of ASL can also be altered as the facial grammar features essential to ASL can be omitted and the linguistic principle of sign formation are violated. Morphemes and grammatical endings essential to English syntax can be dropped (Drasgow & Paul, 1995). Critics also believe that a child must be competent in English morphology and syntax to comprehend and learn from these codes (Drasgow & Paul, 1995).

But supporters of these systems disagree, claiming that these systems make English visible to students, that deaf children will acquire English naturally through seeing it, and that this will lead to written competence in English. They also argue that parents find it easier to learn signed systems. Other researchers see these systems as providing bridges from signing to written English as facilitating English grammar if codes are appropriately used after the child has demonstrated an understanding of the concept (see reviews in Andrews et al., 2004).

And still another English-based system is Cued Speech, a sound-based system composed of eight handshapes representing the consonants, which are placed in four positions around the face that indicate groups of vowel sounds. Combined with the natural lip movements of speech, the cues make spoken language visible (Cornett, 1967). Cued speech has been adapted to more than 60 languages and dialects, and studies show it aids in reading as it provides a visual representation of the auditory phonological code (LaSasso & Crain, 2015). At the Illinois School for the Deaf, cued speech is used in select classrooms to teach language arts (www.illinoisdeaf.org). The Resources section at the end of the book includes Internet sites for Cued Speech.

With the advent of the cochlear implant and inclusive placements with sign language interpreters (Chapter 5), there has been a revival of methods that combine spoken and sign languages in sign bilingual and co-enrollment settings worldwide (see Knoors & Marschark, 2015, for further details). The previous perspective that speech/sign combining methodologies were considered one cause of illiteracy has shifted to studies of the benefits of bimodalism. When two or more sign languages, sign systems, spoken, and written languages come together and are used by deaf multilingual learners, language behaviors such as code-mixing, code-switching, code-blending, cross-modal language transfer, and borrowing between and among sign and spoken languages occur, creating a language resource rather than language detriment (Plaza-Pust, 2014). The issue at hand is whether there are one or two languages being used. Bimodal approaches use two languages while the TC/SC/SSS typically focus on only one language.

Language Teaching Programming

There are three types of programming for language teaching in deaf education: the ASL/English bilingual (dual language) program, the comprehensive approach, and the oral/aural (monolingual) program (Marschark, Lang, & Albertini, 2002). Each differs depending on their language planning—language status, acquisition, and corpus (Knoors & Marschark, 2012). Another differentiating factor is how they allocate or distribute the languages in the classroom (Jacobson, 1995). Each requires teachers to complete a specialized teacher preparation program (Humphries & Allen, 2008; Mitchiner, Nussbaum, & Scott, 2012; Paterson & Cole, 2010; Simms & Thumann, 2007; see also Chapter 5).

ASL/English Bilingual Approach

Historically called the *natural approach*, today, the bilingual approach in deaf education is called *bi-bi*, *sign bilingualism*, *sign-oral*, or *oral-sign (bimodal)*.

Broadly, a dual language user or bilingual is an individual who uses two or more languages for daily usage. Related to Deaf adults, a dual (or multi-) language user is a person who uses the sign language of the Deaf culture and the language of the majority culture in either its spoken or written form. Most are not balanced bilinguals but have different proficiency levels within their two languages, with these levels changing across the person's life span depending on diverse conversational partners and settings (Grosjean, 2010).

Theory, Framework, Goals, and Advantages

ASL/English bilingualism falls under the rubric of theories for bilingual hearing students such as Cummins's Linguistic Interdependence model and Threshold Hypotheses (1979; 1981). The Linguistic Interdependence model proposes that each language contains unique surface features, but underlying these surface features are meanings that are common and can be transferred across languages. The Threshold Hypothesis relates to the idea that students must attain a "threshold" or level of competence in their first language prior to developing proficiencies in their second language to gain cognitive benefits. Related to ASL/English bilingualism, it has been argued that, even though ASL has distinct structural and modality differences from English, meanings in ASL can transfer to meanings in English, particularly in the area of reading comprehension (Ausbrooks, Gentry, & Martin, 2014).

Cummins's theories have been critiqued because ASL does not have a written form that is commonly used in education so the ASL-to-English transfer cannot easily occur (but see description of the Supalla and Cripps sign writing system later), Instead, researchers have suggested that a manual code of English can facilitate the language transfer (Mayer & Wells, 1996).

Others have also noted the similarities and differences between language learning with deaf bilinguals compared to hearing bilinguals (Gárate, 2011, p. 207; Nover & Andrews, 1998, pp. 48–51). More recently, Humphries (2016) has noted the "imperfect match" between bilingual theories and deaf language learners. For example, he claims that deaf students never transition out of ASL; they do not have a heritage language, nor do they begin developing ASL during the sensitive period. Further, hearing bilingual theories does not account for modality differences, and few deaf education teacher preparation programs have fully embraced the bilingual credential, only offering courses in bilingualism. Also, Deaf teachers have been excluded from deaf education, as noted in Chapter 5. But Humphries still sees the strengths of bilingualism for deaf students and notes the value of Deaf culture in the education of deaf children within the context of deaf children learning best in a community of learners with whom they can socially interact and with whom their teachers can mediate learning.

Widely used in schools for the deaf during the 1990s to the present is a tripartite ASL/bilingual language use and teaching model (Nover, Christensen, & Cheng, 1998). This framework has been used in more than 20 K-12 schools for the deaf throughout the United States, including preschools, and in teacher preparation programs. It also has been modified for bimodal bilingual children with cochlear implants (Nussbaum, Scott, & Simms, 2012). The framework emphasizes signacy (receptive and expressive signing); literacy (reading, writing, fingerspelling, fingerreading, and typing for communication); and oracy (speaking, listening and lipreading), with ASL being the language of instruction and English being taught as a second language. The goals are to develop social and academic proficiencies in both ASL and English and give equal status to both languages. It also includes English as a second language

(ESL) instruction and best practices in literacy instructions. Some children, particularly those who are hard of hearing or late deafened, or who began language learning with oral/aural approaches, are successful at learning English as a first language and may learn ASL as a second language, thus becoming dual language users (Grushkin, 2003).

Research has documented that dual language or bilingual individuals have been shown to have cognitive advantages such as creative thinking, mental flexibility, metacognition, communication abilities, and concept development. Deaf and hearing children who are raised with dual languages have metalinguistic awareness, cognitive development, language processing advantages, and higher levels or reading skills compared to those children raised with one language (Allen, 2015; Berens, Kovelman, & Petitto, 2013).

The History of Teaching Strategies

As dual language instruction for deaf children has existed since 1817 and is an approach that has persisted for 200 years, it is important to understand its intellectual roots. Even though nomenclature has changed with theoretical stances over the years (e.g., natural sign/ASL, the manual method/ASL English bilingualism, combined method/bimodalism, manual alphabet/fingerspelling), the central idea is that deaf children can learn and use two languages—their own natural sign and English (Moores, 2010; Nover, 2000).

In the 1800s, Laurent Clerc led his teachers in the teaching of both sign and English. Called the *manual method*, this methodology focused on four modes of communication. The first mode—natural signs of deaf people—was used to teach concepts. The other three modes—fingerspelling, methodical signs, and writing—were used to teach English. The methodical signs method was based on the work of Abbe De L'Epee, the founder of the first school for the deaf in France. He took the natural signs of French deaf persons and placed them in French syntax order. Clerc did the same with English. Nover (2000) notes that methodical signs, including Simultaneous Communication (SC) and manual codes of English as used in the 1980s, were not used for daily communication. These methodical signs provided students with access to patterns of English grammar. Articulation was not taught during that time as it was considered too time consuming. Nover (2000) also documents that early teachers in deaf education used the same bilingual strategies we teach today, such as codeswitching between the language of signs and writing, fingerspelling words, the use of lexicalized fingerspelling, sign writing, and sign language dictionaries (Nover, 2000).

Nover further found that the teaching of articulation emerged in the 1830s when teachers saw the need to teach late-deafened children and hard-of-hearing students. In the 1850s, leaders began debating the role of methodical signs and natural signs as instructional tools. In the late 1800s, Edward Miner Gallaudet advocated a new approach called the *combined method*, which included both the manual method and the oral method. Teachers and leaders published articles discussing the wide variability and flexibility in the allocation of the two languages, signing and English, in oral/aural, lipreading, fingerspelling, and combined method forms. These same communication mode and language allocation issues have continued to re-cycle up to the present time in deaf education.

During the next 60 years in deaf education, from the 1900s to the 1960s, monolingualism played an increasing role in schools for the deaf. Spoken language was the focus of the curriculum in schools for the deaf. Language was taught through structured methods such as the Fitzgerald Key and other visual symbols that corresponded to the structures of English. Oralism continued in the United States (Moores, 2010).

After the rubella epidemic in the 1960s, schools for the deaf could not accommodate the hundreds of deaf children who were born deaf. Consequently, many public preschools were set up, and sign language was reintroduced back into the classroom under the Total Communication philosophy or the Simultaneous Communication methodology. The emphasis remained on spoken language and writing rather than sign language development. Stokoe's linguistic study of ASL enhanced its academic stature. Subsequently, linguists worldwide studied the sign language of their respective countries. The results of these linguistic studies, including the study of bilingual approaches, began to filter into deaf education. For example, in 1968, Judith Williams, a Deaf mother of a young deaf son, published a study related to her son's language acquisition through the use of signs, fingerspelling, speechreading, and auditory training, thus suggesting bilingual approaches.

In 1975, when President Merrill requested proposals on teaching language to deaf students at what was then Gallaudet College, Stokoe submitted a paper, "An Untried Experiment: Bicultural and Bilingual Education of Deaf Children." In this paper, Stokoe called for the use of ASL as the language of instruction with the teaching of English as a second language (Maher, 1996, pp. 125–130). Instead, in the 1970s and 1980s, Total Communication (TC) and Simultaneous Communication (SC) approaches gained popularity within school systems. TC incorporated ASL but also combined signs and speech, similarly to the methodology of Simultaneous Communication (SC).

In the 1990s, bilingual programs were established in Sweden and Denmark (Mahshie, 1995), France (Bovet, 1990), China (Callaway, 2000), and the United States at the Learning Center in Massachusetts led by Marie Philips, at the Indiana School for the Deaf led by Eddy Laird, and at various residential schools for the deaf (Nover & Andrews, 1998). At the present time, however, bilingual programs in Sweden, Denmark and the United Kingdom are declining with more deaf children with cochlear implants being educated in regular schools. But within these inclusive settings, teachers are experimenting with co-enrollment classrooms where both signing and English can be taught (Marschark, Tang, & Knoors, 2014).

Bilingual programming also incorporates elements of current research related to Deaf epistemology, which constitutes the ways Deaf individuals visually learn and process information, resist audism, stay healthy and navigate both the Deaf and hearing worlds (Hauser et al., 2010). "Deaf ways of knowing" can be incorporated into classroom practices (Horejes, 2012), in the formation of deaf-centric research agendas (Andrews, Byrne, & Clark, 2015) and the preparation of audiologists (Andrews & Dionne, 2008), Deaf teachers (Andrews & Franklin, 2011) and Deaf doctoral level leaders (Andrews & Covell, 2006/2007).

A challenge today in deaf education, no matter which placement, whether it be in a special school, in inclusive settings with an interpreter, or in co-enrollment classrooms, is how language planning is conducted, particularly how the two languages (e.g., signs and English), or the one language in spoken and written English formats, are allocated or distributed in the classroom to support each other and to contribute to social, cognitive, and academic development.

Since 1998, teachers and researchers have collected teaching strategies and developed materials based on two bilingual interrelated concepts—language allocation and language transfer—to help deaf students develop their two languages. We present outcome data in the next section.

Teaching Strategies, Materials, and Outcomes

Language separation, allocation, transfer, and ESL (English as a second language) strategies involve different strategies used to teach the two languages (Garcia & Baker, 2007).

Language allocation refers to how the two languages are separated or combined as they are distributed in the classroom by the teacher, curriculum, or instructional materials (Jacobson, 1995). For example, during a series of 2-year inservice with teachers, Nover and his colleagues developed activities that reflected on how much time was spent in instruction in ASL and how much time was spent in using English. Teachers learned how to conceptualize language distribution in terms of topic, person, time, and activity. For example, a teacher may use ASL only when introducing a new topic in a science class, then move to using more English after the child had understood the material in ASL and is ready to write about what was learned. Or a teacher may use more English in a class where the children already understand the topic but need more instruction in English composition skills (Nover & Andrews, 1998).

In both bilingual (sign-print) and bimodal bilingual (oral-sign) programs, the two languages can be separated by subject or topic, person, time, place, activity, curriculum material, function of the lesson, and student (Garcia & Baker, 2007). Teachers will construct a schedule of how deaf children separate their spoken language and sign language with different teachers and in activities throughout the school day (see Nussbaum et al., 2012, for details). Language allocation can also be applied to curriculum materials. For example, teachers observed and interviewed by Crume (2013) created classroom word walls with ASL handshapes for the purpose of building ASL vocabulary. Classrooms also had word walls based on the English alphabet to build English vocabulary. Also, ASL/English bilingual books are examples of allocation of the two languages while reading (Herzig & Malzkuhn, 2015).

Another bilingual methodology used with hearing bilingual students (Jiménez, Garcia, & Pearson, 1996) is language transfer. This strategy has been applied to the teaching of deaf students with some marked differences (Nover & Andrews, 1998). For one, ASL does not have a written form like Spanish, so language interdependence and language transfer cannot occur on this level (see also Mayer & Leigh, 2010, supporting this argument). Another difference is that, unlike ASL, Spanish/English bilinguals who learn to read in their first language, Spanish, can transfer these skills to the learning of English through the use of cognates (*historia*, history; *carne*, carnivorous) (García, Pearson, & Jimenez, 1994). Many deaf children do not have strong ASL skills, so they cannot utilize these advantages that hearing bilinguals have. However, ASL has other features that can assist in vocabulary learning, such as the iconicity in signs, the use of fingerspelling, and the use of initialized signing to map onto English vocabulary (Andrews & Rusher, 2010).

There is evidence that these transfer and translation skills can be taught to young deaf children even if they have low proficiencies in their ASL and that sign-to-print matching can occur at the word, phrase, paragraph, and even story levels (see Andrews, 2012; Andrews & Rusher, 2010). These strategies fall under the umbrella of term of *concurrent use* or *purposive concurrent use* of the two languages in the classroom (Garcia & Baker, 2007).

Researchers are currently concerned with the issue of whether the languages should be separated or integrated through lessons in the classroom (Humphries, 2016). Some advocate for strict separation, and others support the use of integrating the languages within lessons. In the case of bimodal bilingualism, spoken language is presented separately from ASL. In the case of TC, SC, SSS, and MCE, the child uses spoken language with a sign code. The field has not clearly defined these terms as of yet. Some use the term *bimodal* to mean the use of SSS. Others disagree and say bimodal bilingualism separates the two languages and never mixes them (Gárate, 2012).

In daily conversations, Deaf adults frequently will switch between the two languages with an oral/sign, or sign/print, either separately or combined, depending on their comfort level and communication learning histories. In the classroom, codeswitching can be used as an instructional tool and can be combined with spoken language, writing, and print. These codeswitching techniques include translating, chaining/sandwiching, event chaining, preview-view-review, ASL summaries, purposeful concurrent usage, and translanguaging. The Internet provides definitions and examples (see also Andrews, 2012; Andrews & Rusher, 2010; Gárate, 2011; Nover & Andrews, 1998). There are also numerous fingerspelling strategies used in this approach, which we review in the literacy section later.

There are also numerous ESL strategies that have been adapted for use with deaf students. One adaptation is called the *ESL/ASL Bilingual approach* (Evans & Seifert, 2000). These include allowing translation, focusing on comprehension, developing the basic interpersonal communication skills (BICS) and cognitive academic language proficiency (CALP) in both ASL and English, and using the students' sign language as a bridge to the learning of English.

Bimodal Bilingual Approach

Description, Goals, and Advantages

The theoretical framework for bimodal bilingualism is the same as that for bilingualism, except that the spoken language component is emphasized. The goal of this approach is to develop early competence in both spoken and visual languages with children and to develop audition through cochlear implants. This programming is said to decrease the risks of language delay because it provides both languages and allows for phonological awareness to be developed in both languages. It gives the deaf child opportunity to communicate with hearing peers as well as with deaf peers (Mitchiner, Nussbaum, & Scott, 2012). The advantages of this approach are similar to the advantages for dual language learning as stated earlier.

History, Teaching Strategies, and Materials

The history of bimodalism goes back to the early roots in deaf education when articulation was introduced in the schools in the 1830s. Bimodalism continued to evolve more formally into the use of methodological signs and the combined method (Moores, 2010; Nover, 2000).

The Cochlear Implant Education Center (CIEC) at the Laurent Clerc National Deaf Education Center at Gallaudet University offers a model program for deaf children with cochlear implants that utilizes bimodalism. Clinicians and teachers have developed strategies and methods (www.gallaudet.edu/clerc-center/our-resources/cochlear-implant-education-center.html). Proponents claim that parents are comfortable with bimodal approaches because they can use their spoken language to support the learning of signs. They also can feel that they are working with their deaf child to improve their speech. Speech development is a goal that most hearing parents aspire to because the language of the home is spoken. This approach requires careful language planning by teachers using a multisensory approach. Techniques include language immersion in either ASL or English or integrating the languages in different classes or with different teachers (Nussbaum, Scott, & Simms, 2012). Materials for bimodal bilingual children will include materials with sign language as well as auditory components such as talking toys and books. There has been little published documentation on the progress of children in bimodal bilingual programs, although clinical files likely document data on speech, auditory, and sign language development of these children over time.

The Comprehensive Approach

Description, Goals, and Advantages

The comprehensive approach as described earlier is the most widely used educational programming for deaf children in the United States (Gallaudet Research Institute, 2013). The basic goal is English proficiency with signing playing a supporting role rather than being given equal status as a language to be learned. There is no specific curriculum for this approach, and schools will typically use their state standards and modify or differentiate them to meet the levels of the students. The advantage of these programs is that parents and teachers have an easier time learning a signed English system compared to ASL.

History, Teaching Strategies, and Materials

The history of the comprehensive approach is woven into the history of dual language teaching. The idea of Total Communication (TC) became popular because oral methods were not effective for all deaf students. Many children's storybooks and other curricular materials were developed with pictures of signs and later videos of signs placed in English word order overlaid with spoken language. It is interesting to note that many TC teachers use bilingual strategies. For example, codeswitching, translation, chaining/sandwiching with pictures, print and fingerspelling, and translanguaging techniques are used by TC teachers. The difference is that ASL grammar is not emphasized in classroom instruction. However, TC teachers may codeswitch to ASL to expand on a topic if the child has weak English skills and is not following the English discussion. In these programs, typically ASL proficiency skills are not traditionally assessed or even mentioned in the IEP. There is debate among teachers and researchers on whether TC and SC can be considered to be bimodalism. In one sense, they both constitute a language resource (Plaza-Pust, 2014). But on the other hand, since the child is not exposed to a full model of either language and is exposed to this language mixture from an early age, neither language is considered to be a second language (see Gárate, 2011, p. 209, for a discussion).

Monolingual Language Approaches

Description, Goals, and Advantages

Currently called Listening and Spoken Language (LSL), at different times this approach was called *pure oralism/auditory stimulation*, the *multisensory/syllable unit method*, *the language association-element method*, the *unisensory* or *aural approach*, and the *auditory-verbal approach*. Deaf culture, ASL, fingerspelling, or other signing systems are not introduced into the curriculum. Instead, the goal is to develop spoken language with the theoretical assumption that deaf children can acquire spoken language following the same developmental language milestones as hearing children do (see Chapter 4 for information on milestones). The advantage is that parents do not have to learn another language—ASL—to communicate with their deaf children (Northern & Downs, 2014).

History, Teaching Strategies, and Materials

The history of oral education goes back to the Cobbs School in Virginia, established in 1815 (Van Cleve & Crouch, 1989). Other oral schools, such as the Horace Mann School for the Deaf (a Boston public school founded in 1869), the Lexington School for the Deaf in New York City (founded in 1865), and the Clarke School for the Deaf in Northampton, Massachusetts (founded in 1867), have lasted to this day. The John Tracy Clinic (JTC) was established in 1942 to provide correspondence course materials to families of deaf children from preschool to age 5; it continues to provide materials for parents worldwide. The Lexington School for the Deaf incorporates ASL as well as spoken English for teaching purposes. There are monolingual classrooms within public schools that may also have TC as well as ASL/English bilingual classrooms. Theoretical foundations of spoken language development were based psycholinguistic theories of language acquisition for hearing children.

Components include early identification and early intervention, the use of residual hearing to learn spoken language, strategies that incorporate intensive auditory and speech training, and audiological management (Northern & Downs, 2014). Strong parent involvement; amplification technology; developmentally appropriate language instruction; and a range of classroom options (self-contained, mainstreamed, or inclusion settings as described in Chapter 6) are used. Speech training also includes the use of technology such as computer-based visual display of speech production. With cochlear implants in the ascendancy, teachers need training about cochlear implants, how these work, and how to effectively use them in the classroom (Archbold & Mayer, 2012).

Other support services include the use of oral interpreters and computerized note-taking systems such as Communication Access Real-Time Translation (CART), C-Print, or other captioning and speech-to-text software.

Programming Outcomes

Which approach works best? It depends. Various factors enter the equation to predict academic success, but teachers probably pay a large part. We don't have enough evidence-based practices as of yet (Luckner et al., 2006; Marschark, Tang, & Knoors, 2014). There have been some studies that looked at academic achievement. We covered results for spoken language in Chapter 4; here we focus on bilingual, bilingual bimodal, and TC children.

In examining these studies, two points should be considered. One is that deaf learners in all programs are typically not fluent in the language of instruction, be it ASL or English. Second, many of the teaching strategies used in TC/SC/SSS programs are bilingual strategies (perhaps minus ASL grammar). And even though these TC/SC/SSS programs are not teaching two languages (only English), still ASL lexical signs is the mother lode of the majority of signs in these invented systems.

Further, even though they are not exposed to adult Deaf language models, deaf students will use facial expressions, body movements, and a spatial grammar while "signing in English" (see Supalla, 1991, for discussion of ASL-like signing in SC children). Third, although the teachers in the studies mentioned here had taken bilingual classes, none had a bilingual credential[1] with the exception of those in the Myers (2011) study.

Two studies were conducted in day schools and four in center schools. Andrews, Ferguson, Roberts, and Hodges (1997) followed seven deaf children in a kindergarten-1st grade classroom within an ASL/English bilingual school over 1 year. Gains were made in basic concepts, auditory comprehension, picture vocabulary, English grammar, reading, ASL competency, English writing tasks, and mathematics. In another day school program that utilized ASL/English bilingual methods, Gentry, Delana, and Andrews (2007) examined the Stanford Achievement Test, 9th Edition (SAT-9) scores of 25 deaf children, ages 8 to 18, over a 7 year time frame. Relationships were found between reading comprehension achievement and years of ASL usage.

Nover, Andrews, Baker, Everhart, and Bradford (2002) studied 122 children from ages 8 to 18 who attended five schools whose teachers had participated in a 2-year inservice in bilingual methodology. The students (ages 8 to 12) with ASL/English bilingual trained teachers showed significant improvement on the English vocabulary and language subtest of the SAT-9 compared to national norms.

In another center school study, Myers (2011) examined the impact of bilingual programming on reading comprehension using SAT-9 scores. He found moderate relationships between time variables (age when tested, age when enrolled, and number of years spent at a residential school) and performance on the SAT-10.

In still another center school study, Geslin (2007) examined the impact of the bilingual programming on the academic performance of 182 deaf students on reading comprehension and language subtests. He compared deaf children on reading comprehension before his school changed to an ASL/English bilingual approach and found that students ages 13 to 18 years improved their reading comprehension scores compared to students who attended prior to the adoption of the bilingual approach.

Marschark (2011, as cited in Knoors & Marschark, 2012) compared reading achievement scores from a school for the deaf in the United States that used SSS/SC to the Nover et al. (2002) data. The deaf students in his study were 5 to 40 points above the national medians across the same age range and in the same years and also scored at or above the children in the Nover et al. study at all ages except 1 year old. This study confirms the importance of using signs—either through SC/SS or bilingually—in the teaching of reading. This study also confirms the need to further examine language teaching strategies. Could it be that teachers in SC/SSS or TC programs do, indeed, use bilingual strategies such as codeswitching, chaining/sandwiching, and so on? (See Andrews & Rusher, 2010, for a discussion.) Comparing TC/SS/SC programs to ASL/English bilingual programs may be difficult to do because of such confounding factors. To ensure fidelity, it is necessary to go beyond test scores and describe more fully the background characteristics of the participants and the specific strategies the teachers are using.

Two additional studies not only examined reading comprehension but also mathematical achievement in ASL/English bilingual programs longitudinally. Lange, Lane-Outlaw, Lange, and Sherwood (2013) studied 174 participants for reading and 141 for mathematics over a 4-year time span at a charter school whose teachers participated in Center for ASL/English Bilingual Education and Research (CAEBER) training and used a comparison group of hearing same-age peers from national norming studies. The researchers reported,

> [O]ver time the study group's levels of academic growth in both content areas increased and exceeded the performance of the comparison group within a number of years of exposure to the ASL/English bilingual delivery model (8.2 years for reading and 2.5 years for mathematics).

> (p. 541)

Hrastinski and Wilbur (2016) studied 85 deaf students in 6th to 11th grades at a center school to determine the influence of their ASL proficiency on reading and mathematics achievement. Students who were highly proficient in ASL performed better than their less fluent peers in English reading comprehension, English language use, and mathematics.

In sum, these studies illustrate the positive impact that ASL/English bilingualism had on deaf student achievement results in mathematics and reading. If we want to study the efficacy of program types, more controlled studies are warranted that go beyond looking at achievement tests. The studies cited earlier and future studies could be improved upon if 1) control groups are used; 2) a more developed description of the Deaf cultural component is provided; 3) background variables of the children, particularly entering ASL and English proficiencies, are described; 4) specific teaching strategies are outlined; and 5) more rigorous assessment methods of ASL are carried out.

Literacy

Definitions and Achievement Levels

Reading is a complex cognitive, perceptual, linguistic, and sociocultural activity. Reading is also a language process that includes language conventions (including the alphabetic principle) and literacy aspects such as comprehension and composition, ownership and motivation, the school literacy curriculum, the school general curriculum, classroom teaching, the family, and community and society (Taylor, Anderson, Au, & Raphael, 2000). Becoming literate requires strategies that emphasize factors such as comprehension in the act of reading complete text, as shown by the work of Marie Clay and others (Stuart, Stainthorp, & Snowling, 2008). This is not to say decoding is not important. The difficulty with viewing reading as a simple process is that it can misdirect teachers into focusing only on the decoding aspect, rather than focusing on what "reading" really means—comprehending complete texts. A testable hypothesis in teaching reading to deaf children with impoverished language skills would consider comprehension of whole texts in the early teaching of reading whether it's achieved through spoken language or dual languages.

Many Deaf individuals are proficient readers and writers who become professionals (e.g., Andrews, Byrne, & Clark, 2015; Mounty, Pucci, & Harmon, 2014). But for young deaf children, literacy is challenging because they don't have a language base. Reading achievement scores on standardized tests show that they do not do as well as their hearing peers (Traxler, 2000), and this achievement gap widens as they grow older (Marschark & Harris, 1996; Traxler, 2000).

Steven Pinker (1997), a cognitive scientist, wrote, "Children are wired for sound,[2] but print is an optional accessory that must be painstakingly bolted on"[3] (p. ix). To carry this metaphor further, how do we help children "bolt on this optional accessory called reading"? How do we set up instructional environments that foster reading and writing for deaf children?

Factors That Facilitate—Factors That Hinder

Reading starts at birth. Research shows that the amount of time a child spends listening to caregivers is a good predictor of the level of reading they attain later (Wolf, 2007). Studies also show that the brain is most receptive to language acquisition during the "sensitive period" mentioned in Chapter 4. Factors that facilitate early reading development include parents who frequently point out pictures and print on food items, toys, and in the environment to their children and who engage their babies in talk during meal times, bath time, play time, and bedtime storytelling. The intertwining of spoken and/or sign language, cognition, and written language through environmental print and storybooks makes the early years optimal for reading (Wolf, 2007).

Caregivers are often flummoxed in figuring out how to read to their deaf child. For one, eye-contact must be established with the child, the book, and the caregivers' face and hands. Deaf parents can set up sight triangles for their children to assist with eye-gaze synchrony (Clark et al., 2015) and the development of joint attention strategies (Lieberman et al., 2014). Sight triangles refer to having the caregiver, book, and the child's eye gaze form a triangle so child can see the book and the caregiver's signs and have eye contact (Mather, Rodriguez-Fraticelli, Andrews, & Rodriguez, 2006). Limited home literacy experiences and lack of reading and writing materials are factors that restrict early reading experiences (Berke, 2013).

Children begin formal instruction in reading when they enter preschool or 1st grade when they "learn to read" in preschool and elementary school. Following this, they "read to learn" in the later grades. It takes deaf children 3 to 4 more years to learn to read compared to hearing children because they are often learning language at the same time (Hoffmeister & Caldwell-Harris, 2014). Studies show that, as deaf children progress in school, they often have difficulty with reading morphemes, vocabulary (particularly multiple meaning words), comprehending figurative language, verb particles, and syntax as well as accessing world knowledge (Convertino et al., 2014; see reviews in Paul, Wang, & Williams, 2013). Many of these linguistic and cognitive structures are found in children's books, so it can be difficult to find books they can read independently.

Instructional Environments

Some believe that instructional environments should include phonological awareness instruction similar to what is provided for hearing children (Cupples et al., 2014). For hearing children, learning to read an alphabetic script requires children to understand that spoken words can be broken down into parts (e.g., phonological awareness) and that certain letters go with speech sounds (e.g., alphabetic principle). Although not accepted by all scholars, summaries of research compiled by the National Reading Panel (NRP, 2000) and the National Early Literacy Panel (NEP, 2008) suggest that phonemic and phonological awareness is a prerequisite to learning how to read and write.

Sound-Based Phonology and Visual Sign Phonology

The sound-based or auditory phonological orientation has been applied to the teaching of reading to deaf children and in particular the difficulties in decoding words (Paul, Wang, Trezek, & Luckner, 2009; Perfetti & Sandak, 2000; Mayer & Trezek, 2015). This approach has been applied to early literacy learning as more deaf and hard-of-hearing children have access to the phonology of English with cochlear implants or digital hearing aids (see, for example, Johnson & Goswami, 2010; Montag, AuBuchon, Pisoni, & Kronenberger, 2014). However, Mayberry, del Giudice, and Lieberman (2011) counter that language, not phonological awareness, is the key variable to reading for deaf students.

Other researchers suggest that both language-related and auditory code-related skills are needed and that proficiency in face-to-face communication of the target language (English), including its phonological aspects, is critical to the learning of literacy. The *Qualitative Similarity Hypothesis (QSH)* (Paul, Wang, & Williams, 2013) posits that deaf children go through the same process as hearing children, but at a slower rate. Deaf readers use auditory and visual tools such as hearing aids, cochlear implants, lipreading, articulatory feedback, residual hearing, and cued speech or visual phonics—all of which support reading development as these provide access to phonemic awareness and the alphabetic principle. Visual phonics consists of 45 manual representations or hand gestures and 45 written symbols that correspond to the 45 phonemes of English, with a 46th hand gesture used to indicate the silent *e*. Each mouth movement is paired with a hand gesture to represent a single phoneme of English (Paul et al., 2013).

Not all researchers agree that phonological awareness is necessary. Alternative approaches focus on deaf students in the act of reading and documenting their actual reading behaviors using signs and fingerspelling rather than testing the children using phonological tests and then providing instructional environments that remediate their phonological deficits.

Reading researchers have started to experiment with instructional environments that capitalize on deaf students' ASL/English bilingual skills to develop English literacy after a decade of research showing relationships between ASL proficiency and English literacy with young and college-age deaf readers (Ausbrooks, Gentry, & Martin, 2014; Chamberlain & Mayberry, 2000; Padden & Ramsey, 2000; Strong & Prinz, 2000) as well as writing literacy (Singleton, Supalla, Litchfield, & Schley, 1998).

These instructional environments foster the development of reading for signing deaf children that bypass auditory phonologically processing. Through explicit instruction, the children learn to connect meaning to print by going directly from print to meaning or using visual phonology and orthography through mapping signs and fingerspelling. Visual phonology, explained in Chapter 4, is related to ASL linguistics but also English reading. Later, we contrast this approach with sound-based phonology prior to describing these alternative instructional environments.

Both sound-based English phonology and visual sign phonology deal with segmenting the speech stream or the sign stream; these segmentation skills are believed to be critical to early reading because they allow the brain and its memory processes to store more words in addition to activating the reading process. The work of Brentari (1990; 1998; 2001) in ASL phonology has provided a theoretical base and elaboration. Bailes (1998) provides one of the earliest studies that make the connection between ASL phonology and reading in her qualitative study of bilingual deaf children using ASL handshapes and ASL handshape stories as bridges to the acquisition of English vocabulary.

Alternative Instructional Frameworks

Alternative reading instructional frameworks with new testable hypotheses have been suggested by researchers who conceptualize how to teach deaf children reading using their

ASL and fingerspelling (Allen, 2015; Andrews et al., 2016; Hoffmeister & Caldwell-Harris, 2014; Kuntze, Golos, & Enns, 2014; McQuarrie & Parilla, 2014; Supalla & Cripps, 2011). In sum, these sign- and fingerspelling-to-print frameworks suggest that there is more to early reading than mapping spoken language to print. In light of the documented delays in literacy, alternative approaches are warranted for experimentation given the accumulating evidence showing that the early sign language acquisition can facilitate the development of early reading (Clark et al., 2016).

How Fingerspelling Supports Reading

Fingerspelling is more than just 26 handshapes that represent the 26 letters of the alphabet, which are used to spell out English words (see Figure 6.2). Fingerspelling is also a linguistically productive system that allows the user to expand ASL vocabulary through processes such as lexical fingerspelling, making abbreviations, two-word compounds, forming initialized signs, and signed-fingerspelled compounds.

Fingerspelling can also be used as a bridge to English literacy (see review by Baker, 2010). Deaf children use fingerspelling in a variety of ways to recognize sight words and to decode printed texts (Haptonstall-Nykaza & Schick, 2007). Researchers have found correlations between fingerspelling ability, reading vocabulary, and reading comprehension in young and older deaf emergent readers (Andrews & Mason, 1986; Emmorey & Petrich, 2012; Herbold, 2008). Just because there is a relationship between fingerspelling and literacy does not mean that these skills will automatically transfer; children may need exposure and explicit training.

Deaf teachers use fingerspelling more often than hearing teachers and show the links between print and fingerspelled words (Padden & Ramsey, 2000). Researchers have found that directly teaching children the link between fingerspelling and the printed word led to increases in reading vocabulary skills and comprehension skills (Haptonstall-Nykaza & Schick, 2007; Humphries & MacDougall, 1999). Results of a training study with 21 deaf students aged 4 to 14 years showed that students were better able to recognize and write English printed words as well as fingerspelled words when training included fingerspelling that was more lexicalized. The authors believe that fingerspelling helps provide deaf children with a phonological link to English print that becomes a tool for decoding. English mouthing accompanied with finger-spelling may also provide an additional visual phonological link to reading print.

Deaf individuals who use fingerspelling will often chunk fingerspelled letters into sequences that do not always follow the syllable structure of English and use this as a strategy to teach deaf children spelling. For example, Harris (2011; 2013) found that deaf children segment ELE-PH-ANT in this way (e.g., three separate chunks) rather than segmenting the word into three sound syllables, EL-E-PHANT (Harris, 2011; 2013).

Writing

Writing is a practical tool used by Deaf adults to communicate with persons who cannot sign. In the precomputer era, most Deaf adults carried pads and pencils (now smartphones) and write notes to communicate with hearing people. Deaf college students often remarked (to Andrews) that they preferred writing notes instead of using spoken language because not only is it more efficient, but it also eliminates being subjected to the embarrassing startled facial expressions hearing people may unintentionally make if they have never heard a deaf voice before.

Young deaf children can write and should be taught composition skills early on. However, in a review of 17 studies on writing development, writing, instruction, and writing assessment of deaf children ages 3 to 8 years (preschool to 3rd grade), Williams and Mayer (2015) also found that much of the work in early writing focused on spelling rather than composition. Starting deaf children early in learning how to compose messages may help alleviate the low writing achievement levels found with older deaf students. For example, Mayer (2010) reports that, compared to 17- to 18-year-old, deaf students write at the level of an 8- to 10-year-old hearing learner.

A variety of approaches have been used in teaching and evaluating writing skills (Williams & Mayer, 2015). In the 1970s and 1980s, based on Chomsky's transformational grammar theory, after analyzing hundreds of language samples of deaf students from ages 8 to 21, Quigley and his team of linguists and research associates developed the Test of Syntactic Abilities (TSA), writing materials, and a reading series (Reading Milestones and Reading Bridges) to directly teach nine structures that deaf readers and writers had difficulty comprehending (Quigley, Steinkamp & Jones, 1978).

Another writing approach, the bilingual writing program for deaf children, developed by Wolbers and her colleagues (Dostal & Wolbers, 2014; Wolbers et al., 2015), utilizes both the child's ASL and English skills. In a ten-week quasi-experiment study in four classrooms (n = 23 students), deaf students were taught an ASL/English intervention—the Strategic and Interactive Writing Instruction (SIWI). Outcomes included improvement in word identification abilities, increased motivation, and increased writing.

In an unpublished study, Sieben (2014) interviewed six professors of English who taught writing to deaf college students. He found that they all used a variety of communication modes, including ASL, English-based signs, written English, gestures, and ASL/English bilingual strategies, depending on the preferences of the deaf students. One professor emphasized that he used ASL for deep discussions of English grammar and then switched to a signed-English code to highlight inflections (e.g., *-ed*, *-ing*). All noted that most of their deaf students had never written a term paper or lengthy composition until college.

Another study examined the relationship of speechreading to Deaf college students' writing. Language samples were collected after four college students took the Lipreading Screening Test (Aver & Bernstein, 2007, as cited in Bickley, Moseley, & Stansky, 2012). The Deaf writers used function words more correctly, even though they may not have lipread them accurately. Their grammar mistakes were similar to the syntax errors found in previous research such as verb deletions, agreement errors, copula deletion, and nonstandard punctuation.

Literacy Achievement and Cochlear Implants

In a comprehensive review of the literature, Harris (2016) summarizes studies and reports that children who are implanted earlier and who are in spoken language environments have higher achievement in speech production and speech perception. But, she reports that these spoken language skills do not always transfer to early literacy decoding and comprehension studies. Some studies show an increased reading vocabulary and comprehension for deaf children with cochlear implants, but still their scores are not equal to hearing children's scores. And, as the deaf student becomes older, the achievement gap widens (Geers et al., 2008; Marschark, Rhoten, & Fabich, 2007). But findings by Archbold et al. (2008) show that their sample of deaf children with cochlear implants were reading on the same level as hearing peers. Factors such as spoken language skills, language skills, visual word recognition skills, age of implantation, mainstream education, higher nonverbal IQ, auditory memory, visual memory, and parent income were found to impact reading achievement (Archbold et. al., 2008; Connor & Zwolan, 2004; DesJardin, Ambrose, & Eisenberg, 2009; Geers, 2003; Geers, Tobey, Moog, & Brenner, 2008; Vermeulen, Van Bon, Schreuder, Knoors, & Snik, 2007). Children with implants were found to have better reading comprehension scores than children with hearing aids (Marschark, Rhoten, & Fabich, 2007); however, Harris and Terlektsi (2010) found the reverse. In this study, children with hearing aids who attended a school for the deaf performed better than children in the mainstream who wore cochlear implants.

One of the most comprehensive, longitudinal studies on reading achievement was conducted by Geers and Hayes (2011). They studied 112 deaf students with implants who were assessed in elementary school and again in high school. Between 47 percent and 66 percent of the sample scored within or above average range for hearing controls on two tests of reading. Thirty-six percent read at the 9th-grade level or above, and 17 percent read below the 4th grade. The researchers found that deaf students had more difficulty with written expression and exhibited poorer expository writing skills on average compared to hearing peers. The deaf students did not do well on the phonological processing tests and had difficulty with the spelling measures. Those students who were good readers in elementary school were also good readers in high school. Overall, the researchers found that 72 percent of their sample made age-appropriate growth over time and for these students the reading achievement gap between hearing peers did not widen. The researchers conclude that since many of the deaf students did better on literacy measures compared to their performance on phonological processing tasks, other strategies (e.g., visual processing) may provide alternate routes to successful reading acquisition. Explicit instruction in phonological skills has been found to benefit some deaf children with functional hearing (Miller, Lederberg, & Easterbrooks, 2013).

Bilingualism, Neuroscience, and the Deaf Child

What happens in a baby's brain when she or he is exposed to one language or two languages? Neuroscientists use fMRIs and fNIRS brain-imaging technology to study neural activity and examine how these neural systems mediate language and cognitive processes (see Chapter 4). One thread of thought presented throughout this chapter focuses on positive outcomes in dual language programming so as to encourage parents and professionals to expose deaf children to two languages as early as possible. This notion is further supported by the *Perceptual Wedge Hypothesis* model, developed by Petitto et al. (2012). This hypothesis posits that the exposure to more than one language between the ages of 6 and 12 months changes the perceptual and neural processing, thus making the brain more expansive and in ways that are advantageous for the child. Petitto uses the metaphor of the wedge that can open doors. Likewise, the exposure to more than one language, argues Petitto, acts as a wedge and holds open the closing "doors" of the human baby's typical developmental perceptual attenuation processes. In other words, the baby's "sensitive period" for language acquisition stays open longer to facilitate language acquisition in both languages. Petitto's data provides the beginnings of biological evidence for the advantages of dual language exposure for deaf babies.

Standards and Assessments

Language programs are only as good as their evaluations. All states have adopted or created standards for student performance in language arts, including literacy. There are also national standards for language and literacy within the Common Core Standards (CCS, see Chapter 5). There are individual state standards that contain language proficiencies for certifying teachers of deaf students, educational interpreters, and ASL teachers. Recently, the National Association of the Deaf has set up a task force that focuses on strategies to incorporate bilingual bicultural emphases within teacher-training programs and include the development of standards for ASL/English bilingual and bimodal bilingual programming (Diane Clark, personal communication, February 25, 2016).

Assessment in ASL and English are also vital components of the schools' curriculum. The resource section and the Internet provide sources for ASL and English assessments used with deaf students. Measures include the *MacArthur Communicative Development Inventory for American Sign Language* (ASL-CDI) (Anderson & Reilly, 2002), the *Visual Sign*

Communication and Sign Language Checklist (VSCL) (Simms, Baker, & Clark, 2013), and the *American Sign Language: Receptive Skills Test* (Enns, Zimmer, Boudreault, Rabu, & Broszeit, 2013). In addition, the Center on Literacy and Deafness Assessment (CLAD) has assembled a battery of assessments covering cognition, phonological ability, speech perception, articulation, fingerspelling, language, and literacy including letter-sound knowledge, achievement, word identification, reading fluency, spelling, and academic achievement (http://clad.education.gsu.edu/).

For deaf adults, Morere and Allen (2012) provide a battery of tests developed for the VL2 Toolkit to assess both ASL and English in general cognitive functioning, academic achievement, ASL, linguistic function including expressive and receptive language, fingerspelling, and speechreading (see test descriptions in Morere & Allen, 2012).

Conclusions

This chapter presents evidence that dual language teaching in deaf education is not new. Since the beginnings of deaf education in the United States in 1817, leaders such as Clerc and others conceptualized deaf education as the teaching of two languages—signing and English. What is new since the 1960s and 1970s are current theories in linguistic and bilingualism that attempt to take dual language behaviors in hearing children and apply them to deaf children, even though professionals in deaf education are in general agreement that these theories do not always "fit" the language needs of deaf children.

More recently, trends in deaf education show that bilingual programs are declining in the United States and globally with an increase in monolingual (oral/aural) programming. Simultaneously, there is a growing research base for bilingual programming with some positive achievement outcomes. Also, TC/SC/SSS programs are experiencing positive outcomes, which show the robustness of signs as bridges to English (Mayer & Leigh, 2010). However, it is not clear on how these signing programs incorporate bilingual strategies such as codeswitching, chaining/sandwiching, and translanguaging in their English based signing programs. The current state of bilingual education continues to be in flux, and a transformative model is warranted to ensure the equivalence of English and ASL within language programming and that teachers have appropriate bilingual credentials and sign fluency (Humphries, 2016).

A similar situation is occurring in bilingual education for hearing students in the United States. Over a 50-year history of bilingual education within public school settings, starting with the Bilingual Act of 1968 and continuing to the No Child Left Behind Act (NCLB, 2001), there has been a change from the focus on bilingual education to more English-only or all-English language policies for language and culturally different minorities. While critics do not object to bilingualism in general for adults—the ability to use two languages—they believe that dual language instruction detracts from the acquisition of English fluency. And given the wide variety of dual language models, researchers have found it difficult to conduct large-scale studies on their effectiveness, and the research that does exist is inconclusive (Hidden Curriculum, 2014). We are facing similar challenges in deaf education today with the movement toward more English-centered education with cochlear implantation and the exclusion of sign language in early education programs and the wish to allocate more time in the classroom to in general to spoken language instruction, including phonemic instruction in the reading classroom. In light of the fact that most Deaf adults are users of two languages, this trend needs to be reanalyzed and responded to by Deaf and hearing leaders. A positive direction is the establishment of the Bilingual Special Interest Group (SIG) at the Association for College Educators of the Deaf, most of whose 30+ members are active university teachers and researchers in deaf education who have the potential of contributing to the research base (Lons Kuntze, personal communication, February 11, 2016).

Suggested Readings

Everett, Daniel L. (2012). *Language: The cultural tool.* New York, NY: Pantheon.

Is language in our genes? Is it innate? Or is language is a tool invented by humans? Or both? The major thesis of this book is to propose that language is a learned behavior that has been developed by human cultures and societies since the beginning of our species.

Hutchins, E. (2010). Cognitive ecology. *Topics in Cognitive Science, 2*(4), 705–715.

At a Deaf education conference, Tom Humphries recommended we read Edwin Hutchins's work on distributed cognition, cognitive ecology, and cognitive ecosystems to gain insight into new ways of thinking about language learning and language teaching for deaf students.

King, K., & Mackey, A. (2007). *The bilingual edge: Why, when, and how to teach your child a second language.* New York, NY: Harper Collins.

Written by two mothers who are linguists and who have taught their children more than one language, this book takes its readers through the ins and outs of early child bilingualism. This book could be a model for a similar book focusing on ASL/English bilingual children.

Wolf, M. (2007). *Proust and the squid: The story and science of the reading brain.* New York, NY: Harper Collins.

Written by a neuroscientist and professor, Wolf draws on her research in dyslexia to examine what happens to the brain when we read and when children find it difficult to learn to read.

Notes

1   Betty Bounds, assistant superintendent at the Texas School for the deaf, encouraged her faculty to take the Texas bilingual education test after they completed a 2-year ASL/English development program provided by the Center for ASL and English Bilingual Education Research (CAEBER) inservice model for ASL and English bilingual education developed by Dr. Stephen M. Nover, currently at Gallaudet University.
2   Deaf children are also "wired" for sign (Petitto, 2009).
3   Pinker, S. (1997)."Forward. In D. McGuiness (Ed.), *Why our children can't read—And what we can do about it: A scientific revolution in reading* (pp. ix–x). New York, NY: Simon and Schuster. Wolf, M. (2007). *Proust and the squid: The story and science of the reading brain.* New York, NY: Harper Collins.

7   Psychological Issues in Childhood

The dynamics at play between various factors in a deaf child's development are complex, multiply determined, and subject to influences that cannot be predicted.

Brice and Adams (2011, p. 132)

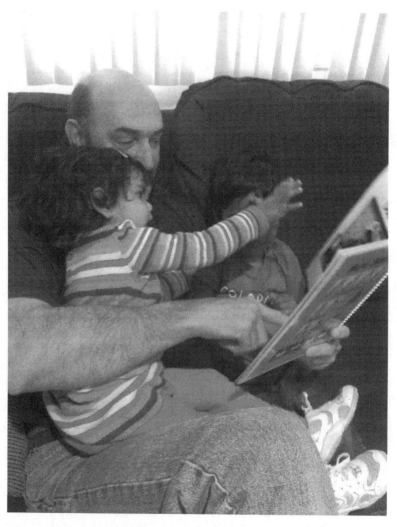

Figure 7.1 Photo of father reading to two children

Source: Used with permission.

Developmental psychologists study the influence of multiple factors on development at every age and stage of life. These include biological, environmental, social, cultural, and behavioral influences. Some aspects of development, such as prenatal development and language development, are closely tied to sensitive periods, which are periods during which a child is maximally ready to process specific kinds of information, language being one, as indicated in Chapter 4. Interactions between the child and the environment, particularly during these critical periods, can profoundly influence how the child develops. With a deaf child, these interactions need to be shaped in ways that can maximize psychological development.

Chapter Objectives

This chapter discusses developmental issues with deaf children. It delves into the parent-child relationship, starting with the importance of positive attachment. The text then looks at the attachment between parents and their deaf children and reinforces the importance of early intervention programs. Subsequently, the socioemotional development, self-esteem, and identity of deaf children and adolescents are addressed. The chapter then considers how childhood psychopathology may be manifested in deaf children. We also present the impact of bullying and child abuse before ending the chapter with a discussion on psychological evaluations with deaf children.

The Parent-Child Relationship

In approximately 95 percent of families with deaf children, the parents are hearing and usually have never met a deaf person nor know anything about what it means to grow up as a deaf person As indicated in Chapter 3, the identification of a child as deaf has an impact on the family as well as on the deaf child (Sass-Lehrer, 2016). It is more than just the absence of hearing that parents of newly identified deaf children are addressing. They may not know what to expect in terms of goals and expectations for their deaf child's future and how to be effective parents (Christiansen & Leigh, 2002/2005). In addition, they may also be struggling with socioeconomic issues, immigration issues, and cultural issues. The nature of their relationship with their deaf child will have bearing on how the deaf child develops.

Attachment

The emotional bond that forms between the infant and caregivers during the first year is called *attachment*. John Bowlby's (1958) attachment theory posits that the infant's ability to thrive physically and psychologically depends on the quality of attachment. When caregivers are consistently warm and responsive to their infant's needs, the infant develops a secure attachment. In contrast, insecure attachment may develop when the caregivers are neglectful, inconsistent, or insensitive to their infant's moods or behaviors. Longitudinal studies have shown that early attachment relationships may in fact have long-term developmental implications for specific socioemotional aspects (see Thomson, Kennedy, & Kuebli, 2011, for details). As reported in related studies (Bohlin, Hagekull, & Rydell, 2000; Sroufe, Egeland, Carlson, & Collins, 2005), for example, children with secure attachments do better in peer group connections and empathy, are less anxious socially, regulate their emotions better, show more solid play behavior and social competency, and are more confident and self-reliant compared to those with insecure attachments, who may be more prone to psychopathology (Sroufe, 2005). Overall, as Sroufe (2005) emphasizes, variations in attachment do not necessarily cause certain outcomes, but attachment itself is critically important for numerous social development aspects such as child adjustment, peer relationships, and even academic test performance throughout life, whether directly or indirectly. For example, if secure attachment leads to good peer play, this in turn can lead to self-confidence. While the external environment can play a strong role in defining the attachment pattern, the internal characteristics of the child can serve as protection from a nonsupportive environment (Young, Green, & Rogers, 2008).

The studies mentioned here most often rely on Ainsworth's Strange Situation (Ainsworth, Blehar, Waters, & Wall, 1978), an assessment procedure that is used with infants between 1 and 2 years of age. This procedure involves a stranger entering a room where a mother and child are playing with a variety of toys. The mother briefly remains with the child and then departs, leaving the child alone with the stranger. Shortly thereafter, the mother returns and spends a few minutes in the room, before departing and returning again. Through a one-way window, observers record the child's behavior during this sequence of separations and reunions with the mother. Attachment quality is assessed based on observations of the child's behavior toward the mother during the entire procedure.

When the mother is present, the securely attached child will use her as a secure base from which to explore the new environment and periodically return to her side (Ainsworth et al., 1978). The child will show distress when the mother leaves the room and greet her happily or be easily soothed on her return. An insecurely attached child will less likely explore the environment, even with the mother's presence. Without the mother, the insecurely attached child may appear either very anxious or completely indifferent. Such children will either ignore or avoid their mothers' attempts to comfort them.

The child's linguistic development emerges out of the almost universal interaction between mothers and their infants that forms the basis for attachment. During this socialization procedure, secure attachment is reinforced when, for example, the infant cries, the mother caresses the child, talks to the child, or picks up the child. The infant will usually cease fussing, look at the mother, who is smiling or speaking, and vocalize back to her. Vision and voice enter reciprocally into play and become part of the early communication swirling around the infants. Such interactions continue back and forth as the dyad give each other cues. Over time, the procedure increases in complexity.

Hearing newborns recognize their mother's voice very early. When the mother leaves physically, infants can still hear her even if they cannot see her. In fact, while hearing individuals appear to rely more on audition in a quality auditory environment, when the auditory signal is less clear, as in a noisy environment, their dependence on vision increases (Binnie, Montgomery, & Jackson, 1974; Dodd, 1977).

If children are identified late as deaf, hearing parents unknowingly deprive the infant of their presence every time they exit the infant's visual field (Montanini Manfredi, 1993). The deaf infants are incapable of hearing an arrival via noise, the sound of approaching steps, or a voice calling from elsewhere. Without compensation through auditory amplification plus ongoing visual and tactile stimulation, the deaf child's sense of isolation can be exacerbated, with potential consequences being language and social delays, though many children can be quite resilient and catch up with appropriate intervention.

Due to universal newborn hearing screening and early identification, caregivers have the opportunity to adapt to the situation and accommodate the deaf infant both visually and auditorially (with auditory aids). Such actions will facilitate the child's linguistic, social, and education experiences if the interactions between caregiver and infant are optimized. In the beginning, caregivers may talk and gesture when their infants are not looking at them. Longitudinal research has shown that, during the first year, with appropriate guidance provided by early intervention programs, hearing mothers can adapt their communication efforts to the needs of their infants by increasing their use of visual-gestural activities in their face-to-face interactions (Koester, Traci, Brooks, Karkowski, & Smith-Gray, 2004).

In comparison, as part of the attachment process, deaf mothers use such activities earlier, including frequent smiling, animated facial expressions, eye gaze, visual-gestural games, waving within the child's visual field, and energetic tactile communication such as tapping their infants to get their attention. They also modify their sign language; this parallels the vocal "motherese" used with hearing children, mentioned also in Chapter 4 (Erting, Prezioso, & Hynes, 1990). Signs are simplified, highly repetitive, and closer to the mother's face rather than within the larger space used among adult signers so that the infants can see the signs when looking at the mother. When the infant looks away or at other objects, the deaf parent tends to sign near the object or within the infant's visual field (Koester, Papousek, & Smith-Gray, 2000). The deaf infants typically respond by mirroring their parents' signs, frequently moving their own hands and arms, with parental praise and encouragement reinforcing these movements. These responses are the precursor to the early gestures and signed communications produced by deaf infants. Additionally, deaf infants alternate their eye gaze between their deaf mothers and the surroundings more frequently. The length of time the deaf infants look at their deaf mothers tends to be longer in comparison to deaf infants with hearing mothers who spend more time looking at the surroundings.

Because deaf parents often intuitively know how to facilitate communication with their deaf infants, they could even be considered "protective factors" in facilitating optimal attachment and socioemotional development in their young deaf children, that is, if they are not dealing with multiple risk factors such as poverty, unemployment, educational deprivation, mental health issues, and domestic violence (Koester & McCray, 2011). The ability of deaf parents to attune with their infants' efforts to convey feelings is based on their experiences in reading "body language," communicating in a visual-gestural modality, and responding to subtle cues regarding the mental and physical states of others, as well as how their own socioemotional needs were met while they were growing up. Their coping skills can be passed on to their children.

The strategies mentioned earlier may at first seem unnatural for new hearing parents, as they are not part of the behavior repertory hearing parents typically assume with hearing infants. However, these parents can eventually arrive at an interactive style that is effective and mutually satisfying, in which each party responds to and influences the other's behavior (Harris, 2010). As this synchronic interaction, so critical for the process of language development, becomes more apparent to the hearing parents, their confidence in their newly found communication skills and their ability to parent their deaf infants will increase (Koester & McCray, 2011). For those who require more guidance, professionals can pass on what has been learned from observing deaf parents.

With auditory stimulation, research suggests that, when infants and toddlers are exposed to conversational-intensity speech through their hearing aids or cochlear implants, together with intensive intervention, their probability for developing spoken language increases (Ertner & Iyer, 2010). Caregivers provide short periods of simple vocalizations at the child's level of development and then progress to more complex vocalizations of speech. They need to associate sounds with objects and do activities that include songs, rhymes, and play within activities (Garate & Lenihan, 2016). Daily routines and play times are opportunities for providing rich auditory information. For example, caregivers can use facial expressions and point to the sound source to direct the infant or toddler's attention to specific sounds in the environment, such as toy noisemakers or whistling kettles. They then communicate what is going on, using either spoken language, signed English, or ASL. The environment needs to be quiet to maximize the focus on the specific sound being highlighted.

As the infant becomes more mobile, caregivers adapt by responding to what the infant is interested in, learning to wait for visual attention or ensuring that the child can hear the communication before communicating, and practicing appropriate strategies for getting the child's attention. Adapting to the infant's needs increases the likelihood for secure attachment. Based on a review of the literature, Brice and Adams (2011) note that hearing level by itself apparently does not contribute to an increased incidence of insecure attachment. In general, the overall attachment patterns between deaf children and their parents do not differ much from those of hearing children and their parents. More critical is how the caregiver connects with the deaf infant and how supportive the environment is, particularly with appropriate resources such as those provided by early intervention programs.

Interestingly, the particular mode of communication is not necessarily the defining factor. Rather, it is the effectiveness of the communication. Hearing parents report that choosing a mode of communication and navigating family communication is one of the most difficult decisions they confront (Mcadow-Orlans, Mertens, & Sass-Lehrer, 2003). Not only that, they may need to re-evaluate communication choices at various points in the child's development, especially if communication needs change, to ensure ongoing optimal communication. Effective communication is influenced not only by the environment (caregivers, peers, teachers, etc.) but also by the characteristics of the child (outgoing, capable of learning, etc.). The evolving language skills of the child as well as the communication match with significant others are both critical for effective growth and attachment (Brice & Adams, 2011). For example, when it is necessary to negotiate the caregiver's departure and return, language often is used to explain the process. If communication is not effective, the security of attachment, quality family relationships, and the child's emotional development may be challenged.

The attachment process may also be influenced by parental attitudes toward their deaf child, as well as their grief and coping responses after the child is identified as deaf (Hadadian, 1995; Spangler, 1988). This could influence the responsiveness of the caregiver and in turn overtly or subtly influence the child's internal sense of security. The process of accepting and supporting the deaf child will foster healthy attachment patterns and enhance the child's capacity for resilience in a world that may not always be accommodating. To accomplish this requires that parents be helped in their grieving process and coping with stress (see Chapter 3 for a brief discussion of parental stress) in order to foster positive attachment.

Hearing Children of Deaf Parents

Most research on hearing infants and toddlers of deaf parents focuses on language and speech acquisition. As a reverse to hearing parents facilitating attachment with their deaf children, how do deaf parents facilitate attachment with their hearing children? How are deaf parents able to respond appropriately to their hearing infants? Technology, such as baby crier systems, enables deaf parents to respond to their infants' calls for attention. Deaf parents can use their intuitive parenting skills to parent their hearing children. But they are not always able to respond to the hearing environment. For example, they may not hear sirens outside that can disturb the infant, and so cannot explain that situation to the child, though they can provide comfort. While the deaf parent may be responding in ways that facilitate attachment, including visual and tactile communication, the child may sense that there is a difference because of parental unresponsiveness to the sound environment, that is, if the parents do not benefit from auditory aids. Based on visual and tactile communication, hearing children may develop early awareness of how to visually get their parents' attention as a means of attunement, thus leading to an acute sensitivity of their environment and an awareness of their difference from their parents (Shultz Myers, Marcus, & Myers, 2010). With parental support, the difference will be accepted, thus facilitating the attachment bond. Research indicates that hearing children of deaf parents are resilient and not overrepresented in the populations of children with social, emotional, or educational problems (Singleton & Tittle, 2000). This demonstrates the ability of deaf parents in general to successfully parent hearing children.

Adoption and Foster Care

Research information on deaf children who have been adopted or are in foster care is scarce. Prevalence statistics do not exist, and much of what is known is anecdotal. Consequently, we know very little about their developmental issues other than the possibility of vulnerability for abuse and its long-term effects (see section on child abuse later in this chapter) for those in foster care. Barbara White (1999) speculates that the entitlement sense that deaf adoptive parents express for deaf children available for adoption is a significant factor based on "goodness of fit" and feelings that they deserve that particular child and know how to encourage bidirectional communication. The seven Deaf parents she interviewed indicated that they put a priority on establishing bonds with their children, providing communication models, and instilling a sense of normalcy as Deaf children. Their adoptees had significant language delays due to previous inaccessible linguistic environments in foster care or orphanages. The parents worked to counteract this with creative approaches to providing ASL and English, such as storytelling and the use of flash cards together with ASL. It also appears that the bonding and attachment processes were closely related to the child's communication needs and the parents' desire to facilitate communication.

Early Intervention Programs

The Individuals with Disabilities Education Act (IDEA) is a law that has evolved from the previous Education for All Handicapped Children Act. This legislation mandates that students with disabilities be provided with a Free Appropriate Public Education (FAPE) that is tailored to their individual needs. Of the four parts incorporated into IDEA, Part C (updated in 2011) mandates services for infants and toddlers with disabilities from birth to age 2 and their families (http://idea.ed.gov/part-c/search/new). Specifically, infants and toddlers need to have a developmental delay or diagnosed condition, including sensory impairment (Raimondo & Yoshinaga-Itano, 2016) in order to qualify for early intervention programs. This covers deaf and hard-of-hearing infants and toddlers who are at risk for developmental delays, including language delays, due to hearing issues. There are early intervention programs for deaf infants and toddlers in each state that provide services in the family's home, or at a conveniently located center or clinic until the children turn age 3 (www.cdc.gov/ncbddd/hearingloss/freematerials/communication_brochure.pdf), after which they transfer to Part B services that focus on providing education within school systems.

For each child and family involved with early intervention, an Individual Family Service Plan (IFSP) has to be developed. The IFSP covers services determined to be appropriate for families and children after the children and their families undergo evaluations, with the primary goal being that of communication and language learning. Services that can be offered include family training, counseling, and home visits; special instruction; speech-language training and audiology; sign language and cued language services; vision services; and assistive technology devices and services. Infants and toddlers with special needs may receive additional services. (See Raimondo and Yoshinaga-Itano (2016) for a review.)

Early intervention programs play a major factor in improving the overall language abilities and educational outcomes for deaf children, essentially by providing families with the tools to maximize the deaf child's integration into the family, the neighborhood, and the school (Sass-Lehrer, 2016). The home needs to provide consistent access to a natural language for deaf children if they are to have the tools they need to use during play, summon help, communicate with their families, become literate, develop in positive ways, and achieve their fullest potential (Sass-Lehrer, 2016).

The ideal early intervention program should serve deaf children and their families from the time the child is identified as deaf. As indicated in Chapter 3, parents/caregivers and other family members need guidance regarding communication approaches and education as quickly as possible. Parents should also receive culturally sensitive counseling and support as they work through their own feelings about having a deaf child and increase their own sense of comfort. At the same time, parents should be developing skills in providing intellectually and socially stimulating environments for their deaf child (Sass-Lehrer, 2016). They may also learn a manual form of communication, or techniques to stimulate spoken communication, depending on the program philosophy of the early intervention program.

The mother of a deaf girl diagnosed at 10 months had this to say about her early intervention program:

> [They were] wonderful. I mean I walked in and I just . . . cried and [they] just listened to me and said there are options, you know, it's not terrible, she's going to be fine, we have lots of kids and . . . they are fine. So that was the next thing that happened and I think that was my ray of hope that things were going to be all right.
>
> (Christiansen & Leigh, 2002/2005, p. 79)

One enabling type of intervention is to ask the family what interventions they think would work for them, keeping in mind the heterogeneity of the families with respect to culture, language, economic resources, genetic makeup, family structure, and their child (Meadow-Orlans et al., 2003; Sass-Lehrer et al., 2016). This involves clarifying parent needs and concerns, identifying questions and supports, minimizing biased information, designing a plan of action, deciding who does what so that both parents and professional partners share responsibilities, and evaluating the process. That will facilitate positive child development.

Professionals should be aware of the importance of including fathers as well as mothers in discussions of and decisions about their deaf children. There is a cultural shift toward fathers being more involved in child rearing as mothers increasingly return to work. Fathers may be at risk for stress just as mothers are, depending on factors such as education, culture, and personal attributes. A study done by Meadow-Orlans, Spencer, and Koester (2004) reports that the reported stress of fathers with deaf infants did not differ significantly from that of their spouses, based on a generally well-educated sample. Additionally, in this study, increased professional support was significantly related to less reported stress associated with their infants.

While it is helpful for caregivers to meet deaf role models early in the identification process in order to learn about the realm of possibilities for deaf individuals, deaf professionals are typically not part of early intervention programs. For this reason, Sass-Lehrer's (2016) book on approaches to early intervention has included an entire chapter on collaboration with deaf and hard-of-hearing communities (Pittman et al., 2016) that supports including professionals who are deaf and can work with colleagues in shaping policies, positions, and services. Deaf professionals provide ongoing critical support in the early years as caregivers learn directly from them how to communicate with their deaf infants and toddlers. They can teach caregivers about the lives of deaf people and provide information on deaf community resources. Interestingly, Jackson (2011) reports that parents of children who are deaf or hard of hearing ranked the benefit of a deaf mentor, role model, or guide among their higher needs.

The position statement of the Joint Committee on Infant Hearing, together with its supplement, provides comprehensive guidelines for establishing strong early intervention systems that are responsive to parent needs and professional competencies (Yoshinaga-Itano, 2013).

However, currently there is no validated ideal comprehensive curriculum for early intervention programs that addresses all the needs of all deaf children and their families, due to the difficulty in incorporating a variety of competencies such as counseling, child development, linguistics, speech and hearing, cultural sensitivity, and instruction. Sass-Lehrer (2016) attempts to remedy this lack of a validated curriculum by outlining ideal components of such programs. Funding is also problematic. States are expected to pick up the extra costs for these programs over and beyond federal appropriations that do not cover all costs.

The Development of Deaf Children

In addition to providing auditory stimulation through auditory aids, enhancing the visual strategies that can maximize reciprocal communication and language development will diminish the problems associated with limited communication, including language delay, and will facilitate play behavior that can lead to enjoyable complex interactions as well as optimal cognitive development and, in turn, healthy psychosocial development (Marschark, 2007; Musyoka, 2015). Chapters 4 and 5 address language development issues. Considering the role of environmental influences, ecological systems theory offers an explanation of how various systems surrounding the deaf child can influence development (Sheridan, 2001; 2008). Sheridan notes the dearth of research on factors external to the personal characteristics of deaf children. Her lifeworld research explored the social environments as well as the internal characteristics of deaf and hard-of-hearing children and adolescents. Focusing on the environment, she uses the term *deaf literacies* to denote an optimal environment involving "multiple systems that are literate in the language, culture, adaptations, behaviors, needs, strengths and resources that deaf and hard-of-hearing people bring to their interactions" (Sheridan, 2008, p. 213). In order to better understand the deaf child's lifeworld, we proceed to take a look at how the deaf child develops psychosocially.

The Role of Play in Early Cognitive Development

Cognitive development is enhanced when children are provided with opportunities to explore their environment in the guise of play (Marschark, 2007; Musyoka, 2015). Vygotsky, a sociohistorical theorist, and Piaget, a cognitive-developmental theorist, see play as enhancing the ability of children to develop and practice adult-like behaviors (Piaget, 1929; Vygotsky, 1978). Marschark (2007) posits that play creates a venue in which children can explore, have fun with various roles, and test out new skills. The process of play, incorporating as it does both reality and pretense behavior, constitutes a critical step in the development of thinking (Vygotsky, 1978). For example, pretending that a box is a car provides a way for children to distinguish between objects and their meanings and facilitates thinking about the mental representations of boxes as other objects, which in turn leads to flexibility in cognitive processing and the ability to abstract. The communities and cultures in which children live will influence how their play evolves and shapes cognitive behavior.

Deaf and hearing children do not differ in how they progress through similar stages of play behavior, but whether they progress depends on their language development (Marschark, 2007; Musyoka, 2015). It is not the deaf child's lack of hearing but rather delays in language development and disruptions in social interaction patterns that may interfere with the deaf child's acquisition and demonstration of symbolic play. The level of sophistication in symbolic play exhibited by deaf children may be a function of their level of language development, social behavior characteristics, and cognitive abilities. Caregivers may feel that they should create as much time as possible in structured learning situations in order to prevent developmental lags.

What they may not realize is that play is equally valuable for communicating various concepts, such as driving to school in a school bus using a box or chairs. If children have diverse experiences, they are in a better position to deal with later social interactions. Keeping in mind that preschool children with age-appropriate language skills get along better with their peers, the cognitive and social aspects of play are critical.

Psychosocial Development

Parents and educators need to attend to the child's psychosocial development since healthy social and emotional development is a critical prerequisite for happiness and success in life. In addition, the emergence of personal identity should ideally allow the child to acquire a solid sense of self in order to develop emotionally and socially and gain a sense of inner security (Calderon & Greenberg, 2011).

What constitutes the process of healthy personal and emotional development? Erik Erikson's (1980) theoretical model of this process postulates eight successive psychosocial stages, each of which is described in terms of successful and unsuccessful solutions to potential crises. The usual outcome is a balance between those two extremes. The successful solution of each stage depends on its level of difficulty and available individual, parental, and social/community resources. The eight stages, beginning with infancy, are (1) basic trust versus mistrust, (2) autonomy versus shame and doubt, (3) initiative versus guilt, (4) industry versus inferiority, (5) identity versus identity diffusion, (6) intimacy versus isolation, (7) generativity versus stagnation, and (8) integrity versus despair. The last three stages cover the adult phases of life and are discussed in Chapter 8. Schlesinger (2000) uses Erikson's psychosocial stages as a framework for tracing the psychosocial development of deaf children and youth. Her observations are incorporated here.

The first stage, that of basic trust versus mistrust, encompasses the early attachment stage. Next comes the autonomy versus shame and doubt stage, which takes place between 18 months and 3 years of age. It encompasses the initial process of learning the behaviors and attitudes appropriate to family and culture. According to Schlesinger (2000), if meaningful reciprocal communication is limited, deaf children show delays. Hearing parents may overprotect their deaf children despite professional advice, thus hindering autonomy. In turn, the children may also initiate power struggles for autonomy through rebelling, such as refusing to maintain eye contact or communicate when, for example, pushed to do something they do not want to do. When parents allow their children some exploratory leeway, these children learn to master new skills in their environments, thereby developing autonomy. Interestingly, Schlesinger (2000) notes that deaf parents with deaf children appear to be more comfortable in allowing more exploration. Power struggles do not appear to be as intense, with these children experiencing fewer eating and toilet training problems.

During the next stage of initiative versus guilt, the task of children (ages 3 to 6) is to develop a feeling of the purposefulness of life and one's own self. Children begin to know whether they are "good" or "not so good" based on feedback. Ideally at this state, parents show the child by example what behavior is appropriate and acceptable. The child, in turn, needs to be able to take some initiative in testing the environment, such as riding bikes down the block and stopping at streets to wait for the caregiver to catch up before crossing.

Deaf children who experience verbal inhibitions because of limited communication will often physically erupt, especially if they are unable to express their feelings in words or signs during a time when children typically have a stream of questions. To avoid diminishing initiative, caregivers need to provide adequate information, establish reasons for external events and for behavior, and establish safety limits that do not overly restrict their deaf children's explorations.

In education settings, the emphasis may be focused on children sitting still and paying attention, thus limiting the various ways to reinforce initiative. But this also provides learning opportunities for new initiatives that can be reinforced during free periods. It is difficult to determine what the optimal teaching situation is for active deaf children with less auditory contact with the environment. Directing visual attention and utilizing good auditory monitoring will facilitate opportunities to encourage initiative within appropriate situations.

Self-concept is evolving during this phase, and deaf children need to be exposed to deaf adults in order to minimize the development of potentially distorted expectations of what happens to deaf children when they grow up. Some children will express the belief that there are no deaf adults because they have never seen any (Pittman et al., 2016). Many only find out about other deaf adults when they are in high school or college. The potential significance of having cultural and ethnic role models available for young people lies in the possibility that these role models can enhance the development of positive social and academic skills. Watkins, Pittman, and Walden (1998) found that, in an early intervention program with deaf role models, more deaf children showed significant improvement in their language skills compared to those in programs without deaf role models. Naturally, this has significant implications for self-concept and quality of life.

For children ages 6 to 11, the task during the school-age period is to develop a sense of industry and accompanying feelings of competency. When children are struggling in school, this may heighten feelings of inferiority that can be difficult to overcome. This can have repercussions for the next stage, which involves internalizing a positive sense of identity, and self-concept may suffer. In order to feel competent, children need to be around people such as teachers who will work at reinforcing their strengths. If parents avoid taking over and do not always tell their children what to do, this will encourage the child's sense of competency. This works when there is sufficient language to explain possibilities that children can choose and what the limits are.

When deaf children are able to converse and socialize at ease with their families and peers, whether through speech or sign, and internalize social rules, this leads to social competency (Hintermair, 2014; Marschark, 2007). Deaf children with hearing parents are not as able to "eavesdrop" or listen to interactions taking place in their environments as do hearing children, who are more aware of events swirling around them. If families develop strategies such as quickly explaining what is going on, or making sure that the deaf child can see everyone in the room, there is less chance for the deaf child to be left out of the loop. Sometimes, unfortunately, even in well-meaning families, it is difficult to remember such strategies in the heat of the moment.

Also, deaf children cannot easily acquire information through television and radio, unless they are exposed to captioned television programs and can comprehend the captions. Deaf children will learn much about the world through the Internet and through books only if their language development and reading skills are up to par. When deaf children are provided with adequate input concerning their social environment, using all sources of information possible, they develop basic understanding of events, social conventions, and typical age-appropriate expectations about relationships. Again, this requires good communication skills (Calderon & Greenberg, 2011). For example, a Danish study involving 334 children with moderate to profound hearing loss demonstrates that if sign or spoken language abilities are good, psychosocial well-being is similar to that of hearing peers (Dammeyer, 2010). If children have language issues or additional disabilities, prevalence of psychosocial difficulties is greater than that for hearing peers. In the U.S., based on a study of 74 young deaf children, deficits in language can have cascading negative effects on the development of social competence (Hoffman, Quittner, & Cejas, 2014).

Deaf children develop social relationships with deaf peers much like hearing children do with hearing peers. These relationships tend to be closer and more interactive, basically because of common understanding and common communication paradigms (Oliva, 2004; Oliva & Lytle, 2014). Marschark (2007) suggests that the social relationships between deaf children differ from those between hearing children, in part because of missing information about the ways hearing children socialize, and in part because of the visual nature of interaction with deaf peers (Marschark, 2007). Whether observed differences in social relationships are deficiencies rather than differences needs to be carefully scrutinized, depending on the age-appropriate nature of the interactions.

Deaf children are also capable of developing good social relationships with hearing peers, but the success of these relationships is very dependent on their social and communicative competence (Oliva, 2004; Reisler, 2002). Such relationships, starting in preschool, tend to be best in a one-on-one situation where attention is more easily focused and the distractions of multiple conversations are minimized (Martin, Bat-Chava, Lalwani, & Waltzman, 2011). Deaf students with or without cochlear implants who are in mainstream schools with no deaf peers have been found to have less positive social and emotional experience, although there is considerable variability (e.g., Antia, Kreimeyer, Metz, & Spolsky, 2010; Hintermair, 2014; Oliva & Lytle, 2014; Punch & Hyde, 2011; Xie, Potměšil, & Peters, 2014). More often than not, they report feelings of loneliness, rejection, and social isolation. It is helpful to note that studies using a loneliness measure report that loneliness levels do not significantly differentiate deaf respondents from hearing peers (Leigh, Maxwell-McCaw, Bat-Chava, & Christiansen, 2009; Schorr, 2006). Additionally, deaf participants scored lower than their hearing peers on prosocial behavior and higher on socially withdrawn behavior (Wauters & Knoors, 2008). We can conclude that responses to measures may differ from narrative responses. If deaf children are not provided with appropriate socialization opportunities, or if they are and still do not develop social relationships, this can be cause for concern. Loneliness and other social problems are potential consequences (Oliva, 2004; Oliva & Lytle, 2014).

Because of the large number of deaf people in my school, I could socialize with my deaf peers. I mainly interacted with two students who were fully mainstreamed. I did not socialize much (if at all) with my hearing peers. I also participated in different organizations and activities, but always shifted to something new each semester or year in hopes of finding a place I could fit in and be accepted by my hearing peers.

(Graduate of a large mainstream program)

I did not socialize a lot during my middle and high school years, especially with hearing peers. I participated in clubs and extracurricular activities, but I never felt comfortable in socializing with my hearing peers. I usually preferred to socialize with the deaf and hard-of-hearing students from the program.

(Fully mainstreamed student at a school where deaf and hard-of-hearing peers were in self-contained classrooms)

I often feel that I have a firm grounding in the hearing side, with a few toes dipping into the deaf side like the hot water from a hot tub, touching it enough to get a feel of the heat, but not needing to immerse myself in the hot water. . . . I spent most of my time with my hearing friends.

(Graduate of an inclusion setting)

With more deaf children in the mainstream, professionals need to work with parents in helping these children establish social connections within their home and school communities that will facilitate healthy psychosocial development. Hintermair (2014) suggests that the socialization problems experienced by many deaf children are due to inadequate environmental accommodations and the limited sensitivity of others to the deaf experience. He recommends programs for deaf students to interact with each other outside of school as well as co-enrollment situations where several deaf students may be part of a class of hearing students. Deaf camps constitute another venue for socialization and exposure to Deaf culture (Oliva & Lytle, 2014; Thomas, 2014). At camps, such as the National Association of the Deaf's Youth Leadership camps; the Aspen winter and summer camps; or even summer computer, reading, and math camps sponsored by state schools for the deaf or the National Technical Institute for the Deaf at Rochester Institute of Technology, deaf students can learn new skills, depending on the focus of the camps, meet Deaf peers, increase their signing and leadership skills, and learn more about their Deaf identity.

Calderon and Greenberg (2011) recommend the use of a comprehensive school-based program known as Promoting Alternative Thinking Strategies (PATHS) (Kusche & Greenberg, 1993). This program, which has been implemented internationally, is designed to improve deaf children's self-control, emotional understanding, and problem-solving skills through teaching social problem-solving behaviors over a period of a year or more (Calderon & Greenberg, 2011). Its effectiveness has been investigated in two major studies in programs and schools with deaf children (Greenberg & Kusche, 1998; National Deaf Children's Society, 1999) and in a study involving children with special needs (Kam, Greenberg, & Kusche, 2004). Overall results revealed more positive social skills.

Moving on, we come to the identity versus identity diffusion stage, which takes place during adolescence when issues of independence enter the picture (Erikson, 1980). The task is to internalize identities through integrating earlier experiences. If the earlier crises of previous stages are resolved, the adolescent is then ready to work on identity explorations.

Identity reflects how people define themselves, what they find important, and what goals they want to accomplish in life. Attachment to parent or caregivers, relationships with peers, and feelings of inclusion in specific social networks contribute to healthy identity development (Calderon & Greenberg, 2011). Social networks can include close friends, extended family members, classmates, and members of organizations or groups. Membership in groups often plays a key role in fostering adolescents' identities. Groups can also endorse values and goals that teenagers may adopt. Before adolescents achieve a true sense of their adult identity, most need considerable time to explore their various options for the different affiliations in their lives. It is important to recognize that identity is multifaceted, with different identity components related to, for example, cultural background, religion, skills, careers, and so on. The Multidimensional Identity Model posits that individuals are constellations of many parts, some of which are more relevant than others depending on situation or circumstance such that identity is centered in context and the nature of interactions (Jones & McEwen, 2000).

Deaf adolescents also need time to explore various options and identities, particularly deaf identity issues. The extent of exposure to deaf adult role models and the perceptions of selves as deaf or Deaf can influence identity development. A deaf person who has attended hearing schools may absorb the standard view of deafness as a disability, while, in contrast, the culture within the school for the deaf may facilitate the construction of identity as a culturally Deaf person (Leigh, 2009). This appears to support Tajfel's (1981) social identity theory, which posits that members of minority groups will achieve positive social identity via two avenues: (1) by attempting to gain access to the mainstream through individual mobility or (2) by working with other group members to bring about social change. Deaf persons may access the mainstream through being "culturally hearing" and assimilating into hearing groups. The alternative is for deaf individuals to get involved with Deaf culture and encourage social changes related to Deaf culture interactions with the majority hearing society. Deaf adolescents will join either group insofar as they benefit from the group in terms of positive self-esteem or self-image. Without this, they likely will leave the group physically or psychologically. Many will connect with both groups and take a bicultural stance. Chapter 8 continues the discussion of deaf identity theories.

I always compare my identity to a line, with the deaf world on one side and the hearing world on the other. . . . My family falls on the hearing side. My friends are mostly on the hearing side. . . . Yet, I can't deny my deaf identity. It has shaped too much of who I am and what I am. My deaf friends are like myself: oral, wear hearing aids or cochlear implants, attend hearing colleges, and work in the hearing world. What we have in common is our deafness, and also our lives in the hearing world. I pass in the hearing world. My deaf identity is equal with my other identities, that of a female, a Jewish person, a resident of the Midwest. My deaf identity has shaped my everyday experiences and the way I see the world. I would not be successful in the hearing world without the support of my deaf friends. I will always remain in the middle, I need both worlds, both sets of friendships to thrive. I will never cross the line completely, since I know I need both sides to be a successful and happy person.

(Graduate of an inclusion setting)

Research that increasingly includes youngsters using spoken language typically shows correlations between hearing or bicultural identity and psychosocial well-being (e.g., Kemmery & Compton, 2014; Leigh, Maxwell-McCaw, Bat-Chava, & Christiansen, 2009; Mance & Edwards, 2012; Moog, Geers, Gustus, & Brenner, 2011). Again, one may reflect more of a hearing identity in one setting, and more of a deaf identity in another setting, depending on communication access, peers, and other factors, thus reflecting a fluid identity (Leigh, 2009; McIlroy & Storbeck, 2011).

Self-esteem and quality of life are constructs that can impact identity. Self-esteem represents judgments about one's worth in different areas, including, for example, interpersonal skills, academics, and athletics. This is based on daily life experiences, whether at home or outside the family, such as school or work where peers play a significant role in providing feedback that can influence or shape one's self-perceptions (Brice & Adams, 2011). Additionally, we need to consider cultural affiliation as well as the internal psychological resources of deaf individuals, including optimism and self-efficacy (Hintermair, 2008). Brice and Adams's (2011) review of the literature suggests that deaf acculturation and bicultural acculturation appear to be advantageous for self-esteem. They acknowledge the importance of parental hearing status, quality of parent-child communication, and the use of sign language for higher self-esteem. Having at least one deaf parent or hearing parents competent in the use of sign language are positive factors in validating the deaf child.

A recent constellation of studies researching the self-esteem of children with cochlear implants reveals a different trend (e.g., Leigh et al., 2009; Moog, Geers, Gustus, & Brenner, 2011; Percy-Smith, Cayé-Thomasen, Gugman, Jensen, & Thomsen, 2008). Overall, the self-esteem of these children is comparable to that of hearing peers, and the trend is to affirm more of a hearing-acculturated identity. Interestingly, bicultural identification was also present for this group. This reinforces the role of fluid identities based on environmental context.

Quality of life is a concept involving multiple dimensions that are based on subjective evaluations of both positive and negative aspects of life (The WHOQOL Group, 1998). These dimensions involve components of well-being, including physical, emotional, mental, social, and behavioral aspects. The quality of life construct can be difficult to measure due to various perceptions of how to define it in measures as well as whether the participant pool involves parents, teachers, or the individuals themselves.

Studies of children with cochlear implants paint a picture of positive quality of life (see Hintermair, 2011, for a brief review). However, as previously mentioned, children and youth with cochlear implants do confront socialization issues that can influence their quality of life, particularly in adolescence. Hintermair (2011) reports on a study done by Gilman, Easterbrooks, and Frey (2004) that revealed scores for global satisfaction and the domains of family, friends, and living environment to be significantly higher for hearing students compared to deaf students. He concludes that important variables that affect quality of life for deaf children and youth include parent-child communication match (either signing or speaking) and whether the educational setting appropriately meets the child's needs. The importance of parent-child communication match is affirmed by a study that found a significant correlation between higher youth perception of their ability to understand parents' communication and perceived quality of life (Kushalnagar et al., 2011).

Bullying of and by children of course is a factor that negatively impacts quality of life. This topic has drawn increased attention in recent years, as witness the special issue on School Bullying and Victimization in the *American Psychologist* (vol. 70, no. 4, May–June 2015). In that publication, an article by Swearer and Hymel (2015) describes bullying as a complex form of interpersonal aggression that involves both dyadic and group dynamics, with negative impacts on not only bullies and victims, but also peer witnesses. They propose a social-ecological, diathesis-stress model that incorporates genetic predispositions to vulnerability or aggression and environmental situations that give rise to bullying. This model underscores the complexities of stressors and risk/protective factors that influence both involvement and intervention.

Bullying is a serious concern for deaf children as well. According to Hadjikakou and Papas's (2012) review of the literature on deaf children and bullying, rigorous research is lacking, with most information being qualitative. It would help to know more about the cognitive processes involved in bullying and how victimization gets perpetuated. As reported, both conventional bullying (causing harm repeatedly and asserting power) and cyberbullying (bullying using technological means) does take place among deaf students as well as their hearing peers (Bauman & Pero, 2011). Bullying may be more evident in schools for the deaf as opposed to mainstream settings, but further research is required to confirm this possibility and understand why that is so. One possibility is that limited exposure to essential social information and social rules may increase vulnerability to bullying behavior or victimization.

The Role of Professionals in Psychosocial Development

With approximately 80 percent of deaf children being educated in inclusion settings, professionals have a responsibility to ensure an optimal educational environment in which these children can flourish. They need to be aware of communication issues and access, environmental distractions such as auditory and visual noise, and how to ensure that children have access to positive psychosocial experiences. They also need to be on top of technology advances that may benefit these students, such as having phones with speech-to-text capabilities for hallways and group situations, for example.

Deaf professionals have a critical role to play in the process of facilitating the process of positive psychosocial adjustment. Again, they usually do not have a major role in providing learning models for hearing parents and their deaf children (see earlier and Chapter 3). Hearing specialists can emphasize the use of deaf role models with whom they can model accessible language acquisition and socialization strategies for the deaf child from birth onward. If parents also hire deaf sitters and invite deaf people, either signing or speaking, to meet their child, the child will have additional exposure to language and social models throughout the developing years. Exposure to the successful lives of deaf people can contribute to the deaf child's and adolescent's sense of self as psychologically healthy.

Childhood Psychopathology

Investigating childhood psychopathology in the case of deaf children can be a minefield because many test instruments used for diagnostic purposes are verbally loaded and lack deaf norms. Also they are often inappropriately administered to children, thus changing the meaning of the questions and hence the responses. Lack of awareness by psychologists of appropriate testing procedures with deaf individuals is at the heart of the problem (Leigh, Corbett, Gutman, & Morere, 1996; Reesman et al., 2014). There have been many cases where gross misdiagnoses have resulted in irreversible psychological and educational damage. As reported in Lane (1999), Matti Hodge and Alberto Valdez spent most of their lives in institutions after having been misdiagnosed as mentally retarded (intellectually disabled) based on low IQ scores that eventually were shown to be invalid after retesting that indicated normal intellectual functioning. (See the next section and Chapter 8 for further discussion of evaluation and psychometric issues.)

There are methodological problems with establishing the prevalence of mental health issues in this population. These problems are similar to those in conducting a poll or making a projection during an election. Different numbers will emerge depending on how the sample is selected, what questions are asked, and how these questions are asked. For deaf children scattered in different school settings, obtaining accurate numbers is a challenge. Problems related to diagnostic criteria, appropriateness of measures for deaf children, evaluator expertise regarding deaf issues and child psychopathology, and whether the sampling studied was truly representative of the heterogeneous population of deaf children, considering that participants tend to be among those motivated to participate, need to be factored in. Heterogeneity is compounded by factors including level of hearing, hearing classification, age of onset, age of identification, communication, cultural affiliation, and immigration status among others.

What we know is as follows: Based on a review of the literature up to 1980, including studies done in the 1970s that assessed the prevalence and nature of psychological maladjustment among deaf children, Meadow (1980) concluded that the prevalence ranged from 8 to 22 percent, compared with rates of from 2 to 10 percent for the general child population. More recently, Brown and Cornes's (2015) (see additional details later) review of the literature covering parent questionnaire and survey reports of deaf children's mental health suggest prevalence rates between roughly 28 percent and 43 percent. Data from children and students themselves reveal varying prevalence rates ranging from 32.6 percent to 54 percent. Even when adjusted versions of measures were used to meet the linguistic needs of participants, the prevalence rates did not significantly shift. Specific to depression, it was noted that deaf adolescents appear to be dealing with higher rates compared to hearing peers. An additional literature review done by Theunissan et al. (2014) notes that "hearing impaired" children and adolescents are more prone to developing depression, aggression, oppositional defiant disorder, conduct disorder, and psychopathy than their hearing peers. Anxiety, somatization, attention deficit disorder (ADD), and delinquency levels varied more. Among possible risk and protective factors were additional disabilities, intelligence, and communication skills.

It has been suggested that deaf children display more behavioral problems because of frustrations in communication (Fellinger, Holzinger, & Pollard, 2012). Considering the earlier-reported findings that communication with family and peers is associated with self-esteem, quality of life, and identity, this assumption is not surprising. Using a sample of 89 deaf and hard-of-hearing students ages 11 to 18 attending different educational settings in Australia, Brown and Cornes (2015) administered the Youth Self Report, written English version, to students using spoken language and the Auslan version (Australian Sign Language) to students using Auslan (note, both versions had similar reliability). This sample reported increased levels of mental health issues (39 percent) compared with hearing peers (14 percent). The authors speculate that these issues start earlier in life and are compounded by limited incidental learning and social difficulties such as misinterpreting social information. Peer rejection may also be a factor, based on a study that reported positive association between that and mental health problems, with a negative association between mental health problems and self-esteem (van Gent, Goedhard, & Treffers, 2011).

Students using spoken English with their families experienced less psychopathology, likely because they were comfortable with spoken English compared to those in families using Auslan or Signed English, perhaps in part because of family members' limited fluency in Auslan (Brown & Cornes, 2015). Additionally, a Swedish study revealed that deaf and hard-of-hearing children as a group showed no significant mental health differences compared with hearing children based on the Strengths and Difficulties Questionnaire (a measure with acceptable reliability) administered to students (Mejstadt, Heiling, & Swedin, 2008/2009). Of this group, 15 percent claimed immigrant status. The researchers explain that Swedish Sign Language exposure starts early and parents are offered sign language courses, so that communication is facilitated.[1] A study that investigated the influences of language, attention, and parent-child communication for predicting behavior problems in 116 deaf and 69 hearing children aged 1.5 to 5 years found that deaf children exhibit more language, attention, and behavioral difficulties and spend less time communicating with parents compared to the hearing sample (Barker et al., 2009). At a residential treatment facility for adolescents, it was found that the deaf adolescents exhibited higher scores than those of hearing peers on psychosocial risk behaviors, including risk to others, aggression, and destruction of property (Coll, Cutler, Thobro, Haas, & Powell, 2009). Looking at all of the studies, the importance of communication ease is apparent. The more restricted communication within families may result in more superficial discussions of thoughts and emotions, thus leading to truncated emotional empathy (Brown & Cornes, 2015). Finally, even though deaf children and adolescents are at increased risk for mental health problems, we must note that approximately two-thirds of the samples reviewed do exhibit positive mental health.

Additional Conditions and Psychopathology

Children with socioemotional issues more often may be sent to schools for the deaf (van Gent, Goedhart, Hindley, Treffers, & Philip, 2007) that may be better equipped to handle this population. These children often will have additional conditions that may exacerbate vulnerability to socioemotional difficulties. In the United States, prevalence rates for these additional conditions (extrapolated from 23,731 deaf and hard-of-hearing students in schools reporting to the Gallaudet Research Institute Annual Survey, Gallaudet Research Institute [2013]) indicate that approximately 40 percent have additional conditions, specifically learning disabilities and intellectual disabilities (most prevalent with 7.2 percent and 8.8 percent, respectively), followed by developmental delay (6 percent), attention deficit disorder (5.4 percent), autism (2.2 percent), and blindness (2.8 percent). The prevalence of emotional disturbance per se was 2.1 percent, a comparatively low prevalence compared to the studies mentioned earlier. It must be kept in mind that schools need a formal diagnosis to list emotional disturbance as primary, while study results are based on parent, teacher, and child responses, which tend to be subjective and are based on observations and feelings, therefore resulting in the higher prevalence rates noted for deaf children.

In recent years, autism has gained increasing prominence as a focus of attention. In addition to the Gallaudet Research Institute statistics mentioned earlier, further study indicated that 1 out of 59 eight-year-old deaf children were receiving services for autism, a higher percentage compared to the national estimates of 1 in 91 (Szymanksi, Brice, Lam, & Hotto, 2012). To be both deaf and autistic creates significant challenges for differential diagnosis since language and communication issues apply to both deaf and autism spectrum disorder diagnosis. The focus is on difficulties in relating with others, using various social behavior criteria (van Gent, 2015). Szymanski (2012) reports on challenging behaviors such as temper tantrums, refusing to participate in activities, and aggression towards others or self. She also provides information on how schools can do a functional behavior assessment to evaluate possible causal factors and suggest how to eliminate these causes in order to prevent behaviors from escalating.

In addition to the problem of determining criteria for various diagnoses, diagnosticians face the complexity of separating the impact of being deaf from the disorder itself (Reesman et al., 2014), such as in the case of learning disability. In fact, there is almost no research on how learning disabilities (LD) or attention-deficit/hyperactivity disorder (ADHD) are manifested in deaf children or on how to separate the problems of limited exposure to stimuli from the standard criteria for learning disabilities. Existing opinions are based primarily on anecdotal evidence, survey opinions, and limited empirical studies. Keeping in mind the sparse nature of the research, current evidence seems to suggest that deaf LD and ADHD individuals have many of the same characteristics as hearing LD and ADHD individuals. However, the primary etiologies of deafness (see Chapter 3) are also etiologies of LD (Mauk & Mauk, 1992). For this reason, the incidence of LD is probably higher in the deaf population than in the hearing population. With ADHD, an additional complicating factor may be the risk of misdiagnosis when deaf children exhibit restless behavior due to limited ability to understand their environment and get bored.

Because of the difficulties with diagnostic criteria, developing validated testing approaches for accurately diagnosing LD or ADHD in deaf children continues to be a difficult task (Reesman et al., 2014). Researchers have to contend with the lack of adequate norms on deaf children; inconsistent control over communication and language factors during evaluation, including how evaluators and deaf children communicate; and the potential reliance of deaf individuals on adaptive attentional and cognitive coping strategies in testing and learning situations that may mask true disabilities. These are all aspects that impact psychological evaluations, which we discuss later in this chapter.

Child Abuse and Its Consequences

Children with disabilities may be more at risk for various types of abuse, with higher incidences compared to that of the general population (Obinna, Krueger, Osterbaan, Sadusky, & DeVore, 2005). Precise figures are hard to come by because researchers use various criteria to determine whether behaviors can be defined as abusive and what constitutes a disability. Abusive behaviors can fall into physical, sexual, and psychological categories (Sebald, 2008).

A review of the literature concludes that, not only in North America (Obinna et al., 2005; Willis & Vernon, 2002), but also in Norway (based on a survey of deaf adults that Kvam [2004] conducted), deaf children may have two to three times greater risk of sexual abuse than hearing children. Findings in general tend to be based on retrospective information asked of deaf individuals. Child abuse incidents in the deaf and hard-of-hearing youth population may be underreported due to various factors. These include fears of retaliation by the perpetrator and by the system in which the abuse occurred (residential schools or/and home), fears of being stigmatized by those who view the reports of child abuse at residential schools as threatening the reputation of residential schools, and lack of understanding on the part of the victim (Schott, 2002).

Many deaf children may not know what abuse is. Thus, they may not understand that they are in abusive situations. They often have difficulty communicating about the abuse and do not know how to explain what has happened to them (Lomas & Johnson, 2012; www.dcmp. org/media/6760-protecting-your-deaf-child-from-sexual-abuse-a-parent-s-guide). They usually do not have the opportunity to learn what good and bad touching are, either from family or school. Since they have less access to information, compared to hearing peers in general, particularly in terms of sexual abuse, they may more readily be victimized. Some may also become perpetrators (http://hawaiifreepress.com/ArticlesDailyNews/tabid/65/ID/9121/March-14–2013-News-Read.aspx).

Abuse prevention and intervention programs will go a long way toward ameliorating any potential consequences (National Association of the Deaf, 2008a). *No-Go-Tell* is an example of a well-known sexual abuse prevention curriculum for schools that provides self-protection training to very young deaf and hard-of-hearing children (Krents & Atkins, 1985). It teaches these children what to watch for and provides standard vocabulary to describe sexual abuse incidents that may have occurred. Since 1985, multiple resources have been developed for parents, professionals, and children themselves on the topic of sexual abuse prevention (www. nsvrc.org/projects/child-sexual-assault-prevention/preventing-child-sexual-abuse-resources). Unfortunately, there are no data on the effectiveness of prevention and intervention programs in preventing abuse or for effective postabuse intervention where deaf children are concerned (Glickman & Pollard, 2013; Sebald, 2008). Sebald (2008) recommends that parents appropriately communicate acceptable and unacceptable behaviors for home, school, and in public.

Treatment Programs

Deaf children in need of psychological treatment, particularly inpatient programs, have few resources (Bishop, 2013; National Association of the Deaf, 2008a). Most treatment is provided by psychologists, school counselors within schools, mental health providers in private practice, or through structuring educational programs to meet the needs of the child as reflected in the IEP (see Chapter 5). Adequate communication with the deaf child is a critical factor for treatment success. Mental health personnel need to be aware of cognitive, linguistic, and psychosocial aspects pertinent to deaf children and youth in order to provide competent services. The use of sign language interpreters should be viewed as a last resort, with so much depending on interpreter competency in the language of children for which little training is provided. Printed resources need to be readable for a population for whom English is less than fully accessible. With the increase in cultural awareness and sensitivity, there is greater attention paid to ensure that reading materials are easily read and understood.

Strategies to facilitate communication and treatment with deaf children and youth who have serious emotional and behavioral challenges resulting from neurological dysfunction, mental illness, or a history of child abuse and/or neglect have been developed by the Walden School, a nationally recognized treatment facility in Framingham, Massachusetts (Bishop, 2013). The language challenges these individuals present with constitute a formidable challenge that contrasts with those at facilities for hearing students.

Psychological Evaluation of Deaf Children

Deaf children are tested periodically throughout the years, as required by IDEA legislation, starting with audiological assessments, intelligence and achievement testing, and psychosocial evaluations, including personality testing. IDEA legislation specifies nondiscriminatory testing and requires that materials and procedures used for the evaluation and placement of special needs children be selected and administered in a manner that is neither culturally nor racially discriminating. The law further states that these materials and procedures must be administered in the language or mode of communication that the child uses (www.wrightslaw.com/idea/law/idea.regs.subpartd.pdf). This means using spoken language; some form of sign communication/language, including ASL or cued speech; or even a foreign sign language, depending on what the child is most comfortable with. Selected tests must be administered in a manner that does not focus only on limitations or penalize deaf children for their linguistic difference. The child's strengths should be taken into account in the evaluation report. (See Reesman et al., 2014, for a review.)

The position statement of the National Association of School Psychologists (2012) on serving students who are deaf or hard of hearing recommends that evaluators understand each student's culture and individuality and that psychologists obtain adequate training and knowledge of language issues as these pertain to deaf children in order to objectively and accurately evaluate them. If psychologists cannot match the linguistic and communication needs of the deaf child, they could render an inaccurate picture of the deaf child's skills and abilities. In this situation, they ethically should take advantage of peer review, consultation with experts, and referral to experts if available. Psychologists who take a few sign language classes or attend inservice workshops are *not* qualified to evaluate deaf children. It takes far more training and experience to deal with the wide variation in which deaf children communicate and use language. Interpreters should be used as a last resort and, again, only if they possess appropriate certification to ensure competence in communicating with deaf children. Interpreters can easily convey incorrect impressions of the child being tested if communication is less than ideal. School psychologists need to be familiar with reliability and validity of psychological assessment measures (see Chapter 8) to avoid misuse with deaf students. They need to be aware of possible additional disabilities or conditions and how to accommodate these during the evaluation process. This needs to be sensitively addressed for reliability and validity reasons (Reesman et al., 2014).

Language-appropriate testing for deaf children is an area ripe for research. More language assessment tools for accurate evaluation of deaf children's language-specific processes are needed. As Reesman et al. (2014) cautions, assessment of the language skills of the child who is deaf or hard of hearing must be differentiated from language-based reasoning skills. The challenge lies in discriminating between language deficits and cognitive deficits when deaf children have varying levels of exposure to English. Many cognitive measures are heavily weighted in English. Therefore, it is important to be sensitive to measurement issues and use multiple forms of assessment (National Association of School Psychologists, 2012). These include assessments in social, emotional, physical, and cognitive areas, keeping in mind that etiological, neurobiological, and social factors may put some students at risk for academic, social, or emotional difficulties. Braden (2001) recommends the following assessment approaches:

1. *Observations* are helpful for developing hypotheses regarding the deaf child's cognitive abilities. Psychologists must be cautious about the inferences they make from observations pending additional evidence.
2. *Interviews* provide a window for assessing the level of cognitive functioning within the parameters of dialogue between the psychologist and the child.
3. *Informal tests* are tests with no deaf norms, which can be utilized as a way of developing hypotheses about cognitive functioning for possible diagnosis and treatment. However, caution must be taken when using such tests due to reliability and validity concerns.
4. *Intelligence tests* are formal standardized tests that provide important information about an individual's functioning and ability levels. The use of nonverbal intelligence tests rather than verbal intelligence tests is recommended due to the limitations many deaf children have in accessing spoken language. Verbal measures should be used only to assess English proficiency, not intelligence.

Information from these multiple forms of assessment, in addition to history, psychosocial evaluations, and achievement testing, should be combined into a total picture of the child's abilities that will generate appropriate recommendations for educational placement and psychosocial development. Recently, tests that examine fluency in ASL have been developed, but establishing deaf norms has been problematic due to the heterogeneity of deaf children in terms of levels of ASL usage. (See www.gallaudet.edu/clerc_center/information_and_resources/coch lear_implant_education_center/resources/suggested_scales_of_development_and_assess ment_tools.html for a list of various assessment measures that are being used to evaluate deaf students.)

Conclusions

Deaf and hearing children have the potential for similar developmental milestones, other things being equal. Being deaf in and of itself is not a causative factor for developmental problems. For these problems we must look to neurobiological, etiological, and environmental factors that can influence development. Unquestionably, based on quality of life and self-esteem research results, deaf children can be resilient even in the fact of multiple obstacles (Zand & Pierce, 2011). Martha Sheridan (2008) focuses on ecological as well as symbolic interactionist perspectives of development to explain how development occurs and how children can view or understand their lifeworlds. Early intervention programs can help parents learn optimal strategies for communicating with their deaf infants and promote positive psychosocial development. Social competence programs such as PATHS can benefit deaf children. Healthy identity development is facilitated when deaf children feel comfortable with being deaf and are exposed to deaf role models. More research into psychopathology in deaf children will facilitate appropriate treatment planning. In order to provide optimal assessment services, psychologists must be knowledgeable about psychological, linguistic, cultural, and social aspects for deaf children and youth and effectively communicate with them.

Suggested Readings

Marschark, M. (2007). *Raising and educating a deaf child*. New York, NY: Oxford University Press.
   This is a comprehensive and entirely readable guide to the choices, controversies, and decisions faced by parents and educators.
Sheridan, M. (2001). *Inner lives of deaf children: Interviews and analysis*. Washington, DC: Gallaudet University Press.
Sheridan, M. (2008). *Deaf adolescents: Inner lives and lifeworld development*. Washington, DC: Gallaudet University Press.
   Both books are about the social development of deaf children and adolescents and their formations of self-concepts. Deaf children and youth were interviewed for these books. Each one comes from a unique background and uses different communication modes. Written by a social worker who is deaf, both books provide rare insights into the minds of these interviewees.
Zand, D., & Pierce, K. (Eds.). (2011). *Resilience in deaf children*. New York, NY: Springer.
   This edited book contains contributions by noted authors that cover multiple pathways for reinforcing resilience in deaf children, starting in infancy and continuing through the emerging adult stage.

Note

1   The increased use of cochlear implantation in Sweden has resulted in less focus on Swedish Sign Language. Whether this impacts mental health prevalence in deaf children and youth remains to be seen.

8   Deaf Adults

Viewpoints from Psychology

I don't care what people call me, labels have the negative value of making smaller boundaries for people.

Michael Graves (1983)

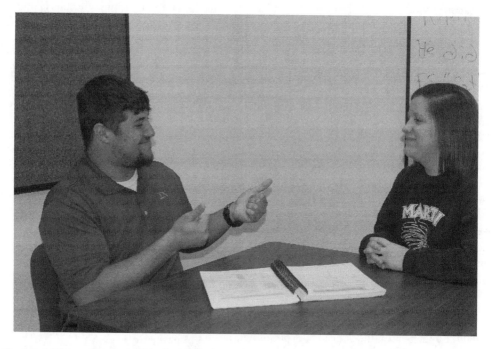

Figure 8.1 Photo of male and female communicating with each other
Source: Used with permission.

The stereotypical image of deaf people as a psychologically homogenous entity, limited in the ability to fully take advantage of the world around them, is changing. Recent publications increasingly show the resilience, strengths, and capabilities exhibited by deaf adults in dealing with life. Their psychological and psychosocial functioning is influenced by innate factors, differences in familial and educational experiences, exposure to varied communication approaches, age of onset, and other variables. Researchers, professional working with deaf persons, and the general public are improving in their ability to recognize the variability in psychological functioning exhibited by deaf persons.

Chapter Objectives

This chapter explores the functioning of deaf adults using the lens provided by models of positive psychology, positive health, and wellness. Adulthood stages and aging are addressed. The meaning of "normalcy" as applied to the deaf population will be analyzed. The roles of deaf identities and self-concept are highlighted as contributory factors to psychological well-being. The reader will be introduced to psychological assessment and mental health issues that are critical for appropriate service delivery.

Positive Psychology and Positive Health

The field of psychology has undergone a transformation. Historically, psychology was preoccupied with negative, pathological, or problem-focused frames of reference such as mental illnesses or the inability of human beings to function as expected. For example, much work was done in the areas of psychopathology, negative emotions such as hostility and depression, and individual deficits (e.g., cognitive factors) that limit one's functional abilities. Starting in the 1940s and onward, luminaries such as Erich Fromm, Abraham Maslow, and Carl Rogers argued that the field of psychology was focusing too much on what the individual was doing wrong or on internal factors that hindered optimal adaptation to daily life, while ignoring the variables that enhance people's ability to actualize their potential in living "good" lives.

Recent publications indicate that the concept of positive psychology has caught the attention of psychologists, who are examining biological, environmental, and cultural factors insofar as these separately and interactively influence positive development or optimal functioning, more specifically how the biochemical, physiological, perceptual, cognitive, emotional, and interpersonal dimensions contribute to the positive psychological health of the individual. (e.g., Carr, 2011; Gable & Haidt, 2005). Positive health models that focus on psychological growth such as Seligman's (2008) model of positive health further specifies that optimal functioning is based on a combination of excellent results using biological, subjective, and functional measures. Seligman concludes that research into positive emotion, engagement, purpose, positive relationships, and positive accomplishments predicts higher achievement, less depression, and better physical health. This has to take into account the fact that obstacles in life do exist, resilience helps, and visualizing obstacles and creating plans can actually enhance motivation (Oettingen, 2014). Strength perspectives have also been considered by the social work discipline (e.g., Saleebey, 1992; Weick, Rapp, Sullivan, & Kisthardt, 1989).

While research and publications in psychology do continue to focus on problematic areas and psychopathology, this positive psychology approach provides a welcome balance to the study of the human condition. We endeavor in this chapter to provide a balanced perspective.

The Deaf Adult: Psychological Perspectives

Research findings have historically depicted deaf persons as being at risk for psychological problems (Pollard, 1992–1993; Vernon & Andrews, 1990). The lack of hearing was blamed for problems in perception, cognition, and interpersonal functioning. In the early 1980s, psychologists such as Edna Levine, Allen Sussman, and Barbara Brauer suggested that it was time to move beyond these inimical and often invalid research findings and look at the survival strengths of deaf adults, many of whom were able to fashion satisfactory lives for themselves. Sussman and Brauer (1999) noted that deaf people have been pathologized rather than seen as healthy personalities. Deaf adults too often encounter naïve professionals who are inadequately informed regarding what it means to be deaf and therefore perpetuate the problems of inaccurate diagnoses. This occurs despite improvements in disseminating information to professionals on how to provide appropriate psychological evaluations of deaf adults (e.g., du Feu & Chovaz, 2014; Fellinger, et al., 2012; Glickman, 2013a; Leigh, 2010; Leigh & Pollard, 2011).

What Needs to Be Done?

Psychological evaluators must consider strengths and specific test factors (described later in this chapter), while still paying attention to deficits in order to minimize negative and inaccurate interpretations for deaf clients. For psychotherapists to work effectively with deaf clients, using strengths models that focus on client assets and abilities in fashioning a positive adjustment to life is strongly recommended.

Normalcy: A Paradigm in Need of Clarification

Normal is a highly ubiquitous word in U.S. society. Few realize that the idea of a "norm" entered the English language only as recently as the nineteenth century (Davis, 1995). Prior to that time, individuals were perceived as imperfect as compared to an unattainable ideal of perfection. Nowadays, *normal* is generally defined as conforming to a standard, usual, typical, average, or expected. From a psychological perspective, *normal* is construed as synonymous with an average psychological trait, such as intelligence, development, personality, or emotional status. The implication is that the majority of the population is expected to fall within the standard bell-shaped curve that reflects probabilities. As such, being "average" or "normal" has become the yardstick as opposed to different, deviant, or abnormal characteristics. Consequently, those who are "different" may be perceived as deviating from what is expected, or what is normal, with concomitant potential consequences, as indicated in the next paragraph.

When parents are told that their child is deaf, this can be a very confusing period since they typically will anticipate a "normal" baby if all goes well. Not only do they have to learn what it means to have a deaf child; they also may have difficulty accepting their child as someone who is "different" (St. John, Lytle, Nussbaum, & Shoup, 2016). Some will write about, for example, their deaf child becoming a "true hearing child" (Parents and Families of Natural Communication, Inc., 1998, p. 33), or "Annie is a joyful hearing child," (Schwartz, 2007, p. 180) as if being labeled as a deaf child implies abnormality. If some of these deaf children end up not following typical hearing communication behaviors as adults, and rely instead on signed communication or use typical Deaf culture behavior such as tapping others to get their attention, they could at times be perceived as not quite normal or as objects of curiosity or pity.

Even though the typical hearing person may see "deaf" as not necessarily "normal," there are many deaf adults who perceive themselves to be normal individuals who happen to be deaf. For example, Sarah Burwell (2015) writes that "being deaf isn't a disability, it's a gift." Related to this, in shifting from the implicit hearing standard of normalcy to a standard of "differentness" as a part of the human condition, she also includes the gift of true friends, of new sounds, and of being appreciative of what she has. With this frame of reference, it is possible to view deaf people as part of the diversity spectrum that encompasses all human beings (Bauman & Murray, 2010; Davis, 1995). Buttressing this point, Tom Humphries (2008) points out that there has been a sociocultural transformation of the narrative that has reframed what "deaf" means, with a new focus on a discourse of language and culture, as embodied in the term "Deaf." This narrative expands on the state of being deaf as a "normal state of affairs" and reflective of a strong, vibrant minority community of Deaf people who live productive lives that involve family, work, and play. This framework counters the notion of deaf as abnormal and deviant.

The Psychologically Healthy Deaf Adult

A multitude of books (see the end of Chapter 2 for a sampling), media publications, and television series that include, for example, Katie Leclerc in *Switched at Birth*, Christy Smith in *Survivor*, Nyle DiMarco in *Dancing with the Stars*, and Marlee Matlin in *The West Wing* are powerful illustrations of how deaf people are taking their place in society. Such publicity has allowed the greater public to learn about how deaf people manage life situations, just like hearing people do. Many understand that deaf people are not necessarily objects of pity or curiosity, but rather people who are competent individuals, pretty much able to take care of themselves like most others. They are more or less capable of parenting deaf and hearing children like their hearing counterparts (Bishop & Hicks, 2008; Mitchiner, 2015; Preston, 1994), and they hold down jobs (Annual Disability Statistics Compendium, 2014; Lang & Meath-Lang, 1995; Schley et al., 2011). It is evident that job possibilities for deaf people have continued to improve over the decades, as witness the emergence of deaf medical doctors, lawyers, emergency medical technicians, psychologists, superintendents of schools, engineers, ad infinitum. We acknowledge the fact that deaf people continue to lag behind their hearing counterparts, particularly those who have not graduated from high school. Research indicates that those deaf individuals who complete vocational or academic postsecondary education increase their likelihood of employment and experience significant earnings benefits compared to those who do not (Schley et al., 2011). In the intelligence domain, Braden (1994) reports on a meta-analysis of the literature that reinforces the similarity between deaf and hearing comparison groups in nonverbal intellectual functioning. Based on a lifetime of observations, Sussman and Brauer (1999) conclude that deaf adults in general have positive self-esteem, are comfortable with being deaf, can assert themselves, ask for help as needed, have effective interpersonal relationships and social skills, and demonstrate a positive zest for life. This happens despite the fact that many deaf adults often have had to deal with the stress of handling negative attitudes in facilitating communication access, as discussed in Chapter 11. Sheridan (2001; 2008) illustrates how deaf children and adolescents rely on their strengths to counter negative stereotypes and situations that they might encounter, strengths that they can carry into adulthood. Zand and Pierce (2011) include chapters that explore the strengths and resilience of emerging adults who are deaf. Yes, there are deaf adults with problems in living and personality issues, which we will discuss when we cover mental health issues later in this chapter, and later in the book related to the deaf offender in the criminal justice system. However, they do not define the entire contingent of deaf people.

Stages of Adult Development

In Chapter 7, we reviewed the first five of Erikson's eight developmental stages that focused on children and youth. In this chapter, we discuss his last three stages, this time focusing on adults.

During the sixth stage of intimacy versus isolation, individuals are grappling less with their identities and focusing more on creating long-term relationships in the form of friendships, love, or inspiration. They are willing to make the sacrifices and compromises that long-term relationships may require. If this does not work, the consequences tend to be distancing and isolation.

In the U.S., 85 percent of deaf people tend to marry other deaf people (Nance, 2004). This can easily be explained by shared experiences and ease of communication that deaf people have with each other, and for those who are members of Deaf culture, a shared language (ASL) and numerous opportunities to engage in social interaction.

Harvey (2003) presents a scenario of Timothy, a Deaf man whose marriage to a Deaf woman represents his efforts to individuate from his nuclear family and shift his loyalties from his parents to his wife. He struggles between loyalty to his wife and loyalty to his hearing parents, whom he sees as authority and guiding figures, in this way reflecting his efforts to work though the intimacy stage. This working-through involves negotiating power, intimacy, and autonomy.

There are deaf people who do marry hearing people. Based on her research findings, McIntosh (2006) opines that the 90 percent divorce rate for deaf-hearing marriages is a myth; her study of 143 spouses from 132 relatively well-educated deaf-hearing couples indicates they experience high levels of marital satisfaction and employ collaborative and partner-oriented conflict-resolution skills. This counters multiple blogs on the Internet that portray such marriages as full of conflict due to hearing privilege (see Chapter 11) and communication issues.

This sixth stage has undergone a reformulation under the rubric of emerging adulthood (Arnett, 2006). This phase covers the period between the end of adolescence and the young adult responsibilities of a stable job, marriage, and parenthood. There are multiple pathways towards these young adult responsibilities. An investigation of the self-reported experiences of a national sample of 44 deaf emerging adults ages 18 to 30 years who rated various life experiences revealed that these highly educated and predominantly Caucasian deaf adults progressed through emerging adulthood similarly to hearing peers with respect to the ability to assume responsibility for themselves, make independent and major decisions, become financially independent, change roles between themselves and their families of origin, and commit to new relationships (Zand & Pierce, 2013). Related to being deaf, these participants endorsed items such as embracing elements of Deaf culture, including having culturally Deaf friends, attending Deaf events, and using ASL. Interestingly, the importance of having hearing friends was highly rated.

Moving on to the next stage, that of generativity versus stagnation, which happens roughly during middle age, Erikson explains that this stage focuses on establishing and guiding the next generation, either through offspring or through other forms of altruism such as giving back to society or doing things to benefit future generations. More specifically, generativity reflects an adult's commitment to promote the well-being of future generations by being involved in parenting, teaching, mentoring, building communities and organizations, passing on traditions, working for positive social change, creating improvements that can impact quality of life, and so on (McAdams, 2006). In contrast, stagnation refers to one's inability to contribute or leave a positive mark, resulting in feelings of unproductivity and uninvolvement in their world. McAdams promotes the idea that generativity is not necessarily confined to the middle-age years but can occur at various stages throughout the life cycle. He reports on research indicating that individual differences in generativity are associated with particular patterns of parenting, social support, and religious and civic involvement. Additionally, highly generative American adults tend to construct life story narratives that reflect topics such as future growth and fulfillment, awareness of the suffering of others, and their own advantages.

What we know about generativity in deaf people comes from their life story narratives, which reflect on their experiences as deaf people with a variety of life experiences that encourage or discourage generativity. The history of deaf people is replete with stories of advocacy for parity with hearing people, equal access, and organizational involvement for both altruistic and social purposes (see Chapter 9 for some examples). Sheridan (1995) explains that this advocacy reflects a process of existential transference over oppressive forces that deaf people may experience in their lives. Here we focus on parenting as a component of generativity.

The role of parenting is a challenge for many. First-time parenthood can be viewed as a developmental phase marked by significant changes in lifestyle, including aspects such as family relationships, financial issues, and socialization patterns. The deaf adult who has not been fully integrated into the hearing family of origin due to difficulties in communication will have to use multiple resources in order to parent a child with warmth and love. Deaf parents who have grown up in supportive, communicatively accessible families will have good foundations for parenting, whether the child is deaf or hearing. Unfortunately, deaf parents report high rates of child removal and loss of custody (Powell, 2014), in general because society views their inability to hear as a sign of inadequacy in parenting. The National Council on Disability (2012) has taken the lead on advocating against such practices for parents with disabilities in their publication, *Rocking the Cradle*.

Erikson labeled his eighth and final stage in his life cycle formulation as "integrity versus despair." It is hoped that, during postretirement, people look back on their lives, come to terms with how they have lived, and feel fulfilled rather than regret or despair over a wasted life. With wisdom comes integrity that comes from having internalized what life is about. This eighth stage covers elderly people, who constitute what we now know to be among the fastest-growing populations in the United States. Elderly people are considered to be a vulnerable group due to the potential of age-related declines in body and mind, although increasing numbers do not experience significant deterioration until the very end of life due to living very active and healthy lifestyles. They can look back appreciatively on their lives. Of those who do experience deterioration, many deal with hearing loss and may experience despair.

Feldman (2010) cautions that we need to separate the elderly deafened and the Deaf elderly, since professionals often conflate them within the geriatric population. The elderly deafened population has attracted more research compared to the population of Deaf elderly individuals (Feldman & Kearns, 2007). We can consider the Deaf elderly population to be a neglected population with minimal resources in medical and mental health service delivery. Feldman (2010) reports that a common perception of Deaf elderly individuals that indicate they feel they have been forgotten. Many of them grew up prior to the ADA of 1990 (see Chapter 1) and thus faced greater discrimination in the workforce and limited access to a variety of services that have encouraged a stance of "certain passive acceptance that involves simply relying on the hearing professional to make decisions" (Feldman, 2010, p. 284; see also Witte & Kuzel, 2000). Isolation is a recurring problem with the decrease in local deaf clubs and the lack of other social opportunities. In comparison, the next generation of elderly Deaf adults (the baby-boomer group) is generally better educated, more into Internet technology, and more aware of Deaf culture and their rights as deaf people. They tend to be less tolerant of situations where accommodations are not provided (Feldman, 2010). They have worked to increase the number of senior resources so that Deaf elderly people can receive culturally affirmative services (https://nad.org/senior-resources). So perhaps we can conclude that, overall, the integrity of this new cohort of Deaf elderly individuals may reveal comparatively greater satisfaction with their lives and less despair over what they have not accomplished compared to previous cohorts. Their identities and self-perceptions may have roles within this domain of integrity, and we explore these constructs in the next section.

Identity and Self-Perceptions

Very often, the word *deaf* appears when deaf adults are asked to describe themselves. *Deaf* (capital *D*) is a characteristic that a good number have internalized in formulating their self-representations or identities, People have different identities depending on their environment and what is most salient at any moment in time. These identities emerge through one's perceptions of similarities and differences in comparison with others, depending on attributes such as gender, ethnicity, occupation, educational level, cultural affiliation, and a host of other variables (e.g., Corker, 1996; Jones Thomas & Schwarzbaum, 2006). The construction of all these identities, both overt and covert (Sheridan, 2001), is created through the process of interaction within different social contexts—for example, the family, the school, the workplace, social settings, religious institutions, the sports arena, and so forth (e.g., Jones Thomas & Schwarzbaum, 2006; Scheibe, 2006). Depending on the setting, people are parents or grandparents, teachers or students, congregants or religious leaders, and so on.

Identity constructs influence personal development. Because of the recent increase in cultural diversity within the U.S. and other countries, interest in cultural or ethnic group membership and social identity has exploded (Sue & Sue, 2015). The goal for current research on the meaning of social identity and how it is measured is that of facilitating individual adjustment between and within cultural groups. What does this mean for deaf persons?

According to Corker (1996), deaf identity is not necessarily a core identity; race or ethnicity takes precedence. How deaf identity develops depends on the extent to which being deaf is salient in one's daily life. If a deaf person is consistently exposed to Deaf culture, whether at school, within the family, or in social settings, the chances for identifying as a Deaf person increases. Those with less exposure may label themselves as *oral deaf, hearing impaired, hard of hearing,* or some other similar term (Leigh, 2009). In the process of exploring how deaf identities develop and the implications for psychological health, researchers have noted that differences in the perceived quality of social experiences are related to one's social adjustment and identity as a person who is deaf (see Leigh, 2009, for details). Generally, the stronger one's deaf identity, the more comfort there is in socializing with deaf peers.

Researchers have taken advantage of different theoretical models to examine the application of deaf and hearing identities. Stinson and Kluwin (1996) used social identity parameters in asking about socialization with deaf and with hearing peers in order to categorize one's social identity as deaf or hearing oriented. Using cluster analysis, Bat-Chava (2000) derived three identity categories—culturally hearing, culturally deaf, and bicultural—based on four criterion variables related to communication and socialization, specifically importance of signing, importance of speech, group identity, and attitudes toward deaf people.

Based on his exploration of cultural and racial identity stage development theories, Neil Glickman (1996) developed a parallel model incorporating four different stages of deaf identity, In Stage 1, the culturally hearing stage, being deaf is seen as a medical condition or disability to be ameliorated, thereby minimizing the need for support services or sign language. Individuals adopt hearing ways of speaking, understanding, and behaving in ways that facilitate integration into hearing society. This stage applies to late-onset deaf adults and deaf persons who grow up using and preferring spoken English, who interact primarily with hearing peers, and who may belong to organizations that advocate spoken language for deaf children. Since Glickman perceives this stage as reflecting some denial of what it means to be deaf, he questions how psychologically healthy this stage is. Later we present research that shows many in this group do exhibit psychological health.

Stage 2, which reflects cultural marginality, includes deaf persons who exist on the fringes of both Deaf and hearing cultures, unable to fully integrate into either. Close relationships with members of both groups are problematic. Interestingly, based on his research with deaf German participants, Hintermair (2008) cautions that some of those identified as marginal may have personal resources other than connecting with hearing/deaf groups and may do well in life. Deaf individuals in Stage 3 immerse themselves within Deaf culture, identify as Deaf, and behave as they think authentic Deaf people are supposed to. Hearing values and deaf people with "hearing minds" who speak English are denigrated. In Stage 4, the bicultural stage, the deaf person can integrate the values of both hearing and Deaf cultures and positively relate with deaf and hearing people. In this stage, both ASL and English are respected.

Theoretically, the Stage 4 integrative stance reflects enhanced psychological health. Deaf individuals starting off in the culturally marginal stage may progress to the bicultural stage as the final one in the process of deaf identity development, whereas Deaf children of Deaf parents, who usually reflect pride in being Deaf and can demonstrate comfort in dealing with both Deaf and hearing worlds, typically assume a bicultural identity early on. Because not every deaf person starts at the first stage, progression through the various stages is not necessarily linear.

Glickman (1996) developed the Deaf Identity Development Scale (DIDS), a 60-item measure that consists of four scales, each reflecting one of the stages just described. Follow-up studies indicated that the bicultural scale did not differentiate between deaf and hearing respondents, including those who may have never met a deaf person (Fischer, 2000; Leigh, Marcus, Dobosh, & Allen, 1998), possibly due to social desirability factors emphasizing biculturalism. Fischer and McWhirter (2001) shortened the DIDS to 48 items and demonstrated acceptable reliability for all 4 categories. Nonetheless, their Bicultural Scale demonstrated the lowest, albeit acceptable, reliability score. As deaf people interact more often with hearing peers at work, through the Internet, or via other avenues, biculturalism is increasingly seen as socially desirable.

Taking another approach, Maxwell-McCaw (2001) developed a deaf identity model with theoretical groundings in the acculturation process. The acculturation framework posits that acculturation patterns for immigrants will vary according to the level of psychological (or internalized) identification with the culture of origin and the new host culture, as well as the degree of behavioral involvement and cultural competence in each culture. Paralleling this, Maxwell-McCaw theorizes that the acculturation patterns for deaf persons can vary in terms of the level of psychological identification with Deaf culture and with the culture of their hearing society and the extent to which they are behaviorally involved and culturally competent in each culture. To test this idea, she developed the Deaf Acculturation Scale (DAS) and demonstrated its reliability and validity with 3,070 deaf and hard-of-hearing adults. It is made up of two acculturation scales—a Deaf Acculturation Scale and a Hearing Acculturation Scale—each consisting of five subscales that are parallel to each other and measure acculturation across five domains covering psychological identification, cultural behaviors, cultural attitudes, cultural knowledge, and language competence related to deaf and hearing environments (see also Maxwell-McCaw & Zea, 2011). Individuals can score as hearing acculturated (high scores in hearing acculturation and low scores in deaf acculturation), marginal (low scores in both hearing and deaf acculturation), deaf acculturated (high scores in deaf acculturation and low scores in hearing acculturation), and bicultural (high scores in both deaf and hearing acculturation). Maxwell-McCaw (2001) found that deaf acculturation and biculturalism were equally associated with higher self-esteem and satisfaction with life, more so than for those who were hearing acculturated. Marginalism was found to be the least adaptive of the four acculturation styles.

As this book emphasizes, the deaf community is increasingly multicultural. Identity formulations cannot ignore the ethnic dimension (Leigh, 2009; 2010; 2012). In fact, Corker (1996) claims that ethnic identity takes precedence over deaf identity because of family influences in the early years. Those individuals to whom the deaf child is exposed depend very much on whom the family members interact with in daily life. Usually, these are members of the family's ethnic group. With increased exposure to deaf people in later years, one can expect an interactive effect between ethnic identity and deaf identity categorizations depending on the situation. Interestingly, recent preliminary research based on the DAS suggests that Black Deaf identity may be factored differently from White Deaf identity and recommends that future research examine the intersections of Deaf identity and racial identity (Nelson Schmitt & Leigh, 2015).

The multicultural deaf person tends to integrate membership in diverse communities: the larger deaf community, the ethnic hearing community of origin, the ethnic deaf community, and the predominant majority community (Corbett, 2010; Wu & Grant, 2010). This requires altering behaviors to fit the specific community as explained by the alternation model, which focuses on codeswitching or alternating behaviors appropriate to the cultural situation. Theoretically, the stress level would be lower than for the assimilation mode, which requires giving up one culture (and identity) in order to assimilate into the other culture (LaFromboise, Coleman, & Gerton, 1993). With the changing ethnic composition of the deaf community, the topic of cultural identities in deaf persons, the intersectionalities of these identities, and psychological adjustment related to interactions of various identities is an area ripe for research (Leigh, 2012), considering that a general review of publications in mental health research indicates unacceptably low reporting rates of race, ethnicity, and culture in research participants (Lewis-Fernández et al., 2013). In fact, the topic of intersectionality has gained prominence in the literature, ever since Crenshaw's (1989) article, which elaborates on how intersecting social identities overlap with related systems of oppression, dominance, or discrimination. Systems that can be explored include racism, sexism, homophobia, ableism, and so on.

Moving on to the self-perception domain, researchers have long been interested in the self-concept or self-esteem of deaf people and how these might be influenced by relatively negative attitudes about deaf people. Both terms have often been used interchangeably in the literature, although their meanings differ (Harter, 1997). *Self-concept* is defined as a relatively stable cognitive structure that reflects subjective awareness of one's stable attributes such as beliefs, moods, intentions, and actions or, in essence, self-perception or self-knowledge (Kagan, 1998). *Self-esteem* reflects the emotional and judgmental view of one's own self or, in other words, the feeling that comes from the experiences of feeling accepted, competent, involved, and recognized (Brice & Adams, 2011). These mental representations of the self regulate and influence psychological well-being (Harter, 1997).

Based on a review of studies covering self-concept and self-esteem continuing into the 1970s, Vernon and Andrews (1990) concluded that the self-concept of deaf people tended to be more negative compared to the general population. However, the validity of many studies from that period is questionable because of measurement issues (as mentioned in Chapter 1 and explained later in this chapter).

The theme emphasized in more recent studies is that the self-perceptions (self-concept, self-esteem, self-image, etc.) of deaf adults vary depending on different contextual factors. There have been numerous studies on the self-esteem of deaf children and adolescents (see Chapter 7 for a brief review), but very few have focused on deaf adults. In a seminal meta-analysis of 42 empirical studies investigating self-esteem in deaf children, college students, and adults, mostly from the late 1970s through the early 1990s, Bat-Chava (1993) notes lower self-esteem in comparison to hearing people. Higher self-esteem in deaf adolescents and adults appears to be associated with several contextual variables: having deaf parents, communicating with one's family using sign language, and using sign language in school. Also, as mentioned earlier, higher self-esteem is associated with culturally Deaf as well as bicultural identities in comparison to hearing or marginal identities (Bat-Chava, 2000; Hintermair, 2014; Maxwell-McCaw, 2001). These findings represent a significant change when one considers earlier studies such as Sussman's (1974), which noted lower self-esteem in those deaf adults who felt they did not speak well in contrast to deaf adults who felt good about their use of spoken language. Additionally, Hintermair's (2008) study of deaf German adults noted that, in addition to cultural affiliation, psychological resources such as life optimism and self-efficacy are also significant factors for the development of self-esteem.

Bat-Chava (1993) interprets her findings to mean that deaf people are not necessarily passive recipients of the majority's negative attitudes. Rather, they may adopt psychological mechanisms that facilitate positive self-esteem, such as comparing themselves with deaf peers and not with hearing peers, or valuing sign language and other deaf community attributes. Seminal events, including the recognition of ASL, increased awareness that a Deaf culture exists, and the Gallaudet University Deaf President Now movement of 1988 had a profound influence in reshaping the self-perceptions of many deaf people in a more positive direction (Leigh, 2009; Maxwell-McCaw, 2001). More recently, the inclusion of Deaf people in movies, theater, and TV series (e.g., *Switched at Birth*) as well as publicity about successful Broadway plays including Deaf people (*Big River* and *Spring Awakening*), Carol Padden as one of the 2010 MacArthur Genius Award recipients, and the selection of Roberta "Bobbi" Cordano as the first female Deaf president of Gallaudet University, among other events, all serve to highlight the achievements of notable Deaf people and reinforce self-pride/self-esteem.

Bat-Chava (1993) found that the level of self-esteem in the studies she reviewed varied as a function of the measure, its format, and the way in which instructions were conveyed to research participants. Unmodified measures or written instructions (even if supplemented by sign language) resulted in lower self-esteem scores for deaf participants, whereas modified measures or instructions administered in sign language yielded similar scores for hearing and deaf participants. This leads directly to the consideration of psychological measurement issues and how these impact on the portrayal of deaf adults.

Psychological Assessment of Deaf Adults

Psychological assessment is essentially a process during which individuals are evaluated for the purpose of describing behavior and obtaining a diagnosis that will lead to some type of intervention or recommendation for services (Braden, 2001; Framingham, 2013). Psychological assessments are typically performed by psychologists whose training involves administering and interpreting psychological tests. For deaf adults, these evaluations are usually requested by social or vocational service agencies to determine eligibility for social, vocational, or educational (remedial or postsecondary) services, to assess mental status and the capacity to take care of oneself, or to evaluate competency to stand trial (Braden, 2001). When deaf adults themselves request psychological assessments, this is usually because they are concerned about conditions such as learning disabilities or attention deficit disorders There may also be medical concerns related to the aging process or some form of trauma that affects one's behavior (Braden, 2001).

Deaf adults differ from hearing counterparts to varying degrees in hearing acuity, age of onset, parental hearing status, communication method, linguistic use, educational background, social experience, ethnicity, cultural identity, gender, and the presence of additional disabilities depending on etiology, among other things. These diversity factors all influence how the psychological evaluation is conducted, which psychological tests are used, and how they are interpreted (Maller & Braden, 2011; Maller & Immekus, 2005; Sligar, Cawthon, Morere, & Moxley, 2013).

The Assessment Process

Psychological evaluations typically involve observation of the client to determine behavioral characteristics; interviewing the client to obtain a history that covers information on medical, developmental, and past as well as current functioning; administering psychological instruments that will address the referral question; and interpreting the results. With the client's permission, information can also be requested from educational, medical, or social service agencies with which the client may have been involved. Psychologists who do not have a strong knowledge base of deaf people, their issues, including education, language and communication, diversity variables including culture, and issues related to assessment effectiveness for this population, do their deaf clients a serious disservice through inaccurately interpreting test results (Sligar, Cawthon, Morere, & Moxley, 2013). We explain further in the following sections.

Effectiveness of Psychological Tests

Tests are selected depending on the purpose of the assessment (e.g., cognitive, socioemotional, vocational, or neuropsychological) and individual characteristics such as age, language and culture, and ability to understand questions and respond as required. Pollard (2002) identifies five factors that determine whether specific tests are appropriate for deaf individuals: 1) relationship to the evaluation question, 2) how instructions are communicated, 3) the nature or content of items/tasks, 4) response modality, and 5) scoring methods and norms. If there are problems with any of these factors, results may be biased.

No psychological evaluation can take place without checking psychometric aspects, specifically whether tests consistently or *reliably* measure the constructs being assessed (e.g., depression, identity, or performance-based intelligence) and whether these tests are *valid* for different groups of people (i.e., they actually measure the constructs they are supposed to measure in those different groups). For example, intelligence tests may play a critical role in making high-stakes decisions related to classification, diagnosis, competency, and educational placement (Maller & Braden, 2011). It has been documented that deaf examinees tend to score approximately one standard deviation below the mean of hearing examinees on verbal measures of intelligence (Maller & Braden, 2011). This is likely due in part to limited access to the English language. In comparison, deaf examinees tend to obtain performance intelligence scores that are comparable to hearing peers. However, a review of recent studies on intellectual functioning does not cast much light on the significance of differences between deaf and hearing groups or within deaf groups that emerge over a variety of tests, subtests, and samples, perhaps in part because of small deaf sample sizes and how these are constituted that may exacerbate or mask differences (Hu, 2015). Not only that, current tests of intelligence such as the popular Wechsler tests (WAIS IV and WISC IV) and other intelligence tests have performance tests or subtests that may or may not penalize deaf examinees (see Maller & Braden, 2011; Sligar et al., 2013, for details). We also need to ask whether integrating verbal and performance intelligence scores accurately reflect the deaf examinee's intellectual functioning. It is not uncommon to see test reports doing exactly that; the impression these reports give is of lesser intellectual functioning than what the deaf person may be capable of, unless mastery of English is not an issue.

TEST RELIABILITY

Test reliability refers to the degree of stability, consistency, predictability, and accuracy of tests (Maller & Braden, 2011). With good reliability, one can assume that a test score will not significantly change if the person is tested at different times, even though results will vary depending on mood, alertness, or problems in test administration. Usually, the variability is greater for personality measures than for ability measures such as academic achievement, aptitude, or intelligence. Test manuals rarely have information on reliability results for samples representing special populations, including deaf examinees (Maller & Braden, 2011). This can make interpretation of test results for deaf individuals less definitive. We note that journal editors are now expecting reliability results for measures administered to deaf participants in research studies to ensure that these measures were reliably measuring the constructs being researched.

TEST VALIDITY

A test is valid when it accurately measures the construct or variable it is supposed to measure (Maller & Braden, 2011). Establishing test validity is difficult, particularly when the constructs are abstract concepts, such as intelligence, anxiety, or creativity. For example, do items on an intelligence test actually reflect the deaf test-taker's intelligence? Three main methods of establishing validity are as follows:

1. *Content validity* involves comparing new items with the content of similar tests or check-ing that the items clearly reflect the skills or knowledge area being measured. For example, a test on handling money needs to match the person's actual skills in handling money. Experts in assessing deaf individuals are rarely consulted during intelligence test devel-opment to determine the appropriateness of item content or format for this population (Maller & Immekus, 2005).

2. *Concurrent or predictive validity* is determined by comparing test scores with performance on a related measure, either at the same time for concurrent validity or some time later, as in comparing test scores of job applicants with job status 1 year later, for predictive valid-ity. For example, deaf examinee results on one measure of intelligence has been compared with results on a different measure of intelligence to see of both measures are tapping into the same construct (Maller & Braden, 2011; Maller & Immekus, 2005). Results overall have shown moderate correlations.

3. *Construct validity* reflects the extent to which a test actually measures a theoretical construct or trait. This requires analyzing the trait and how it should relate to other variables and testing whether these relationships hold up. Good engineers should be able to obtain high scores on a test of spatial relationships, for example. This would indicate that the test actu-ally reflects a construct necessary for good engineering. The factor structure of a test should result in similar scores for deaf and hearing samples if the test measures the same constructs for both samples. If there are factor structure differences, there may be test bias because scores are less likely to mean the same thing for both samples (Maller & Braden, 2011).

Reliability and validity continue to be thorny issues for individuals from different cultures and for deaf individuals in general. When deaf people are members of different cultural groups, interpretation of test results becomes that much more complicated.

The Use of Norms

To evaluate and interpret the meaning of scores on a psychological test requires comparing these scores with test norms. Test norms are scores obtained by large numbers of individuals who represent the population being studied. One frequent difficulty is that different norma-tive samples from the same large population may result in different interpretations for any one score on specific tests because of lack of uniform representation within each sample. The *Standards for Educational and Psychological Testing* (American Educational Research Association [AERA], American Psychological Association [APA], & National Council on Measurement in Education [NCME], 2014) has issued guidelines for test developers and users. For members of special populations, their test scores should be scrutinized to ensure that these accurately represent their functioning. Unfortunately, only a few test developers provide evidence that their tests are reliable and valid for deaf and hard-of-hearing examinees (based on small sam-ples), likely due to the lack of group homogeneity, the costs associated with work concern-ing low-incidence populations, difficulty in obtaining large samples, and limited knowledge regarding this population (Maller & Immekus, 2005; Sligar, Cawthon, Morere, & Moxley,

2013). While tests with deaf norms are believed to be more fair in that deaf individuals are compared to other deaf peers rather than hearing peers, Maller and Braden (2011) believe that deaf norms may be neither representative of the deaf population or useful because this population is so heterogeneous with respect to hearing levels, communication, parent hearing status, ethnicity, educational levels, and so on. Since deaf and hearing nonverbal intelligence norms do not differ significantly, Braden (2001) argues that deaf norms are unnecessary for nonverbal intelligence tests but are more appropriate for academic achievement tests. If a deaf woman reads better than most deaf people, and her reading level is comparable to the average hearing reader, we can infer that her English comprehension is exceptionally adequate considering the circumstances and make relevant recommendations.

Linguistic and Communication Factors

Knowing the deaf adult's linguistic and communication preferences will facilitate test selection and administration with the goal of understanding the person's current functioning. Responses based on the deaf person's "best language" or primary mode of communication will also more accurately reflect individual strengths as opposed to deficiencies or weaknesses (Braden, 1994; Sligar et al., 2013). The use of verbal measures of intellectual functioning, memory, and personality are most often inappropriate unless reading and writing test scores provide evidence of adequate English proficiency, even if the person prefers spoken language, signed English, or some combination of sign and speech. On the other side of the coin, it can be important to assess the deaf adult's competency in English language usage (whether it is the first or second language), depending on the referral question. For any deaf adult, including ASL users, the clinician must weigh the need for careful evaluation of a deaf person's skills in verbal information against the possibility of creating misleading impressions about the client's cognitive limitations because of verbal difficulties (Braden, 2001). Evidence of competency in other domains of intelligence and achievement should be emphasized. Generally, for cognitive assessment, language-reduced measures meeting one's language level are most appropriate.

Test Accommodations

Test accommodations are defined as a change in format, content, or administration that does not change the construct the test is measuring but rather makes the test accessible to those who might otherwise be penalized without these accommodations (American Psychological Association, 2012). Psychologists need to determine whether accommodations are appropriate for clients to yield a valid test result. For deaf examinees, accommodations may include gestural administrations, signed instructions of nonverbal tests, and translations of items on verbal tests, including the use of sign language interpreters.

REVISING OR TRANSLATING TESTS

Measures that are either linguistically revised or translated into ASL to meet the needs of deaf adults must be reassessed for reliability and validity to gauge if the constructs being measured are still being tapped, since linguistic changes can result in changes in the meaning of test items. When translating, it is essential to follow the following steps to ensure adherence to the true meaning of test items: 1) initial translation from, for example, English to ASL by a native or near-native expert user of both languages; 2) blind back-translation from ASL to English by another expert; 3) careful comparison of both versions to identify discrepancies; and 4) redoing the first two steps to resolve discrepancies and ensure that equivalent constructs are being measured in both languages (Bracken & Barona, 1991, as cited in Maller & Braden, 2011). This can be a challenging process. For example, Cohen and Jones (1990, p. 46) write that "It's alright for my child to have an imaginary friend" could be translated using ASL signs for *fantasy, pretend,* or *not real* to represent the imaginary friend concept. However, after back-translation into English, the sentence became "It's ok if my child doesn't have any real friends." To correct for the lack of conceptual equivalence, signs for *imagine + envision + friend* could be used.

There have been suggestions that deaf adults would be better served with the use of ASL-based psychological measures developed specifically for ASL users, based more on the deaf experience, thereby avoiding the pitfalls of translations. This is an area in need of research.

Computer-Assisted Assessments

Computer testing is now available to assess for various conditions, including attention deficit hyperactivity disorder and executive functioning (defined as a set of mental skills such as organization, planning, and reasoning that help you get things done). Computer simulation tasks are also used for the assessment of intelligence (Kröner, Plass, & Leutner, 2005). Test publishers now offer web-based test administration. According to Groth-Marnat (2009), computer-based tests are advantageous in terms of administration and scoring efficiency as well as evidence of reliability and validity when compared with traditional paper-and-pencil versions.

Whether these computer tests are accessible and appropriate for deaf individuals depends on how verbal and visual these are, whether there is access to captions or ASL, and whether results are reliable and valid for deaf people. With the advent of video capabilities, researchers are now turning to computers to create assessments in different domains directed specifically towards deaf individuals. Noteworthy examples include the development of an ASL-accessible health survey that was presented using film clips of the translated items and answer choices incorporated into a touch-screen computer interface (Barnett et al., 2011) as well as a culturally and linguistically specific deaf depression screener using ASL that is delivered via computer (Eckhardt, Goldstein, Creamer, & Berry, 2013). Additionally, the VL2 (Visual Language and Visual Learning), a National Science Foundation Science of Learning Center, has created a variety of neurocognitive assessment tools that involve the use of computer tests utilizing ASL (http://vl2.gallaudet.edu/resources/asl-assessment-toolkits/). A caveat, however, is that there are challenges due to the variety of communication needs and regional signs in ASL, not all of which can be captured via computer format compared with humans who can be flexible in matching the communication needs of different deaf examinees.

Using Sign Language Interpreters in Assessment

The consequences of communication problems during the psychological evaluation can result in invalid conclusions about individual functioning. Therefore, it is best to check with the deaf client or referring agency to ascertain communication needs and make appropriate arrangements. If the psychological evaluator is not a fluent signer, or is not easily understood by the client, certified sign language or spoken language interpreters should be recruited. Direct signing or interpreted administration is preferable to poorly spoken, written, or gesturally based communication (Sligar et al., 2013). Certified interpreters are trained to assess the client's communication needs, adjust communication to suit client preferences, provide ongoing English-ASL translations, and maintain confidentiality. Administering psychological measures with the use of a sign language interpreter carries some risk because of the lack of standard ASL procedures that could compromise test integrity and test results. Even if certified, interpreters may vary in how they interpret test instructions without a standard protocol. In mental status evaluations of deaf individuals (discussed later), distinguishing ASL variations from language issues or psychotic distortions requires specialized mental health and assessment training, which certified interpreters do not necessarily have (Leigh & Pollard, 2011). Sligar et al. (2013, p. 113) provides the following examples: 1) the interpreter may present the signed language of a deaf examinee in a clean way, masking the language deficit of the examinee, and 2)

> [A] test administrator may ask, "How are two items alike?" and the test taker may sign "not" with a back and forth head movement. The interpreter may then voice "I do not know" when the test taker's response of "not" may indicate either that the two items are not alike or the answer is not known.

The field lacks methodologically sound studies that indicate whether the use of interpreters is equivalent to direct signing with the client in assessment situations.

Mental Status Examinations

Mental status exams are observations and interviews conducted by qualified mental health service providers in order to assess one's current cognitive, emotional, and interactive functioning for psychiatric diagnosis purposes (Brannon, 2015). To avoid misdiagnosis, assessing the mental status of deaf adults requires special considerations, including communication skills and an awareness of the day-to-day realities of deaf persons (Leigh & Pollard, 2011). Specifically, deaf people do not necessarily behave and think the same way hearing people do, and issues related to literacy levels (see Chapter 6), limitations in fund of information due to lack of access, and language dysfluency make mental status exams a minefield for the average mental health clinician with limited knowledge about what it may mean to be deaf. Behavior such as flailing hands or hysterical outbursts have been cited as confirming evidence for psychiatric diagnoses when in fact such behavior may represent frantic attempts to communicate in situations where the deaf adult is feeling very misunderstood. Training of mental health clinicians is covered in Chapter 1. Certified sign language interpreters can facilitate accurate diagnosis if they are trained in mental health interpreting and can accurately convey, for example, psychotic productions within ASL discourse.

Socioemotional Assessment Issues

The personalities of deaf adults have historically been portrayed as causing significant problems in daily functioning due to immaturity, egocentrism, impulsivity, concreteness, and similar negative appellations (e.g., Lane, 1999; Pollard, 1992–1993; see also Chapter 1). Professionals now know that the psychological functioning of deaf clients in mental health agencies is not the same as that of the psychologically healthy deaf adult (Lane, Hoffmeister, & Bahan, 1996; Leigh & Pollard, 2011). Considering the fact that most socioemotional measures are English based, their use in differentiating deaf individuals with varying degrees of psychological problems and psychopathology from the "normal" deaf adult requires understanding of the psychometric and linguistic issues that we have already described. Because of this lack of understanding, tests of personality tend to yield biased results. Recent research in this area is sorely lacking compared to the relative wealth of studies up until the 1970s, studies that for the most part suggested pathology. What we now know is that less complex, English-based socioemotional measures may be useful for deaf examinees who are comfortable with English. For example, the reliability (internal consistency) of the Beck Depression Inventory II (which did not require linguistic revision due to item clarity) for a sample of deaf college students was .88, which is good (Leigh & Anthony-Tolbert, 2001). In contrast, an exploratory study done by Cole (2003) confirmed that the abbreviated version of the Minnesota Multiphasic

Personality Inventory-2 (MMPI-2), which was administered to 89 nonclinical deaf adults who met the MMPI-2 minimum reading level requirement, found that the written English version of this measure was not a valid measure for her sample of deaf adults. This is an illustration of the potential problems with English versions of psychological measures that psychological examiners have to deal with.

Projective methods are an alternative procedure for assessing socioemotional functioning or personality in deaf adults. These are designed to elicit information on how one responds to ambiguous stimuli. Unfortunately, there are significant issues related to psychometric validity (Groth-Marnat, 2009; Shapse, 2015). For this reason, Framingham (2013) considers projectives to be part of the informal assessment process rather than formal assessment, which relies more on psychometrically stronger tests.

The use of drawings, such as the Draw-A-Person test, the House-Tree-Person test, and the Kinetic Family Drawing test, are among the most popular of the projective techniques because they can be done quickly and are useful for global ratings of socioemotional functioning despite the fact that questions about validity persist, not only for these measures, but also for the projective measures mentioned later. A pilot study of the House-Tree Person test with a small sample of deaf adults demonstrated encouraging reliability and validity results (Ouellette, 1988).

Other projective tools that are frequently used with deaf adults include the Thematic Apperception Test (TAT) and the Rorschach Inkblot Test. Both instruments require that the examiner write down responses to test items made by the examinee. For this reason, examiner bias becomes a problem when responses are translated from ASL to English or filtered through a sign language interpreter before being written down, heightening the danger of inaccuracies. Schwartz, Mebane, and Mahony (1990) compared signed and written administrations for a small group of deaf adults with a college-level education who were administered the Rorschach. They concluded that signed administration was preferable to the participants writing responses, since the latter could lead to underreporting of several Rorschach variables. They noted visual-perceptual differences between deaf and hearing persons and provided deaf sample mean scores for the variables investigated. Based on experience, Siedlecki (1999) considers the Rorschach useful for deaf psychiatric patients with limited ASL skills and recommends additional research.

Advances in Neuropsychology

Neuropsychology involves the study of brain-behavior relationships that are elicited through the use of neuropsychological test batteries (Groth-Marnat, 2009). Behavioral responses as well as brain scanning techniques in response to test items or stimuli help neuropsychologists extrapolate information about brain activation and how it influences a person's ability to perform certain tasks. The ability to create computer-based stimuli for research projects such as computer-generated visual imagery tasks has made it possible to create exciting avenues for exploring how deaf people process information neuropsychologically.

There is evidence that deaf persons demonstrate different cortical functions in comparison to hearing peers as a function of hearing status and degree of familiarity with sign language (e.g., Emmorey, 2002; 2015; Poeppel, Emmorey, Hickok, & Pyikkänen, 2012). Research has also demonstrated that there are neurological similarities between signed and spoken languages, such as left hemisphere lateralization (Poeppel et al., 2012). This highlights the universal nature of language.

Considering specific neuropsychology tests, validity and bias challenges also apply. A variety of neuropsychological tests have been evaluated for their usefulness with samples of deaf adults, with some measures showing evidence of ability to separate neurologically intact deaf adult users of sign language from those suspected of having neurological impairment such as dementia (University College London, 2015; see also Leigh & Pollard, 2011, p. 219, for a brief review). In the future, functional neuroimaging research will eventually influence neuropsychological test development, test norms, and interpretation, not only for hearing people, but also for deaf people.

Multiple Sources of Information

Finally, it is important to realize that testing is only one part of the assessment process. Multiple sources of information need to be gathered to provide the most useful data (Framingham, 2013). Information that should be obtained prior to formal testing includes medical, audiological, linguistic, educational, and vocational histories (Sligar et al., 2013). More specifically, information on age of onset, use of assistive technology, type of communication, and access to early intervention among others, if available, should be obtained. Sensitivity to ethnic and cultural background is critical for fairness. During the assessment process, interviews and observations provide an opportunity to gather background information, observe how the client behaves during the assessment process, and assess how well the deaf client provides background details that will help to interpret test data and respond appropriately to referral questions such as those asking about the client's potential for higher education or the impact of head trauma on the client's functioning. In the end, a well-written report includes all of this information and addresses the client's current functioning while responding to the referral question.

Psychopathology

Demographics

Deaf adults are affected by mental health problems, just as the rest of humankind is (e.g., du Feu & Chovaz, 2014; Estrada & Sleeboom-Van Raaij, 2015; Fellinger, Holzinger, & Pollard, 2012; Leigh & Pollard, 2011). Unfortunately there are few epidemiology studies. The information we have is based on extrapolations from incidence rates of mental illness for the general population combined with incidence data for all levels of hearing loss, not necessarily specifically for the Deaf or hard-of-hearing population (du Feu & Chovaz, 2014; Leigh & Pollard, 2011). It appears that rates are higher for deaf adults based on a review of several European-based studies (Fellinger et al., 2012), with at least one Norwegian study reporting rates more than double that for the general population (Kvam, Loeb, & Tambs, 2007). It is important to note that these rates are not due to deafness per se (Fellinger et al., 2012), considering the presence of many psychologically healthy deaf adults, but rather to risk factors such as environmental impact (psychological, social, or abuse) or biological/neurological vulnerability (most commonly nongenetic causes such as prematurity or intrauterine infections) (du Feu & Chovaz, 2014). Many of the affected deaf adults, previously termed *low functioning*, are dealing with language and learning challenges that can easily lead to behavioral and emotional disorders (Glickman, 2009).

Based on previous reviews of epidemiological studies and clinical observations, the general perception is that the prevalence rates for deaf adults with specific psychiatric diagnoses appear to be quite similar to those for hearing adults, particularly for psychotic disorders such as schizophrenia (Fellinger et al., 2012; Leigh & Pollard, 2011), although one study reports higher rates for their inpatient psychiatric population (Landsberger & Diaz, 2010). When deaf people experience formal thought disorders, this needs to be deciphered from their signs. Auditory hallucinations, most often described as "hearing voices," tend to be experienced more through language or "feeling" stimuli rather than sound stimuli (Paijmans, Cromwell, & Austen, 2006). There is a significantly higher diagnostic rate for impulse control disorders, learning disabilities, and pervasive developmental disorder, while the frequency for personality disorder diagnosis is lower (Fellinger et al., 2012; Landsberger & Diaz, 2010). There is a propensity towards endorsing more symptoms for anxiety and depression compared to the general population (Fellinger et al., 2012). Data regarding the prevalence of intellectual disabilities (formerly known as mental retardation) and neurological disorders such as dementia have varied from greater to less prevalence (Landsberger & Diaz, 2010; Leigh & Pollard, 2011). As for autism, the prevalence is significantly higher for deaf people compared to hearing individuals (Fellinger et al., 2012; see also Chapter 7). As a caveat, appropriate diagnosis depends on separating symptoms for autism from those due to hearing differences, especially language delay, socialization difficulties, or repetitive behaviors.

Interestingly, it appears that there is a restricted range of psychiatric diagnoses for deaf population samples, meaning that the less common psychiatric disorders were less frequently diagnosed (Leigh & Pollard, 2011). Additionally, deferred or missing diagnoses are likely to be more frequent. This is likely due to clinician error based on unfamiliarity with deaf clients as well as differences in the way these clients use mental health services. As mentioned earlier in the mental status examination section, experienced mental health clinicians who confront communication barriers with deaf clients are not as able to do thorough diagnostic interviews, even with sign language interpreters, unless they have some knowledge of how deaf people communicate and view the world. In the case of psychiatric disorders such as schizophrenia, a thorough understanding of deaf ways of communicating will facilitate the recognition of language atypicalities in the signing of deaf persons that can better ensure correct diagnoses (Leigh & Pollard, 2011).

Substance abuse rates reportedly are similar to that of the general population, if not higher, but appear to be lower in psychiatric settings (Fellinger et al., 2012). Risk factors include heightened stress levels, alienation from family, low self-esteem, limited peer support, and particularly trauma/victimization (Guthman, Sandberg, & Dickinson, 2010; Titus, 2009; 2010). A significant proportion of deaf and hard-of-hearing clients in the Minnesota Chemical Dependency Program for Deaf and Hard of Hearing Individuals, the best-known such program in the U.S., exhibits dual diagnoses of substance abuse and psychiatric conditions that make it easier to identify those in need of treatment, even though access to treatment continues to be difficult (see next section) (Guthman et al., 2010). Interestingly, the desire of the deaf community to present a positive image may mask the true level of substance abuse. This is also compounded by limited exposure to information, such as the lack of captioned televised public service announcements or inaccessible prevention curricula in mainstream education programs (Guthman et al., 2010).

Based on evidence suggesting that children with disabilities may be at higher risk for sexual abuse or child maltreatment (see Chapter 8), available information suggests that the incidence figures may be high for deaf persons in comparison to the general population. Deaf victimization that can result in long-term sequelae, such as physical, emotional, cognitive, and social consequences and includes physical and sexual abuse, neglect, emotional abuse, and communication isolation (Bishop, 2013; Sebald, 2008), particularly if the abuse is ongoing. A study by Schenkel (2010, as reported in Dube, 2011) found a direct correlation between childhood maltreatment and higher rates of negative cognition, depression, and posttraumatic stress in adulthood. Victimization histories of deaf and hard-of-hearing youth admitted to substance abuse treatment include more widespread and higher severity abuse compared to hearing peers, with deaf females reporting significantly greater prevalence of sexual and emotional abuse (Titus, 2009; 2010). Drinking and drug use may be used to reduce the stress of abuse or deal with difficulties in the environment.

Recent reports present sobering research evidence on physical assault, sexual coercion, sexual harassment, psychological abuse, and intimate partner violence against Deaf women, with prevalence rates generally exceeding that for hearing samples, even as much as twice the rates for hearing samples (e.g., Anderson, Leigh, & Samar, 2011; Barnett et al., 2011; McQuiller, Williams, & Porter, 2010). Victims will often experience significant psychological sequelae, including posttraumatic stress disorder, major depression, dissociative disorders, substance-related disorders, eating disorders, and borderline personality disorder (Barber, Wills, & Smith, 2010).

Service Delivery

Gournaris, Hamerdinger, and Williams (2013) estimate that, in the U.S., approximately 130,000 users of ASL will require mental health services, with 30,000 of this number dealing with severe mental illness. Historically, specialized mental health services for deaf persons were nonexistent before the 1950s (see Chapter 1 for details). Even though the percentage of deaf clients per se who actually receive mental health services continues to be a very low percentage of those in need of such services, perhaps as low as 3 percent (Raifman & Vernon, 1996), current levels of service have improved due to the increase in trained clinicians, as noted in Chapter 1. However, most services continue to be minimally available to this most underserved population in the U.S. and tend to be provided through ASL interpreters rather than directly with ASL-fluent clinicians despite the fact that there are issues of concern regarding interpreters, as noted earlier (Leigh & Pollard, 2011; National Association of the Deaf, 2008a). The number of inpatient units for Deaf patients has decreased to the single digits compared to previous years. Many deaf inpatient programs are now "integrated" into larger hearing programs with the use of sign language interpreters (M. J. Gournaris, personal communication, November 13, 2015). Gournaris also advises that, overall, there are fewer inpatient programs for hearing patients as well due to current emphasis on shorter length of stays in hospitals and the advancement of outpatient treatment. In view of historical evidence that deaf inpatients experience longer stays compared to hearing counterparts due in large part to insufficient community-based services, lack of staff who sign plus lack of 24/7 sign language interpreting (Fellinger et al., 2012; Trumbetta et al., 2001; Vernon & Daigle-King, 1999), this only serves to compound the problems deaf people have in accessing mental health services. Specialized group homes for deaf residents are also in short supply.

Although there are many mental health outpatient clinics, psychiatric services, and private practitioners advertising services for deaf clients, as indicated in *Mental Health Services for Deaf People: A Resource Directory, 5th edition* (2015), published by the Department of Counseling and the Gallaudet Research Institute, both at Gallaudet University, these are located mostly on the East and West coasts. Most areas continue to be underserved and accessibility to community mental health clinics serving local communities, including deaf communities, is limited. The National Association of the Deaf (2003) has a position paper covering standards of care that emphasize culturally affirmative approaches.

Pollard (1994) considers the use of small community mental health centers specializing in deaf clients to be discriminatory, even though they do provide valuable services. The valuable services provided in these specialized centers incorporate Deaf culturally affirmative approaches, with most of them attempting to follow practices such as those for mental health settings described in Gournaris, Hamerdinger, and Williams (2013) as well as those for Deaf residential treatment programs described in Glickman and Heines (2013). However, in contrast, the perception of discrimination is related in part to the fact that these clients are not referred to larger centers with more comprehensive services that are available to the general public, such as staff psychiatrists on site, or different programs that match individual treatment needs by offering different therapy options, including medication, various types of individual psychotherapy approaches family/group therapy, day treatment, and evening activities, to name a few. The low incidence of deaf persons makes it difficult for general mental health clinics to recognize the need for accommodations such as videophones to communicate directly with deaf clients. Cost factors complicate the use of sign language or spoken language interpreters.

Johannes Fellinger (2015) describes his concept of health centers for deaf people in Austria using a one-stop framework, one objective of which is to offer high-quality, specialized mental health services by trained providers. These centers are affiliated with general hospitals for more readily accessible medical services. He notes that focused and consumer-oriented health care reduces the numerous risk factors Deaf people have to cope with. This approach appears to counter the limitation of small community-based centers.

Outside the U.S., in countries such as Mexico, specialized mental health services for deaf people are almost nonexistent (Estrada, 2015). Estrada views this as a violation of the World Health Organization recommendation that approximately 10 percent of a national health budget be devoted to mental health, with Mexico at 2 percent and nothing allocated to deaf mental health services. García and Bravo (2015) note that such health laws that guarantee access to health services may exclude, discriminate against, or treat deaf people less favorably through lack of accessibility and accommodation.

Adult Deaf survivors of abuse (including domestic violence, sexual assault, and harassment) are no longer as "invisible" as they were in the past, thanks to the establishment of organizations such as ADWAS (Abused Deaf Women's Advocacy Services) in Seattle, Washington, and DAWN (Deaf Abused Women's Network) in Washington, DC. They provide services to help these women get back on their feet and gain some semblance of mental health. ADWAS, founded in 1986, has helped to establish 19 agencies for Deaf survivors across the country (Anderson, Leigh, & Samar, 2011). This is an illustration of how dire the situation has been for Deaf survivors.

Considering the substance abuse statistics for deaf and hard-of-hearing people mentioned earlier, substance abuse treatment facilities for Deaf people are woefully lacking. In fact, there has been a decrease in such facilities, primarily due to lack of funding and specialized staff (Guthman & Sternfeld, 2013). Mainstream facilities may provide interpreters, but the complex issues of substance abuse, mental health, cultural sensitivity, and limited access 24/7 make the efficacy of such programs subject to question. Current technology, such as videophones and online webcam meetings has improved the level of care.

Psychotherapy approaches include psychoanalysis, psychodynamic approaches, cognitive-behavioral therapy, dialectical behavior therapy, humanistic-oriented therapy, clinical hypnosis, and group therapy, among others. Being deaf does not preclude any of these approaches (Sussman & Brauer, 1999). It is crucial to recognize that to be culturally affirmative and empowering for individuals and families, therapeutic approaches must be matched to individual needs, sociocultural factors, and individual communication requirements, whether the person is deaf or hearing. Relying on medication alone, although tempting when there are communication problems, is not sufficient in most cases without psychotherapy to reinforce emotional self-regulation and more positive ways of functioning (e.g., Cuijpers et al., 2013). If medication is indicated, Sleeboom-Van Raaij (2015) emphasizes the need to understand the impact psychotropic medication may have on deaf patients, carefully assess these patients, and clearly communicate medication effects before prescribing such medications.

While the mental health field is increasingly focused on evidence-based practice (treatment approaches that are supported by research evidence and clinical expertise), research projects directed at evidence-based practice for deaf clients is sorely lacking. Clinicians have developed approaches that work with specific deaf populations based on experience (e.g., Glickman, 2013a).

Deaf adult perceptions of mental health service delivery can provide insight into areas in need of improvement. Steinberg, Loew, and Sullivan (2010) interviewed deaf adults about their beliefs and attitudes regarding mental health and found that communication issues were seen as central to mental health, with respondents recognizing that effective service delivery is facilitated when communication barriers are dealt with appropriately. Many do anticipate communication barriers and prefer signing mental health personnel for direct communication. However, respondents are generally willing to work with sign language interpreters but were concerned about the ways in which interpreters might convey information that would facilitate diagnosis and therapy. How these interpreters may affect the diagnosis, psychotherapy, and outcome continues to be a subject for investigation. The presence of a third party (the interpreter) in situations privy to confidentiality and emotions will alter psychotherapy dynamics (e.g., Harvey, 2003). When psychotherapists get training in how to handle interpreter influences during the course of psychotherapy, they can use these influences to facilitate the process of therapy. Additionally, specialist training in mental health interpreting will minimize the potential for misrepresenting the statements made by deaf adults.

Teletherapy or distance counseling using video for sessions is a promising new avenue that can facilitate services for Deaf clients in areas where accessible mental health services are few or nonexistent (Gournaris, Hamerdinger, & Williams, 2013). According to Gournaris (2009), there is increasing evidence to support the equivalency of video and face-to-face communication. A majority of Deaf clients using one Deaf-centered counseling practice report a strong preference for videophone sessions with Deaf counselors who "get" the Deaf experience over meeting in person with hearing clinicians and interpreters or even with hearing clinicians who sign (Whyte, Aubrecht, McCullough, Lewis, & Thompson-Ochoa, 2013). Gournaris (2009) has reported on appropriate provider procedures, including informed consent and practicing within state regulations, which vary from state to state.

Diversity Issues

Because of immigration and the increasing multicultural nature of the deaf population in the U.S., mental health service delivery to deaf persons must take the ethnic dimension into account. Pollard (1994) has documented that deaf persons who have received public mental health services are less likely than hearing persons to be from racial/ethnic minority groups. Whether this continues to be true today in view of current U.S. multicultural demographics remains to be seen. In any case, the lack of cultural sensitivity and the presence of racism, either conscious or unconscious, on the part of service providers as well as the negative implications of being labeled as one in need of mental health services detracts from the feeling of safety and support that mental health professionals would like to convey to clients (Corbett, 2010).

Professionals should examine their racial psychohistory in order to understand their attitudes toward their own and other race/ethnic groups (Corbett, 2010). This will help them to work productively with deaf persons of diverse cultural backgrounds. Such a process represents the first step toward cultural sensitivity and, in turn, cultural competence. Cultural competence includes awareness, not only of Deaf culture, but also the deaf person's culture of origin as well as the multiple identity aspects of that person, in order to provide culturally appropriate mental health treatment.

Specifics on treating African Americans, Asian Americans, Latinx, and American Indians can be found in Leigh's (2010) *Psychotherapy with Deaf Clients from Diverse Groups*. This book additionally addresses aspects of diversity other than race and ethnicity. Diversity also encompasses those deaf adults who are DeafBlind; elderly; in college; gays, lesbians, bisexual, transgender, or questioning; abuse survivors; substance abuse users; and a myriad of additional identity categories such as, for example, deaf adults who use spoken language, deaf adults with cochlear implants, and gender. Each of these groups has unique issues in addition to being deaf, thus emphasizing intersectionalities that clinicians need to be attuned to. It is a tall order for mental health clinicians to be sensitive to each of these aspects of diversity, but this is necessary for culturally affirmative service delivery.

Conclusions

Deaf adults run the gamut from those who are psychologically healthy, with positive self-perceptions and strong identities, to those who struggle with psychopathology. Instead of focusing on a deficit model, the current stance is to identify the strengths of those individuals and their ability to manage in a complex world, while taking into account areas where they need support or help. As noted in Chapter 1, mental health, psychology, and research training programs specializing in deaf populations are now graduating professionals who are well prepared to advance the understanding of the psychological makeup of deaf adults and improve service delivery to this group. This understanding will be enhanced by the addition of researchers who are deaf and trained to critically examine the ways in which psychological constructs are applied to deaf populations. It will be a long time, however, before there is a decrease in the urgent need for these professionals.

Suggested Readings

The books listed here provide overviews of mental health, psychotherapy, cognition, deaf identities, and resilience as indicated by their titles.

du Feu, M., & Chovaz, C. (2014). *Mental health and deafness*. New York, NY: Oxford.

Estrada, A. B., & Sleeboom-Van Raaij (Eds.). (2015). *Mental health services for deaf people*. Washington, DC: Gallaudet University Press. (*International focus*)

Glickman, N. (Ed.). (2013). *Deaf mental health care*. New York, NY: Routledge

Leigh, I. W. (2009). *A lens on deaf identities*. New York, NY: Oxford.

Leigh, I. W. (Ed.). (2010). *Psychotherapy with deaf clients from diverse groups*. Washington, DC: Gallaudet University Press.

Marschark, M., & Hauser, P. (2008). *Deaf cognition*. New York, NY: Oxford.

Zand, D., & Pierce, K. (Eds.). (2011). *Resilience in deaf children: Adaptation through emerging adulthood*. New York, NY: Springer.

9 Deaf Adults
Viewpoints from Sociology

[T]o be deaf is to stand at multiple intersections of language, culture, disability, society, politics, ethics, and the body.

Young and Temple (2014, p. 2)

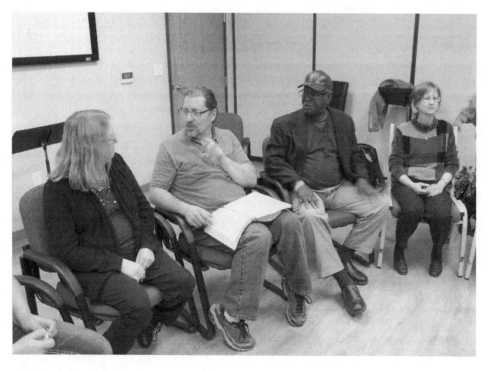

Figure 9.1 Photo of group of people signing
Source: Used with permission.

How do deaf people live their lives as part of a larger society? Their collective consciousness and broadly shared understandings have served as a basis for their coming together as a sociological entity, even taking into account the heterogeneity of this group. Communities of deaf people have been documented since at least the 1700s (Van Cleve & Crouch, 1989) and probably earlier. When deaf persons come together, they do not necessarily feel weighted down by inadequacy. Rather, throughout time, they have been able to internalize a dynamic sense of identity and comfort in themselves as a minority group with their own traditions and organizations. The 1988 Deaf President Now movement (see Chapter 1) highlighted the coming of age of the deaf community as a proud sociopolitical entity (Christiansen & Barnartt, 1995).

Chapter Objectives

This chapter briefly outlines sociological perspectives of the deaf community. It explores the role of the Deaf President Now movement in influencing the deaf community's sociopolitical evolution. The chapter then presents information on different groups of deaf people, various deaf organizations, their roles in the lives of deaf people, and the political context for some of these organizations. It is important to recognize that the deaf community, as a microcosm of society at large, is not immune to sociocultural and technological changes. Those will be described as the text looks at deaf clubs and other avenues for socialization, deaf venues for athletic and religious activities, the influence of technology, and employment and health care issues.

Sociological Perspectives of the Deaf Community

Sociology involves the study of how humans interact and the evolving values and ideas that form the basis of these interactions. Both the medical/disability and sociolinguistic models (see Chapter 2) have sociological elements that shape the self-perceptions of groups of people.

Within the medical model, the sociological implication is that the deaf person needs to accommodate to the larger hearing society in the interest of *better* social relationships with hearing peers. This requires changing the nature of the hearing loss by altering or minimizing it through the use of speech lessons, auditory training, and technology assistance such as hearing aids, cochlear implants, and other listening devices. This model reinforces the concept that deaf individuals (or individuals with disabilities) rely on professional authorities with the goal of creating a pathway to some sort of recovery or amelioration of the disabling condition. This is part of a larger framework in which these authorities sometimes impose a benevolent paternalism (tendency to protect) on those who differ, do not fit society's expectations, or who appear unable to fend for themselves (Lane, 1999). According to Lane, when professionals with vested interests take on the mantle of paternalism, it becomes very difficult for deaf persons to throw off this paternalistic shield and take charge of their own lives. Sociologically, this creates the notion that the deaf person who "overcomes" deafness is more acceptable in society. However, to give the medical model its due, there are many deaf individuals who use professional help well and function very independently in hearing society with effective compensatory tools, even when they or those around them perceive being deaf as a significant disability that entails struggling at times (e.g., Christiansen, 2010; McDonald, 2014; Reisler, 2002).

In exploring the sociopolitical implications of disability definitions, activists are challenging the notion that disability is an individual problem (see Albrecht, Seelman, & Bury, 2001; Swain, French, Barnes, & Thomas, 2005, for reviews). From their perspectives, society's typically negative attitude toward people with disabilities and its failure to accommodate them by enhancing environmental access has created the problem of disability. Sociologically, instead of welcoming individuals with disabilities as individuals with different notions of environmental access, society generally sees them as problems. In other words, Olkin (1999) writes that people without disabilities cite physical limitations as major problems for people with disabilities, whereas people with disabilities themselves tend to focus on social barriers and negative attitudes.

In the case of culturally Deaf people, being Deaf has very little to do with one's ears. For these individuals, being Deaf means enhancing visual access and relocating the limits and barriers from inside the body to outside the body and the public sphere (Humphries, 2014). If society cooperates in enhancing visual access, social barriers will then be eliminated. Since deaf persons know what they need in order to manage daily lives, it is they, not the professionals who "serve" them, who are the ultimate authorities on their needs. (See Chapter 11 for additional discussion.)

For these reasons, many deaf people see themselves as a minority group, struggling to gain equal opportunity with nondisabled citizens. Increasingly, this group is defined more as a sociolinguistic group of people who are culturally Deaf and less as individuals with disabilities. Through their language, cultural traditions, and organizations, they have coalesced into a community of people, many of whom see being deaf as part of the spectrum of diversity. Together with other deaf and hard-of-hearing people who do not identify with Deaf culture, they have created social and political momentum in critical arenas with the goal of obtaining social justice. For example, they work together to fight for parity in civil rights, access to optimal educational environments for deaf children, upward mobility in employment, and communication access (including interpreter services, functional equivalence in access to telecommunication, etc.). The implications of the 1988 Deaf President Now (DPN) movement go beyond the recognition that a deaf person could successfully take the helm of Gallaudet University (Greenwald, 2014; Humphries, 2014).

Deaf President Now: Implications for the Deaf Community

During the 1988 DPN movement at Gallaudet University, the only liberal arts university for deaf students, the Board of Trustees' choice of a hearing rather than a deaf candidate to head Gallaudet sparked a campuswide uprising against what appeared to be a prejudice on the part of the Board. Those who participated in the uprising wanted to validate the inherent capabilities of qualified deaf candidates as a means of counteracting the traditionally low expectations held of them by hearing decision-makers (Christiansen & Barnartt, 1995). Their collective action took the needs of deaf people out of the disability framework and reframed these as a civil rights issue (Armstrong, 2014). Nationally and internationally, this event was widely publicized by the media.

The ability of deaf persons, both within Gallaudet University and throughout the nation, to get information, communicate with each other and the media, and collaborate as a community during this movement was enhanced by demographic, social, and technological influences (Christiansen & Barnartt, 1995). The 1964–1965 rubella epidemic swelled the ranks of deaf people. Sign language interpreting changed from the stop-gap measure of using family members or friends to a professional service (see Chapter 11 for further details). Legislation directed at improving access emerged, as discussed later. This allowed deaf people the opportunity to understand and participate when interacting with hearing persons in schools, on the job, and with medical and other service providers. Technology, too, played a prominent role. In the 1970s and 1980s, television captioning drastically increased the amount of information deaf people could access (this was before the Internet age). Deaf people were more directly exposed to media portrayals of groups fighting for self-determination. This heightened their sense of unfair treatment and oppression when being continually passed over for increased employment and policy-making responsibilities. Additionally, at that time, instantaneous communication was finally possible due to the proliferation of text telephones (TTYs), which provided deaf people with access to telephone communication (Peltz Strauss, 2006). Previously, the major means of communication had been via face-to-face and postal contact.

Through widespread media publicity, DPN awoke the nation and the world to the existence of a vibrant deaf community and increased the awareness of U.S. society regarding the needs of deaf people. As Jankowski (1997, p. 131) states, "Indeed, for Deaf people, a victory meant the creating of a new image. A new vision for Deaf people and the world watching them was that, indeed, Deaf people 'can.'" This translated into more positive self-images and increased feelings of empowerment.

The political involvement of deaf people began in the late 1800s, when the National Association of the Deaf (NAD) was organized (Armstrong, 2014; Van Cleve & Crouch, 1989). There were intermittent periods of effective political activity, but after DPN, the political acumen and strengths build up by the NAD and other deaf organizations came of age as more deaf people learned to capitalize on the political process to campaign for a variety of goals and objectives. More frequently, they engaged in political action (Humphries, 2014). Various protests were held to emphasize the need for additional deaf administrators, teachers, and staff at residential schools throughout the country, to defend ASL usage, to lobby for the use of deaf instead of hearing actors for deaf roles in films, and to fight for emergency information captioning on TV stations (Christiansen & Barnartt, 1995; Jankowski, 1997). Deaf groups gained more influence in shaping social policy to incorporate barrier-free environments, most notably with reference to the Americans with Disabilities Act of 1990 and the Telecommunications Act of 1996, among others. Deaf groups have advocated for states to set up systems of social services or community service agencies, and in some states and countries, they have gained official government recognition of ASL or their local sign languages (Humphries, 2014).

Sociopolitically, in the eyes of deaf people, the most important thing about these laws (which legislated different types of accommodations) is that society acknowledges their right to the various types of access enjoyed by the majority society. Now, legislators and others are more willing to work politically both with deaf organizations and with organizations of people with disabilities. For example, in order to win support from both the deaf community and groups of people with disabilities, sponsors of the Telecommunications Act of 1996 agreed that provisions mandating the accessibility of telecommunications for all people with disabilities would be included in the act (A. Sonnenstrahl, personal communication, November 16, 2015; see also Peltz Strauss, 2006 for details). As Humphries (2014) writes, "DPN seems to have awoken a community used to acquiescence and propelled its members into action. The legacy of DPN is still felt whenever the Deaf community believes it must act to gain the equity it craves" (p. 68). This applies not only in the U.S. but also internationally (Druchen, 2014). For example, Druchen writes that in South Africa, DPN galvanized Deaf people to work on gaining civil rights for themselves, including the recognition of South African Sign Language as the official language of Deaf South Africans and having the South African Council for the Deaf run by Deaf people instead of hearing people.

Yes, progress is being made. However, the struggle continues. Mandating accommodations does not necessarily guarantee their implementation. Architectural accommodations for individuals with mobility disabilities involve a one-time cost, but communication accessibility requires ongoing economic support (e.g., Task Force on Health Care Careers for the Deaf and Hard-of-Hearing Community, 2012). This becomes a disincentive that can easily engender "hidden discrimination" for Deaf people applying for jobs. Proving that it exists is no easy task. The amount of money devoted to attempts to "eliminate" hearing loss remains greater than the amount spent to ensure equal access for deaf persons. For example, more funds are directed toward a cure for deafness than toward enhancing accessibility of 9-1-1 emergency centers for deaf persons. It took years until wireless carriers in the U.S. agreed to implement a nationwide, interim text-to-9-1-1 solution by May, 2014, pursuant to the passing of The Twenty-First Century Communication and Video Accessibility Act of 2010 (www.apcointl.org/resources/next-generation-communications-systems/text-to-9-1-1.html). This act updates federal communications laws to increase access of persons with disabilities to twenty-first-century technologies (www.fcc.gov/guides/21st-century-communications-and-video-accessibility-act-2010). Within the framework of universal access, when finalized, this will be a boon not only for deaf people, but also for hearing people caught in violent situations when it is not advisable or possible to make voice calls to 9-1-1.

At the time of this writing, the Deaf community in Milton, Ontario (Canada), was protesting the selection of a hearing superintendent at a local school for the deaf and stating that no deaf people were on the panel selecting candidates (Stevenson, 2015). It has been suggested that revealing a disability in an interview should be avoided if possible and should not be mentioned on a résumé (Bouton, 2013). Because of cost factors, medical settings have often limited the hiring of sign language interpreters for deaf patients seeking medical consultation, ADA provisions notwithstanding (Interpreting in Health Care Settings, 2015). Deaf patients have continually instigated complaints and lawsuits in order to remedy the lack of equal access in hospital settings, most of which have been decided in their favor. The critical point to be made is that deaf people are advocating for themselves in ways not seen prior to DPN.

The deaf community that instigated the 1988 DPN movement had a largely White face. There were no African American deaf leaders, even though Washington, DC, (where Gallaudet University is located), has a large African American community. Many minority deaf people and their leaders did not perceive themselves to be a significant part of this historic movement. However, the infusion of multiculturalism into the deaf community in recent years, fueled by the increase of multicultural students in settings where deaf children and youth are educated (Gallaudet Research Institute, 2013), has reinforced the need to acknowledge diversity in the deaf community. The publication of books such as *Sounds Like Home: Growing Up Black and Deaf in the South* (Wright, 1999); *Psychotherapy with Deaf Clients from Diverse Groups* (Leigh, 2010); *Still I Rise* (Anderson, 2006); *Moment of Truth* (Lang, Cohen, & Fischgrund, 2008); *Signing in Puerto Rican* (Torres, 2009); and *Deaf in D.C.* (Vasishta, 2011), as well as various chapters on multiculturalism in deaf-related texts show that the deaf community is changing, as American society is changing. The empowerment message emerging from the DPN protest now involves multicultural deaf individuals. Dr. Glenn Anderson, a prominent African American Deaf leader, became Chair of the Gallaudet University Board of Trustees after the resignation of Phil Bravin, a well-known deaf community member who was the first deaf post-DPN Chair. Dr. Robert Davila, of Mexican origin, was Assistant Secretary for the Office of Special Education and Rehabilitative Services in the U.S Department of Education before becoming Gallaudet University's 9th president. Claudia Gordon is the first Deaf female African American attorney in the U.S.; she presently works in the U.S. Department of Labor's Office of Federal Contract Compliance Programs. And the list continues.

Deaf Organizations

The commonality of being deaf does not override the pluralism of U.S. society, which is also reflected within the deaf community (Leigh, 2009; 2012). Existing groups of deaf people have different interests and different goals, various communication beliefs and cultural backgrounds, and multiple understandings of how to be deaf. We now provide brief descriptions of some of the major deaf organizations that have shaped the nature of the deaf community and highlight how these have contributed to quality of life. These organizations have united for common causes but have gone their separate ways when consensus fails. Many of them are connected with local chapters or groups.

- In 1880, the National Association of the Deaf (NAD, www.nad.org), the oldest organization in the U.S. founded and run by people with disabilities, came into being (Van Cleve & Crouch, 1989). At that time, the goal of the NAD was to bring deaf people throughout the U.S. together to deliberate on their needs and advocate for basic rights. Today, it is a civil rights organization with a national board and affiliates that are state associations of the deaf. As a nonprofit federation, its mission is to preserve, protect, and promote the civil, human, and linguistic rights of deaf and hard-of-hearing Americans. Politically, its ability to advocate successfully throughout the years is a reflection of the empowerment Deaf people have experienced as a result of DPN and the ADA of 1990 (see earlier in this chapter and Chapter 1). Currently, the NAD works on the federal level to ensure that the accessibility and civil rights of deaf and hard-of-hearing persons are safeguarded. It advocates for the educational, vocational, legal, and social concerns of its deaf constituents. Its website (www.nad.org) and *NADmag* publication have reported on a wide range of issues that the organization has been involved with, such as social justice, educational policy, telecommunications access, emergency warning systems, senior resources, health care, sign language interpreter certification, access to quality sign language services, fairness in employment, and the changing nature of vocational rehabilitation services. The NAD founded the National Center for Law and Deafness, now known as the NAD Law and Advocacy Center, in 1976, and hired its first attorney in 1977 (National Association of the Deaf, 2015). The NAD Law and Advocacy Center provides legal advocacy, assistance, and education related to the rights of deaf people. To achieve its political goals, the NAD works closely with both state and national deaf and disability organizations and coalitions. Its membership base was historically White male. It is now shifting to a more diverse base that reflects U.S. demographics; this can be seen both at the board level and in outreach work. There is also a youth division, the Jr. NAD, which uses leadership training activities in different venues, including the highly successful four-week-long NAD Youth Leadership Camp for deaf and hard-of-hearing high school students, with the goal of focusing on self-determination, sense of community, and thirst for knowledge to encourage the development of new Deaf leaders among young deaf students from both residential and mainstream programs.

- On the international front, the NAD is affiliated with the World Federation of the Deaf (WFD, www.wdeaf.org; Rosen, 2009), which is made up of associations of deaf people from all over the world that contribute to the enhancement of cultural, social, and economic status of deaf persons. It is one of the oldest international organizations dedicated to advocacy of, for, by, and with Deaf people. The WFD was established in 1951 with the goal of increasing global cooperation and currently represents approximately 70 million Deaf people, 80 percent of whom are in developing countries. Its primary mission is to ensure the human rights of Deaf people in every aspect of life, including the right to their sign language and education. It has consultation status with the United Nations and holds international congresses every 4 years. See the Deaf International Connections section for additional details.

- State associations of the deaf carry on political activities to ensure that legislation and services are favorable for deaf people. For example, a number of these associations have worked to establish permanent state offices or commissions to serve deaf and hard-of-hearing citizens who require better access to state programs and services, to improve television captioning, and to institute local emergency warning systems. These associations started off by keeping deaf people within each state linked as a social community and then branched off into advocacy. Opportunities for political action are often combined with social events at biennial conferences.

- The Alexander Graham Bell Association for the Deaf and Hard of Hearing (AGB, www.agbell.org) is an organization devoted to the support of listening and spoken language for parents and the provision of training for professionals. AGB provides educational resources, advocacy, and career development for its members. It used to have a deaf and hard of hearing section for deaf adults who use spoken language, in addition to a professional and a parent section. These sections were recently disbanded in favor of a more cohesive organization where all members intermingle. AGB is part of several coalitions, of which the NAD is also a part, devoted to shaping public policy, including policies related to early intervention, reauthorization of IDEA (see Chapter 5) and improved movie theater access. As of this writing, deaf AGB members and other deaf individuals have banded together to file a class-action lawsuit against studios that do not caption song lyrics in major movies and TV shows, including those in which the dialog is captioned. One of AGB's most successful programs is the Leadership Opportunities for Teens (LOFT), a four-day sleep-away program geared towards high school teens who primarily use listening and spoken language. The LOFT goal is to develop or strengthen skills in individual leadership, teamwork, group dynamics, public speaking, and self-advocacy. Participants are often the only deaf students in their mainstream schools and have gained immeasurable benefit from sharing their experiences with peers and gaining advocacy skills. Although this organization is historically seen as opposed to the use of sign language for educational purposes, it has a position statement on ASL that recognizes its importance in Deaf culture and supports parent choice regarding language or communication method.

Specialized Organizations

In recent decades, a number of organizations have emerged in response to specific needs expressed by diverse groups of deaf people, reflecting different constituencies, different life issues, and different goals, paralleling what happens in the hearing community. This attests to the commonality of social interaction processes and the push toward banding together for similar purposes within deaf and hearing communities. The following is a description of some of those specialized organizations, most of which also have local chapters or associations.

- People deafened after childhood banded together in 1987 to form the Association of Late-Deafened Adults (ALDA, www.alda.org). It enables members who are seeking a community that understands what it means to lose hearing later in life to band together and "find a family." In addition to encouraging a sense of community, the ALDA's mission is to support the empowerment of late-deafened people by serving their needs through support, education, and advocacy activities for legislation related to, for example, captioned media, telecommunication and relay services, and job accommodations. It holds annual conventions where attendees can hang loose about their communication issues and use whatever works. Its website includes testimonies from ALDA presidents about what it means to become deaf and how ALDA has helped them feel connected. There is also an Internet organization for people dealing with hearing issues called the SayWhatClub (www.saywhatclub.com) that is dedicated to helping those who are deafened, hard of hearing, or have an interest in hearing issues to communicate with each other, share coping and "life" skills, reduce feelings of despair and isolation, and enhance self-concept and optimism. This provides one way for individuals to learn about the ALDA.
- The World Federation of the DeafBlind (www.wfdb.eu) was formally organized in 2001 with a focus on improving the quality of life for DeafBlind people and the services they need worldwide. It has links to DeafBlind organizations around the world. Delegates get together at general assemblies in conjunction with Helen Keller World Conferences every few years. Enabling DeafBlind members to be full participants requires the presence of tactile interpreters and guides or SSPs (Support Service Providers), who provide access in the environment and help them make logistical decisions. The American Association of the DeafBlind (AADB) was a U.S. consumer advocacy organization devoted to encourage independent living for its DeafBlind members. Unfortunately, as of this writing, it

is moribund due to lack of personpower and funding. There is technology that enables DeafBlind individuals to connect with each other (see brief description in the Technology section below).

- Deaf Seniors of America (DSA, www.deafseniorsofamerica.org) reflects the presence of a large group of deaf seniors, paralleling the increasing number of Americans who are elderly. They need support in dealing with aging issues, similarly to their hearing peers, and want to know more about issues such as dementia, retirement savings, communication access in assisted living and nursing homes, and so on. Many seniors look forward to socializing and learning at DSA biennial conventions, where DSA performs its mission of providing seminars dealing with issues impacting their well-being and safety and informing members about advocacy efforts and national, state, and local resources to improve their participation in deaf and mainstream societies. Current plans include joining with the NAD to ensure national attention is paid to senior citizen needs such as accessible technology, emergency access, and the establishment of accessible senior citizen housing focused on ASL users. It is largely composed of White Deaf individuals. See the following for commentary regarding the formation of ethnic groups.
- Deaf Women United (DWU, www.dwu.org) is an organization of, by, and for Deaf women. It functions as a system of communal support that also provides information and training in the areas of organizational management, personal growth, and empowerment. Deaf women are unique to the extent that they encounter double discrimination and oppression based on gender and being deaf (Barnartt, 2006; Wax, 2010). Barnartt suggests that gender takes precedence over being deaf as the "master" status, meaning that being a woman may create more negative consequences in life compared to being deaf, at least for educational attainment and occupational status. DWU endeavors to affirm these deaf women's experiences in a positive light. It is involved in advocacy, education, and outreach to ensure that gender and access issues do not deprive deaf women of the opportunities available to others. Biennial conferences provide a platform for deaf women to network and provide support. This is an organization that redresses the historical neglect of the contributions Deaf women have made in advancing sensitivity to the interface of gender and Deaf with its recounting of their accomplishments. DWU also has an annual Youth Interchange program for Deaf girls to network and attend workshops to get ideas on implementing social change in their community and to develop confidence and personal growth.
- Hearing Loss Association of America (HLAA, www.hearingloss.org; formerly known as SHHH) defines itself as a consumer and advocacy organization that focuses on consumers with hearing loss. It aims to counteract the effects of untreated hearing loss that has the potential of impacting one's overall health and quality of life, sometimes leading to social isolation and depression. Its members tend to be primarily individuals who do not see themselves as part of the Deaf community. The HLAA's mission is to open the world of communication through education, information, support, and advocacy. It aims to provide assistance and resources for these individuals and their families to adjust to lives with hearing loss, eradicate the stigma associated with hearing loss, and raise public awareness about the need for prevention, treatment, and ongoing hearing screenings throughout life. The areas of communication access, public policy, research, and service delivery related to hearing loss are prime targets for their advocacy efforts. The HLAA collaborates with deaf organizations when common goals such as telecommunications access are identified. It provides chat forums and annual conventions to bring members together.
- Rainbow Alliance of the Deaf (RAD, www.deafrad.org) is a national organization established in 1977 that focuses on the educational, economical, and social welfare of deaf GLBTQ (gay, lesbian, bisexual, transgender, and questioning) individuals. These

individuals will often struggle with the coming-out process and self-acceptance as rites of passage (Gutman & Zangas, 2010; Leigh, 2012). They also need to navigate the worlds of hearing people, heterosexuality, work, differing ethnic communities, and GLBTQ communities. Each setting represents differing contexts for discrimination or acceptance, particularly in areas where heterosexuality is seen as the norm (Gutman & Zangas, 2010). Several research studies support the possibility that Deaf community traditions of cohesiveness, openness, strong interpersonal connections, and GLBTQ visibility may create more positive attitudes compared to hearing communities in general (see Leigh, 2012, for a brief review). Support such as that provided by RAD facilitates the acquisition of skills needed to manage the situations and issues that may emerge in these different settings. The organization fosters fellowship opportunities through biennial conferences, which enable members to discuss solutions to problems related to social and legal issues. Some major metropolitan areas also have deaf GLBTQ communities that facilitate networking and social support (Gutman & Zangas, 2010). The website http://planet.deafqueer.com provides up-to-date information on events, advocacy, and education for deaf GLBTQ individuals.

- TDI (www.tdiforaccess.org), formerly known as Telecommunications for the Deaf, Inc., appeared on the scene in 1968 when deaf members of AGB and NAD joined forces to contribute and service teletypewriters for deaf people (Peltz Strauss, 2006). Members of the deaf community volunteered to condition and distribute the first machines. Since then, TDI has evolved into a national advocacy organization that promotes equal access to entertainment, media, information technology, emergency preparedness, and telecommunications through education, networking, collaboration, advocacy, and national policy development. In this capacity, TDI has been politically active in collaborating with various organizations and coalitions to push for legislation and regulations with various federal agencies. TDI disseminates information via the Internet about up-to-date news and action alerts and holds biennial conferences for networking and policy review purposes.

Ethnic Deaf Groups

Ethnic groups emerged as the deaf community became more diverse and as deaf people of different ethnic origins sought each other out. For example, deaf African Americans established their own social clubs and sports teams even though similar clubs for deaf people were nearby (Burch, 2002; Jankowski, 1997). This reflects their "unseen" status, with exclusion from all-White deaf schools due to segregation before the historic *Brown v. Board of Education of Topeka* Supreme Court decision to end legal segregation in public schools, as well as from Deaf-sponsored recreational activities, based on lack of connections with Deaf peers, all of which illustrates the pervasive influence of White skin privilege and experiences of discrimination (Corbett, 2010). Many Deaf individuals of color experienced racism, both overt and subtle, and exclusion from the dominant White Deaf society despite the common bond that being deaf implies (e.g., Leigh, 2012). Based on these experiences, Black Deaf individuals often view themselves as being part of a Black Deaf culture distinct from the White Deaf and Black hearing cultures, with its own standard ways of relating and its Black ASL. The linguistics of Black ASL as a dialect of ASL is now beginning to be studied extensively (McCaskill, Lucas, Bailey, & Hill, 2011; Ogunyipe, n.d.).

Because people with common ethnic origins tend to bond together and affirm their unique cultural heritages, local and statewide groups were formed. The next logical step was to establish national organizations. It is important to consider the fact that such organizations encompass individuals with multiple heritages and countries of origin. For example, Black Deaf individuals may consider themselves to be African American, African, or Caribbean, each of which may reflect unique cultural heritages and differences. Deaf Latinx and Deaf Asian Americans count multiple countries with their own unique heritages and languages, including sign languages, as part of their background, while Deaf Native Americans/American Indians collectively are from multiple tribes, each of which has their own language and cultural traditions.

- National Black Deaf Advocates (www.nbda.org), founded in 1982, was the first ethnic entity to appear on the scene. It was created partially in response to the NAD's reluctance to address the concerns of the Black Deaf community and is the leading Black Deaf organization in the U.S., with 30 chapters in its fold. Its goal was to create role models and a vision of success for Black Deaf youth in the process of empowering this group, as based on its mission to promote leadership development, economic and educational opportunities, social equality, and safeguard general health and welfare. It is involved with advocacy efforts to ensure civil rights and equal access to education, employment, and social services for Black Deaf and hard-of-hearing individuals. There is also a Black Deaf Senior Citizen program to support the unique needs, concerns, and challenges faced by this group, as well as the Collegiate Black Deaf Student Leadership Institute, which provides intensive one week leadership training opportunities for minority college students, and the Youth Empowerment Summit, which offers one week leadership training and challenging activities for Black Deaf and hard-of-hearing youth in mainstreamed, home schooled, and deaf institutions.
- National Asian Deaf Congress (www.nadcusa.org) was established in 1997 as part of its second National Deaf Asian Congress. It has as its goals empowerment, leadership skills development, and dissemination of resource information while also recognizing and preserving Asian Deaf cultural heritage, identity, and history for Asian American Deaf people. Because the Asian American and Deaf population is small in comparison with the African American Deaf and Latinx Deaf populations, it is not common to find an Asian American Deaf cultural group to identify with except in a few large urban settings (Wu & Grant, 2010). For this reason, it is typical for members who represent multiple Asian countries to interact and bond with each other, as they do in biennial conferences and chapters/affiliates. As its website states, it is strengthened by the diversity of its members who represent various geographic regions, languages, religions, cultures, and generations.
- Sacred Circle (www.deafnative.com) is an offshoot of the earlier Intertribal Deaf Council, founded in 1994 with the goal of carrying out traditions and cultures of Native American Deaf people and improving the appreciation of these cultures on the part of members and the public at large. It provides education, information, and training about American Indians, Alaska Natives and First Nations Indians who are Deaf, DeafBlind, hard-of-hearing, and late deafened to tribal councils and interested parties in order to improve the social, educational, vocational, health, and spiritual well-being of this population. These individuals will often have tenuous connections with their communities of origin depending on their level of communication and integration within their hearing families (Eldredge, 2010). Being educated in schools for the deaf strengthens their connection with the majority White Deaf culture but weakens their tribal connections. Organizations such as Sacred Council and Deafatives (www.deafatives.com) foster their ability to take pride in their ethnic heritage.
- National Council of Hispano Deaf and Hard of Hearing does not have an active website but has recently hosted biennial conferences. There are local organizations such as the Latino Deaf and Hard of Hearing Association of the Metropolitan DC Area, Inc., (www.ldhhamdc.org), which was founded in 2005 and provides opportunities for networking and advocacy for equal access, similarly to the NBDA. Again, the Hispanic/Latinx Deaf population is a mixture of individuals from diverse Central and South American countries, and

as such represents a significant component of diversity. Nonetheless, they also face the commonality of discrimination and language barriers due to the nature of their experiences in emigrating to the U.S. and living in various U.S. communities.

Religious Groups

Religious interest in deaf people goes back to the time of the Old and New Testaments and includes the possibility that there may have been a deaf community in Athens as far back as the fifth century BC (Bauman, 2008a; Van Cleve & Crouch, 1989). Starting with Spanish Catholic monks in the 1500s, and in succeeding centuries proceeding to European and American Protestant clergy, a major motivation for establishing educational programs was to provide deaf students with access to religion and redemption (Van Cleve & Crouch, 1989). During the 1800s and well into the 1900s, residential school administrators required chapel services and religious classes for their deaf students (Burch, 2002). These services, often run by deaf ministers, were usually conducted in sign language, which was viewed as a means of direct access to religious doctrine for deaf people who had been created by God. Deaf religious leaders, including Catholic priests, Jewish rabbis, and Protestant ministers, have been trained to take their place along with hearing religious leaders, including imams, in organizing religious-based events and services. A search on the Internet indicates that Deaf religious centers are scattered throughout the U.S. National religious organizations such as the Lutheran Church Deaf Mission Society, United Methodist Congress of the Deaf, Deaf Ministries, International Catholic Deaf Association-U.S. Section, Jewish Deaf Congress, Chabad, and Global Deaf Muslim collaborate with local religious settings and organizations to serve Deaf people. According to Burch (2002), such deaf religious organizations reinforce a sense of normality parallel with hearing religious offerings and simultaneously afford deaf congregants a unique sense of identity. With the influx of immigrants, the deaf community is now taking notice of deaf members who follow Buddhism, Hinduism, Islam, and other religions that are now taking root in the U.S.

Religion cannot be divorced from spirituality. While religion is typically perceived as related to organized movements, spirituality refers more to feelings based on based on private prayer, meditation, quiet reflection, and yoga, although some do see spirituality as tied to organized religion (Psychology Today, 2015). Nonetheless, there is a dearth of research on spirituality in the Deaf community (Delich, 2014). Spirituality is seen as important in one's sense of purpose and self-awareness. For example, an interview study involving 14 African American parents raising deaf children indicated that their relationship with God through the use of spirituality was a powerful source of support and hope (Borum, 2008). There are Deaf groups that band together to connect with their spiritual selves. A phenomenological interview study of five American Indian Deaf women suggested that a healthy sense of balance in mental, emotional, physical, and spiritual aspects led to their development as leaders (Paris, 2012).

Deaf Clubs

Deaf people have maintained contact through national, regional, and state organizations, but it was the Deaf clubs throughout the U.S. that historically formed the mainstay of local Deaf communities (Lane, Hoffmeister, & Bahan, 1996). Those clubs provided opportunities for Deaf friends to continue socializing after they had left the environs of residential schools. Not only did the clubs provide opportunities for activities that encourage interaction, such as dances, celebrations, sports, events, workshops, and so on, they also provided a means for the transmission of Deaf culture, customs, history, and worldviews. At these clubs, Deaf members served as mentors and educators as they welcomed young members. These clubs also created supportive environments, or a safe haven without the communication barriers that typically existed beyond the club settings. These clubs were also separated by race, with Black Deaf clubs coexisting with White Deaf clubs (Padden, 2008).

An obvious explanation for the decline of Deaf clubs is that the advent of television captioning and the Internet, as well as accessible telecommunication devices, including smartphones and videophones, seems to have created less of a need for Deaf clubs, with deaf persons no longer strongly feeling the need to convene in Deaf clubs to maintain the sense of community (Padden, 2008). However, Padden presents evidence indicating that the decline began even before new technology took off. When Deaf people were predominately in mundane, repetitive factory jobs, they needed a place to socialize outside of work. With the changes from manufacturing to service industries and the movement towards more expanded work opportunities, the need to find a centralized place to meet lessened. Deaf people began splitting off into professional associations (e.g., teacher associations, mental health associations) or groupings based on race, class, gender, and ethnicity. Consequently, many Deaf clubs have closed or are on the decline, with remaining members mostly elderly. Deaf clubs in Europe are experiencing decline as well and are increasingly populated by elderly members (Padden, 2008). Occasional events such as Deaf Awareness Days or Deaf Expos are now serving as new venues for Deaf community interactions. The boundaries that separated Deaf events from the hearing community are no longer as firm, as Deaf events take place in hotels, convention centers, and sports arenas where hearing people mingle as well. With deaf persons having more opportunities to interact with hearing peers because of improved telecommunications and sign language interpreters at work, in school, and at recreational activities, the boundaries of Deaf groups have become more permeable, even while these individuals maintain strong Deaf culture orientations.

Deaf Sports

The role of sports looms large in the lives of deaf people (Ammons, 2009). Deaf community publications and media devote sections to sports events organized by deaf schools or organizations and deaf sports competition results. There are numerous international, national, state, regional, and local organizations that sponsor deaf sports activities. For example, go to www.usdeafsports.org, the website for the USA Deaf Sports Federation, for a listing of sports and events that deaf athletes can participate in. This federation is the premier national sports organization in the U.S. Founded in 1945, the USA Deaf Sports Federation is linked with regional and local sports groups as well as with the International Committee of Sports for the Deaf, which has 96 member countries (www.sportsanddev.org). It sends U.S. teams to the Deaf equivalent of the Olympics, namely, the Deaflympics (www.deaflympics.com) every 4 years for winter and summer games. There is also a European Deaf Sports Organization (www.edso.eu), formed in 1983. But even before that, there were numerous European Deaf Championship events.

Through managing the sociocultural contexts of sports, deaf athletes and volunteers are able to ensure social gratification and self-actualization, as well as a sense of belonging and ease of communication, when everyone understands everyone else. Deaf sports also provide venues for self-determination in an area that is not bound by the negative expectations deaf athletes may face in hearing venues where their participation may be limited (e.g., Ammons, 2009; D. Stewart, 1991). Deaf athletes can be mentors and role models within a wide variety of sports, including baseball, basketball, skiing, snowboarding, soccer, and wrestling. Consequently, they serve as athletic inspirations for deaf youth. Some deaf athletes have broken into big time. To cite a few examples, Curtis Pride was a former Major League Baseball outfielder. Derrick Coleman was the first deaf American footballer to win the Super Bowl. Matt Hamill, wrestler, has won Ultimate Fighting Championships.

Deaf International Connections

Go to a Deaf international conference, and you will see amazing communication between people from different countries with different signed languages. As hearing people have noted, Deaf people manage language barriers better than their hearing counterparts when traveling in foreign countries. With body language, basic signs, and gestures, communication happens. International conferences such as the WFD's (www.wfdeaf.org; see also earlier discussion) World Congress conferences have been held all over the world every 4 years, starting in 1951[1] with 25 national associations of the Deaf participating. The 2011 Congress was held in South Africa and the 2015 Congress in Turkey. There are now 134 national associations of the Deaf represented in the WFD. Their conferences tend to be well attended and give Deaf people a chance to get together, share experiences, and provide insight and support in dealing with national and transnational civil rights, educational, and cultural issues.

Gallaudet University has hosted two highly successful Deaf Way international conferences established for the purpose of bringing Deaf people together to celebrate their way of life as opposed to conferences that focused on how to solve problems that Deaf people have (Goodstein, 2006). Ten thousand people attended the Deaf Way II Conference in 2002. This conference focused on language, culture, history, and art in addition to celebrating the visual, performing, and literary arts though a Cultural Arts Festival. People went home determined to make changes in their countries.

On a more limited scope, Deaf-related international conferences such as the Deaf History International Conference and World Congress on Mental Health and Deafness also bring Deaf people as well as hearing peers together. E-mail and the Internet have served to greatly facilitate Deaf people coming together transnationally, but as Murray (2008) emphasizes, Deaf people also took advantage of international connections in the nineteenth century, using ships that crossed oceans and railroads that crisscrossed Europe. At these conferences, meeting places become temporarily Deaf-centric where being Deaf is a standard way of being.

International gatherings are not only face-to-face; these are also virtual, thanks to technology that crosses the globe. For example, Deafzone (www.deafzone.com) was created to advertise Deaf events in various countries, allow for the exchange of e-mail and text addresses, and encourage online discussion of various issues. This has created Deaf-centric sites that are temporary, fluid, and situational (Murray, 2008).

Countries all over the world have deaf communities that are working towards achieving language, educational, and civil rights for themselves. Only recently have efforts in South America (Hidalgo & Williams, 2010) and sub-Saharan Africa (Cooper & Rashid, 2015) come to light. This attests to the persistence and motivation on the part of international deaf communities in making progress

There are organizations run by Deaf people that endeavor to create opportunities for Deaf citizens of developing countries where efforts are wanting due to lack of support and training. Discovering Deaf Worlds (www.discoveringdeafworlds.org) is an example of one such organization whose goal is to advance the self-determination of signing Deaf communities through local capacity building in developing countries. This organization "trains the trainers," who then can empower their own people to improve standards of Deaf education, communication accessibility, employment opportunities, and human rights.

Technology

While we have touched on how technology has facilitated international connections, it is also evident that today's technology has created new avenues not only for how deaf, DeafBlind, and hard-of-hearing individuals interact with each other but also with hearing persons. The communication and geographical boundaries that create distance between these individuals have been breached by e-mail; text and videophones; captioned telephones; the Internet with its chat rooms, blogs, and v-logs (blogs in video format); instant messaging; FM systems; CART (Communication Access Real-Time Translation); captioned television and film; digital hearing aids; cochlear implants; and more (Leigh, 2009). Video relay services connect deaf and hearing persons, with a sign language interpreter displayed on a monitor via computer or smartphone handling calls between both parties, signing the hearing person's spoken language to the deaf person and voicing the deaf person's sign language to the hearing person. Adaptations are being made for DeafBlind individuals through the use of, for example, software that utilizes an interface compatible with screen/braille reader technology. The development of technology that facilitates live communication between Deaf or hard-of-hearing people and individuals who do not know sign language is evolving now with sign language recognition apps. Visual alerting systems enable deaf people to know when others want to connect with them, either via telecommunications or in person via doorbell signals, and so on. This ongoing transformation in ways of interacting with others reinforces the continual reshaping of Deaf cultures and communities as participants increasingly connect with each other and with hearing people virtually. For example, two decades ago, Deaf students at Gallaudet University could be seen signing with each other while walking through campus. Today, you will see many of the students texting or checking their smartphones as they cross campus. And you likely have bumped into hearing people texting or checking their smartphones outdoors. In the twentieth century, deaf people were instrumental in creating a culture of universal and equitable design in the creation of "deaf technologies" such as with the video relay system and captioning access (Humphries, 2014). How this virtual communication is changing Deaf individuals and national or international Deaf communities (as well as hearing communities) is a topic for ongoing study (Murray, 2008).

The World of Work

One only has to pick up the book *Deaf Persons in the Arts and Sciences* (Lang & Meath-Lang, 1995) to see that occupational possibilities for deaf persons were plentiful in previous decades. Nowadays, occupational possibilities have continued to expand, thanks to increased awareness about the capabilities of deaf people and their determination to enter occupations previously impervious to their entry. Stockbrokers, physicians, cooks, architects, engineers, printers, lawyers, woodcarvers, baseball players, poets, actors, museum curators, chemists, janitors, computer technicians, software developers, administrators, business owners—deaf women and men have entered these fields and more. There are more college-educated deaf individuals than ever before. Deaf individuals have climbed into the upper echelons of government, a premier example being Dr. Robert Davila (see earlier in the chapter). Deaf individuals have been elected to parliaments in their respective countries, including Gary Malkowski, Canada's first Deaf parliamentarian; Wilma Neuhoudt-Druchen, the first Deaf woman to be elected to the South African Parliament; and Helga Stevens (Belgium) of the European Parliament. Numerous deaf people are employed in various U.S. federal government capacities and many of them have joined Deaf in Government (DIG, www.deafingov. org), an organization that assists members in working to resolve communication barriers, deal with accessibility issues, and promote fully inclusive work environments through networking and fostering professional growth. Deaf workers are also found in settings ranging from those specialized in providing services to deaf children and adults, where they may have numerous deaf coworkers, to those settings where they may be the only deaf employee. Success stories of breakthroughs in fields originally perceived as closed to deaf persons are legion. For example, in the Obama administration, White House Receptionist Leah Katz-Hernandez, Deaf herself, was responsible for greeting anyone who had an appointment with the president or his aides and handling meeting rooms.

But not all is rosy. Robert Buchanan's book, *Illusions of Equality* (1999), outlines the struggles deaf people have had in trying to achieve stature or even employment in the workforce, benefiting primarily from times of economic expansion such as those following both world wars. All too often, when deaf people access entry-level jobs, they are not provided the same opportunities for advancement available to hearing peers, even if they are university graduates (Kelly, Quagliata, DeMartino, & Perotti, 2016; Task Force on Health Care Careers for the Deaf and Hard-of-Hearing Community, 2012; Winn, 2007). Additionally, Deaf minority career success stories are few, although the number of minority Deaf individuals with successful careers is increasing.

Historically, deaf people have more frequently been found in jobs ranging from unskilled to skilled labor (Buchanan, 1999). One popular and prestigious occupation was printing, in part because residential schools for the deaf had strong vocational training programs in printing (Van Cleve & Crouch, 1989). Today, skilled printing positions have disappeared due to industry changes, with advanced technology taking over printing functions that formerly required experienced workers.

Another previously popular work area was the postal service (Lane, Hoffmeister, & Bahan, 1996). This field became feasible for deaf workers when training was provided to prepare deaf applicants for civil service examinations (Deaf American, 1969; 1970). Going back to 1906, access to these examinations had been limited for deaf people due to guidelines excluding them, among others. It took years of strong political action on the part of deaf leaders to overturn these guidelines for various federal positions and to remove examination barriers (Buchanan, 1999; Van Cleve & Crouch, 1989). For example, Al Sonnenstrahl (personal communication, November 16, 2015) recalls that the civil service examinations for post office positions included questions about music and vocabulary that essentially were unrelated to job performance abilities.

Today, there is no specific vocational area that deaf people are flocking to, illustrating how occupational choices and opportunities are currently well diversified. Education has become increasingly important, with job requirements demanding higher skill levels and ability to deal with rapid technological change for those desiring advancement. So how do deaf and hard-of-hearing people fare in this type of work environment? Unfortunately, information in this area is limited (Appleman, Callahan, Mayer, Luetke, & Stryker, 2012). Also, information on ethnically diverse deaf workers is sorely lacking.

It has been reported that hearing loss is associated with significant unemployment and underemployment compared to the general population and earnings are significantly lower than for hearing counterparts (Garberoglio, Cawthon, & Bond, 2014; Kelly et al., 2016; Task Force on Health Care Careers for the Deaf and Hard-of-Hearing Community, 2012). There are numerous stories of unsuccessful attempts by deaf and hard-of-hearing individuals to enter health care training and employment or achieve promotion. A compounding factor is that automation of many work functions has hurt the deaf unskilled worker (Buchanan, 1999). Barriers to employment include inadequate academic skill development and technical training, difficulties with communication, misunderstandings about how deaf and hard-of-hearing employees function, and employer attitudes based on pervasive beliefs that these employees cannot perform on par with hearing employees and may be costly in terms of accommodations (see further discussion in Chapter 11). Employer perceptions about the communication competence of potential deaf employees are a significant problem, specifically with speaking, writing, and listening (Kelly et al., 2016). Kelly et al. review communication strategies that could help these deaf employees. In a study done by Punch, Creed, and Hyde (2006), hard-of-hearing high school students noted that other people's lack of understanding regarding their hearing issue constituted the greatest potential barrier to their educational and career goals. Another issue that needs attention is that of upward mobility for minority deaf persons.

On a more positive note, Garberoglio et al. (2014) report on recent statistics indicating that 37 percent of deaf individuals are enrolled in postsecondary institutions (representing a significant increase from data collected almost 30 years earlier) and that 57 percent of deaf young adults who were up to 8 years out of high school are currently employed. This, however, is qualified by the fact that 1) only about 25–30 percent of deaf students complete their postsecondary programs and 2) the population researched did not include those who have worked longer and have not been able to advance in their careers or jobs, even when they have received the same career training, academic degree, and job experience as their hearing counterparts.

The Americans with Disabilities Act of 1990 (ADA) and the American with Disabilities Act Amendments Act of 2008 limits the ability of employers in settings with 15 or more employees to exclude job applicants on the basis of disability (National Association of the Deaf, 2015). Although the explicit message is that of encouraging employers to learn that persons with disabilities do make good workers with reasonable accommodations, enforcement continues to be a problem. Intent to discriminate can be difficult to prove. Willingness to hire deaf people exists, as does resistance, the ADA notwithstanding. Even though deaf workers as a group have long since proved themselves to be good workers, the struggle for equality in accessing the workplace continues.

Those deaf persons who remain unemployed have recourse to Social Security Disability Insurance (SSDI) and Supplemental Security Income (SSI). As of 2004, approximately 154,000 persons with *vertiginous syndromes, other ear disorders, and deafness* received either SSI or ASDI. Considering the fact that many deaf people can hold jobs, simply adhering to the criteria of average pure tone hearing threshold of 90 decibels in the better ear (Social Security Administration, 2015) is untenable. However, more comprehensive evaluations to assess ability to work are not cost-effective in the eyes of the Social Security Administration. It is important to keep in mind that a good number of Social Security recipients may have additional disabilities or are unable to internalize work requirements and thus cannot function effectively on the job. Also, the rules for SSDI or SSI are a disincentive to work when entry-level or manual-type jogs may not pay more than what SSDI or SSI provides or if the worker runs up against the minimum allowable earnings to qualify for SSDI or SSI benefits.

Deaf people have resorted to peddling when they were unable to obtain jobs, and campaigns against peddling were instituted by deaf organizations in order to dispel the notion that deaf people collectively needed charity (Buck, 2000). Current perceptions are that peddling is less frequent due to greater awareness of training and employment options for deaf people in need. Self-respect and pride in the deaf community are also mitigating factors. The widely publicized 1997 discovery of an illegal network of deaf Mexican peddlers in the New York City borough of Queens who were subject to threats and violence in order to produce cash for the ringleaders testifies to the ongoing lucrative nature of peddling (Hidalgo & Williams, 2010).

Training for Work

To address the employment disparities that have been reported here requires that educational programs serving deaf and hard-of-hearing students incorporate transition efforts in their master plan. Critical juncture points include those from secondary schools to postsecondary education or employment and from postsecondary education to employment. State vocational rehabilitation programs, employers, and community representatives, as well as the students and their families, need to be involved in chartering career and vocational pathways, creating learning opportunities in the community to facilitate the transition process and ensuring employment opportunities (Reichman & Jacoby, n.d.; Task Force on Health Care Careers for the Deaf and Hard-of-Hearing Community, 2012). Fostering job-related skills and a work ethic are integral parts of this process.

The Final Report of the Task Force on Health Care Careers for the Deaf and Hard-of-Hearing Community (2012) includes a list of recommendations for education and training that starts in the school system with promoting career awareness and academic skills development for middle and high school students. Additional recommendations include providing postsecondary educational opportunities at a variety of degree and training levels together with effective strategies for supporting effective career learning in relevant disciplines, and enhancing employer practices to support the success of their deaf employees. The Task Force also recommended setting up a national resource that would provide guidance and consultation about interpreting services, access services, assistive technologies, and universal design possibilities; sponsoring partnerships among postsecondary institutions, private industry, and the federal government in the development of new access services or devices; and generating certification standards and procedures regarding the provision of access. The focus of these recommendations was on health care training, but these recommendations could also be applied to other career sectors.

Businesses

Business owners have included enterprising deaf people eager to make their own living. There are probably upwards of 639 such businesses in the U.S. (Atkins, 2013). Technology has been a boon in that deaf business owners now can access the Internet, e-mail, smartphones, and video relay and captioned telephone services, thereby broadening their business base, not only in the deaf community, but also in the hearing community. These technological advances have enabled them to increase collaboration, networking, and strategizing and to take advantage of market forces (Atkins, 2013). Atkins's interview study of 14 deaf business owners revealed that many of them started their own businesses due to "push factors," meaning that they ventured on their own after being laid off or underemployed. Deaf-owned businesses were often based on areas of interest or, in other words, "lifestyle businesses." Mentorship was seen as critical in the development of human and social capital required to get a business going. Because of recent interest in deaf business ownership, Gallaudet University has added training in this area. However, barriers remain. For example, people still do wonder about how capable deaf people are of running their own business. Also, it is difficult to get mentors, loans, training, or technical and government assistance, all of which are more readily available to minorities and women (Atkins, 2013; Rosenberg, 2015). Added to that, few online videos and seminars are designed for small businesses using ASL (Rosenberg, 2015).

Health Care Issues

Deaf and hard-of hearing individuals are subject to significant health care disparities and are less likely to have access to outreach programs and mass media health care messages about various conditions such as HIV/AIDS, not only in the United States, but also in other countries (e.g., Brown & Mkhize, 2014; Pick, 2013). Because of cultural and linguistic barriers, they are at high risk for low health literacy (Brown & Mkhize, 2014; Kuenburg, Fellinger, & Fellinger, 2016; McKee et al., 2015) and inequitable access to medical and behavioral care, which then results in poorer outcomes (Barnett et al., 2011; Pick, 2013). They are less likely to have seen physicians compared to the general population and more likely to encounter communication barriers during medical-related contacts. Despite legal mandates, hospitals are often remiss when asked to provide ASL interpreters for deaf patients (see earlier in the chapter). Results from an ASL-accessible health survey administered via a touch-screen kiosk, which allowed for selection of English text or ASL via video for item presentation, identified a low prevalence of current smokers and three glaring health inequities: obesity leading to increased rates of cardiovascular risks and possibly diabetes, partner violence, and suicide (Barnett et al., 2011). Due to the high educational levels of the deaf participants, who were recruited from a well-educated Rochester, New York, deaf population, the researchers believe the findings underestimate the magnitude of health disparities that may manifest in other ASL populations. In another study, this time in Chicago, deaf participants were additionally found to be at higher than anticipated prevalence of high blood pressure (Sinai Health System and Advocate Health Care, 2004). By linking National Health Interview Survey data that included information from deaf people with the National Death Index, Barnett and Franks (1999) found increased mortality rates for deaf adults. HIV/AIDS continues to be a significant problem with one study suggesting that deaf people are twice as likely as hearing people to test positive for HIV/AIDS (Monaghan, 2008). Deaf college students were found to engage in risky sexual behavior at higher rates compared to hearing counterparts; this has implications in terms of potentially contacting HIV/AIDS (Zodda, 2015).

Even taking into account the multiple reasons for the health problems reported here, including family history, medical problems at birth, education, socioeconomic status and income, ethnicity, and race, English literacy and lack of access to information about healthy practices and healthy relationships that counteract stress are critical factors as well. Research has mostly been done on White Deaf individuals, and research on the health care needs of minority deaf persons is sorely needed. The fiscal costs of providing accessible health care should be compared with the long-term costs of failing to provide accessible health care information. If health care providers were sensitive to the communication needs of their deaf and hard-of-hearing patients, and aware of how to modify written communication and when to utilize sign language interpreters, they would do a far better job of addressing their obligations to serve those in need of good health care services. The website www.Deafmd.org provides ASL videos on various diseases and understanding medical tests. Information on advanced directive care in ASL format is also provided by www.healthbridges.info.

Like their hearing counterparts, aging deaf persons require increased contact with health care professionals. In the U.S., where old age tends to be devalued, these deaf individuals are at an even greater disadvantage because of communication barriers to health information and emotional support. Results from a focus group study confirmed feelings that providers are ill-prepared to care for them (Witte & Kuzel, 2000). They seemed resigned to prejudice and practical problems, reflecting attitudes prevalent prior to the Deaf President Now movement and its galvanizing effect on the deaf community's movement towards civil rights and social justice. Companies now provide in-home medical alert systems, including personal emergency response and health monitoring system solutions that keep these elderly deaf individuals safe and independent in their own homes. But when they require assisted care or health care facilities, including nursing homes and hospice, there are few facilities designed specifically for elderly deaf persons where deaf community connections are maintained, although the list of accessible and Deaf-friendly facilities are increasing as of this writing (www.aplaceformom.com/senior-care-resources/articles/deaf-assisted-living, and https://nad.org/senior-resources). Many of these needing residential placements will end up isolated in mainstream facilities where daily they deal with staff misconceptions about their ability to comprehend information. In other words, staff will assume they are being understood when in fact this may not necessarily be the case.

When facing challenges related to the dying phase of life, elderly deaf people and the deaf loved ones who are dealing with dying relatives face confusion and uncertainty based on limited information about physical conditions or services in hearing health care facilities due to inadequate communication. However, on a more positive note, their resilience and patience during this phase because of their lifelong experiences in coping with communication barriers helps them as they navigate this phase. When death happens, deaf community members tend to rally around the deaf families of the deceased and provide support.

Considering all of this, it is possible that communication barriers on the part of physicians may be a result of conditioning to negative stereotypes about deaf people, which are based on limited knowledge. Decisions to limit communication accessibility are often based on cost, ADA requirements notwithstanding. It is believed that addressing language barriers will result in improved medical care for deaf ASL users. As stated in Barnett, McKee, Smith, and Pearson (2011), this is a social justice issue that the medical community needs to address. The National Association of the Deaf (n.d.) has a position statement that deplores the problems Deaf people face in accessing health care and notes that most medical training programs do not adequately prepare medical staff to effectively communicate with this population despite the existence of federal laws requiring health care providers to ensure that effective communication takes place. The scarcity of providers versed in ASL, the monetary challenges concomitant with providing language/communication services, and the limited awareness of the needs of the deaf population all contribute to the health care disparities of this population. This position statement includes a list of recommendations that focus on the importance of effective communication and how this can be achieved as well as a list of legal mandates that stipulate the provision of appropriate, effective, and quality communication for deaf people seeking health care.

Conclusions

The sociology of the deaf community is highly reflective of the larger society in terms of its complexity and its susceptibility to the dynamics of social policy that influence the ways in which society members interact. The more one understands about sociological factors as these apply to deaf people, the more one is able to develop strategies that will enable deaf people to optimally manage their lives. Considering the struggles of deaf people to achieve parity with hearing peers through the decades, their efforts to test the limitations imposed by hearing society, and their inherent resilience, deaf people have come a long way. More work remains to be done in order to lower barriers to opportunities that deaf people desire.

Suggested Readings

Bragg, L. (Ed.). (2001). *Deaf world*. New York, NY: New York University Press.
   This book provides a comprehensive and balanced selection of historical sources, political writings, personal memoirs, and critical essays that present a kaleidoscope of topics that relate to what was covered in this chapter.

Cooper, A., & Rashid, K. (Eds.). (2015). *Citizenship, politics, difference: Perspectives from sub-Saharan signed language communities*. Washington, DC: Gallaudet University Press.
   Not many know that sub-Saharan Africa is one of the most linguistically, culturally, and geographically diverse regions of the world, with 2,000 languages within its borders. This book covers local deaf people's perspectives on citizenship, politics, and differences and in so doing also addresses aspects of culture, gender, language use, race, ethnicity, sexuality, and ability.

Friedner, M., & Kusters, A. (Eds.). (2015). *It's a small world: International Deaf spaces and encounters*. Washington, DC: Gallaudet University Press.
   This book covers how the concept of "Deaf-Same" has impacted deaf spaces locally and internationally, including countries in the global North as well as global South. Relations between deaf people in these countries are analyzed.

Moores, D., & Miller, M. (Eds.). (2009). *Deaf people around the world: Educational and social perspectives*. Washington, DC: Gallaudet University Press.

Researchers from 30 nations describe the shared developmental, social, and educational issues facing deaf people as well as current trends and reveal that deaf people generally have gained a sense of confidence, empowerment, and awareness of what their experiences mean.

Note

1   As reported by Murray (2008), the earliest World's Congress of the Deaf was held as part of the Chicago's 1893 World's Fair. Over 1,000 Deaf people from the U.S. and Europe attended as part of this congress, which was viewed as "co-equal" to 225 other congresses on topics ranging from temperance to religion to women's progress.

10 The Deaf Defendant
Legal, Communication, and Language Considerations

What I need to know
To get beyond
The "I don't know"
And the death it brings,
To the life of knowing
Which is freedom.

Mark Ehrlichmann
(2013)

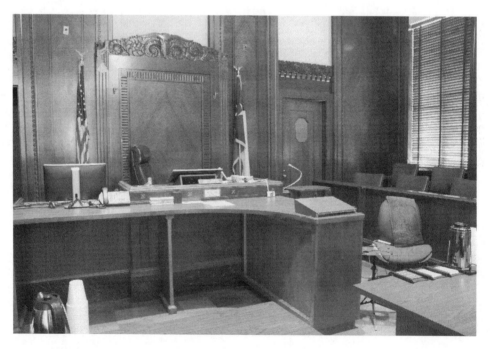

Figure 10.1 Photo of courtroom

Source: Stanley Hatcher (with permission).

Introduction

When hearing loss, language delay, and mental health issues combine and Deaf individuals become ensnared in the criminal justice system, they face a web of difficulties in obtaining due process and their constitutional rights. Multiple legal, communication, and language factors impact their treatment from arrest to incarceration. Frequently, communication breakdowns occur at the police station, in the jails, and in the courtroom, creating a perilous situation. At one end of the spectrum, Deaf individuals are treated harshly by a system that does not understand their cultural and linguistic needs. But on the other end, Deaf individuals may be treated more leniently and dismissed, particularly for misdemeanors. This reflects a kind of paternalism, which is neither helpful nor safe for the Deaf suspect, nor for society (Bramley, 2007; Vernon & Vernon, 2010).

Chapter Objectives

In this chapter, the skeins of legal, communicative, and linguistic factors that surround Deaf defendants are unraveled. We provide information on the prevalence of Deaf offenders and the types of crimes they commit, together with the challenges they face in accessing the criminal justice system. The components of a communication and language assessment, resources, and a research agenda based on the needs and experiences of Deaf defendants are also provided.

The Deaf Defendant

As reflective of the Deaf population, Deaf suspects and prisoners are diverse related to ethnic background, hearing levels, age, cognitive levels, education, communication and language preference, use of technology, and gender orientation. Many Deaf defendants have even more impoverished linguistic skills in ASL and in English compared to many other Deaf individuals (see Chapters 4 and 6). This linguistic deficit significantly reduces their world knowledge and general information fund (LaVigne & Vernon, 2003). This condition, which has been termed as *language dysfluencies*, *minimal language proficiencies*, or *semilingualism*,[1] means they lack fundamental communication skills in both American Sign Language (ASL) and English (Glickman, 2009). While they may have some social ASL and English skills to communicate about bodily functions, routine activities, foods, objects, and so on, they do not comprehend abstract or complex legal information. When they become entangled in the criminal justice system as a suspect, defendant, or prisoner, they are denied their basic rights as granted by the Bill of Rights and the 14th Amendment of the U.S. Constitution, and state constitutions and statutes as well (LaVigne & Vernon, 2003). And even though these protective federal and state laws exist, Deaf defendants face discrimination, abuse, and neglect (Vernon & Andrews, 2011).

A Legislation Framework

Deaf people who are incarcerated do not lose their basic civil rights such as freedom of speech and religion. They have the right to be free from inhumane treatment and cruel and unusual punishment. Further, they have the right to be free from physical and sexual assault and to receive medical and mental health care (HEARD[2] Deaf In Prison FAQ, www.behearddc.org/images/pdf/deafinprison%20fact%20sheet%20.pdf).

And even though laws such as the 504 of the Rehabilitation Act of 1975 and the American with Disabilities Act of 1990 were written to protect people with disabilities, these laws are often ignored, with many convicted Deaf defendants having no concept of their basic rights or even why they are in jail in the first place (National Association of the Deaf, 2015).

The Bill of Rights and Due Process

Constitutional protections for Deaf citizens include the Bill of Rights and the 14th Amendment. The Bill of Rights, which consists the first ten amendments, was ratified and added to the Constitution in 1791 (Cullop, 1999, as cited in LaVigne & Vernon, 2003). The 4th Amendment protects citizens from unreasonable searches and seizure, including arrests or the taking of belongings. In one case, defense attorneys mounted a challenge when the state used as evidence seized transcripts from TTY[3] conversations between a Deaf suspect and his girl-friend who was later murdered. The defense team argued that seizing these transcripts of a TDD call between Rewolinski, who threatened the woman he later murdered, violated their client's 4th Amendment rights (*State v. Rewolinski*, 1990). The court ruled that the TDD call was not protected by the 4th Amendment. The jury found Rewolinski guilty of first degree, premeditated murder.

The 5th Amendment provides protection from self-incrimination and the right to remain silent. The 6th Amendment provides the right to have an attorney, the right to a speedy and public trial, the right to a trial by jury, the right to present a defense, and the right to confront the accuser and witnesses. When the 14th Amendment was ratified in 1868, the U.S. Supreme Court incorporated parts of the Bill of Rights into the "Due Process Clause" of the 14th Amendment, thereby ensuring that citizens when suspected of crimes have protections when encountering state and local law enforcement agencies and in court (LaVigne & Vernon, 2003).

Deaf people cannot be asked to give up their rights or be punished for failure to meet obligations without notice of the rights they are giving up. Deaf people with low levels of reading and ASL proficiencies do not understand these rights. Police will often show preprinted forms to convey this information, and deaf persons are asked to sign a waiver that stipulates they understand their rights. But even with an ASL interpreter, deaf persons with minimal language or language dysfluencies may not understand the legal concepts.

Rights to due process was seen in the case of *Miranda v. Arizona* (1966), where the United States Supreme Court ruled that suspects had to be advised of their right to an attorney during in-custody interrogations (6th Amendment), the right to remain silent, and that anything that was said could be used against the suspect. Furthermore, statements made during police questioning could not be used unless certain safeguards were followed. This changed on June 1, 2010, when the Supreme Court's majority severely curtailed the Miranda Waiver (*Berghuis v. Thompkins*, 560 U.S. 370 [2010], www.oyez.org/cases/2009/08–1470).

Under the new law, once Miranda rights have been read to the suspect or defendant, he or she must explicitly invoke their right to remain silent in order to end police questioning. The new interpretation of Miranda hurts Deaf defendants far more than hearing defendants because it requires them to articulate their wish to remain silent and their request for a lawyer. However, it also requires that the arresting officer or the interrogator inform the suspect or defendant of these two requirements. In most cases with Deaf people, federal law requires that a qualified sign language interpreter be present. The majority of the time when apprehended by the police, however, an interpreter is not provided (Andrews, Vernon, & LaVigne, 2006; 2007). The case study of Gerald P.[4] in the Case Studies section of this book illustrates the challenges Deaf suspects and defendants face. Next, we review two laws that are designed to protect deaf suspects and defendants.

The Rehabilitation Act of 1973 and the Americans with Disabilities Act of 1990

Two federal laws, Section 504 of the Rehabilitation Act of 1973 and the Americans with Disabilities Act of 1990 (ADA), as amended by the ADA Amendments Act of 2008, prohibit discrimination against qualified people with disabilities in pretrial detainees, persons accused of a crime, and prisoners who participate in or benefit from federally assisted or federally conducted programs and in any state public accommodation, respectively, including correction and probation offices, jails and prisons, and most of the judicial system. Auxiliary aids, including sign language interpreter services, are listed in the United States Department Section 504 regulations, which require that communication with deaf and hard-of-hearing individuals be effective. Despite this mandate, Deaf defendants in court hearings and in jails and prisons frequently are not provided with sign language interpreters or other auxiliary aids (Miller, 2001; National Association of the Deaf, 2015). Also mandated are equal access to medical, psychiatric, or psychological assessments and court proceedings. The *Aikins v. St. Helena Hospital* (1994) case deals with the court system in a hospital situation. The *Mayberry v. VonValtier* (1994) and *Vacco v. Mid Hudson Medical Group* (1995) cases pertain to health care providers and aspects of the admissibility of TTY tapes. In one case (*Tugg v. Towey*, 1994) related to therapists, the court ruled that therapists for Deaf clients must be fluent in sign language and knowledgeable about Deaf culture, rather than having a therapist who uses an interpreter. This case raises liability issues with psychologists and psychiatrists, particularly in cases involving homicides and other felonies as well as legal issues related to the ADA (National Association of the Deaf, 2015; Vernon, Steinberg, & Montoya, 1999).

Prevalence and Types of Crime

There are an estimated 2.5 million prisoners in state and federal prisons (Bureau of Justice Statistics, 2014). While precise numbers are not available for deaf and hard-of-hearing persons, data indicate there is an overrepresentation of prisoners in county jails and state prisons with an estimation of 35 to 40 percent who may have some degree of hearing loss (Jensema, 1990; Miller, 2001).

Data from HEARD suggest that there are tens to hundreds of thousands of deaf, hard-of-hearing, DeafBlind, and deaf-disabled prisoners nationwide, noting that the 500 it has been able to find over the past 3 years is a mere fraction of the numbers of deaf prisoners across the nation (considering the fact that Louisiana alone has found more than 2,000 deaf and hard-of-hearing prisoners). HEARD created the only national database of deaf prisoners because most local, state, and federal governments still do not track or index the location or accommodation needs of deaf prisoners (www.behearddc.org/images/pdf/deafinprison%20fact%20sheet%20.pdf).

In England and Wales, there are 86,000 prisoners, of whom approximately 400 have some type of hearing loss (HM Inspectorate of Prisons, 2009; Young, Monteiro, & Ridgeway, 2000). McCulloch (2011) found that prisons in England and Wales lacked services for deaf prisoners. In one study, ten deaf prisoners reported they did not feel safe, suffered loneliness and isolation, could not understand the booking process or the prison schedule, and felt cut off from fellow prisoners due to the lack of sign language communication (HM Inspectorate of Prisons, 2009; McCulloch, 2011).

Studies show that Deaf offenders commit the same types of crimes as hearing offenders do, such as murder, rape, assault, arson, child molestation (pedophilia), child pornography, soliciting minors for sexual encounters through chat rooms and the Internet, car theft, writing false checks, theft, larceny, and burglary (Miller, 2001; Bureau of Justice Statistics, 2014). However, studies indicate differences in prevalence among the different types of offenses. For example, in a Texas sample of 97 prisoners, 64 percent of the deaf prisoners were incarcerated for violent offenses in comparison to 49 percent of the overall state prison offender population (Miller, Vernon, & Capella, 2005). Sexual offenders comprised 32.3 percent compared to 12.3 percent of the hearing prison population. Murder was committed by 10 percent; assault, by 9 percent; robbery, by 7 percent; and child injury, by 3 percent. Another 18 percent committed crimes of property and 18 percent had drug-related crimes. Related to education, 68 percent of the Deaf offenders had not graduated from high school. Deaf prisoners read on average at the 3.1 reading grade level or below with 61 percent reading below the 4th grade. In contrast, Texas hearing offenders read at about the 7.1 reading grade level. Clearly, most of the deaf prisoners do not have the language skills to participate in their arrest and courtroom proceedings or participate in treatment programs in the prison environment (Miller, 2001).

Homicide

Deaf individuals who commit homicide raise unique forensic issues. On the one hand, it is difficult, if not impossible, to give them a fair trial. On the other hand, they pose safety issues for society. For example, in a clinical study of 28 deaf murderers, a significant percentage had severely limited communication skills in both ASL and English (Vernon et al., 1999). Thus, they were linguistically incompetent and therefore could not understand the charges against them, nor did they know how to participate in their own defense. The researchers noted links between neurological impairment associated with the underlying etiology of deafness and violent behavior. Eighteen of the 28 subjects had medical or psychodiagnostic evidence that suggested neurological involvement. Fifty percent of the sample was diagnosed with antisocial personality disorder, which is associated with criminal histories in addition to homicide. Alcohol and drug abuse was found in 64.3 percent of the cases, and 11 of the 14 individuals diagnosed with antisocial personality disorder also had a history of addiction. Four of the defendants had psychiatric disabilities when the murder occurred, and three of them were diagnosed with paranoid schizophrenia. The researchers note, "In many ways, this population underscores the manner in which biological, environmental, and social factors converge in the genesis of violence (Vernon et al., 1999, p. 514). There is also a lack of mental health and support services for this population (Vernon & Leigh, 2007).

Sexual Crimes

Sexual crimes include pedophilia, rape, sexual assault, downloading child pornography, and texting in chat rooms for the purposes of soliciting sex. Pedophilia is defined by the DSM-V as a sexual preference for prepubescent children that is manifested by persistent and recurrent thoughts, fantasies, urges, and sexual arousal and behavior; it is found almost exclusively in men (American Psychiatric Association, 2013; Berlin & Krout, 1986; Seto, 2008). Pedophilia is believed to be due to a medical condition rather than an ethical defect in character, but nonetheless the lay public typically responds with revulsion to pedophiles (Vernon & Rich, 1997).

As a result of publicized accounts of crimes committed against children, Congress and state legislatures have passed harsh legislation such as the Adam Walsh Child Protection and Safety Act (AWA, 2006). The AWA established a national sex offender registry law, expanded federal jurisdiction over existing crimes, and increased the statutory minimum and maximum sentences. Upon release, sex offenders are barred from specific locations and may be forbidden to go to swimming pools, schools, churches, parks, and bus stops. Almost every residential area is off limits. This forces many of them to be homeless, to live out of cars, or set up tents or trailers in the woods (Farley, 2008). Pedophiles adjudged to be dangerous have to wear electronic monitoring devices for the rest of their lives. There are also state laws that include sentences for rape and child molestation of from 10 years to a mandatory of 25 years (Farley, 2008).

Data from two studies, one with 22 cases (Vernon & Rich, 1997) and another with 41 deaf sex offenders suffering from pedophilia, showed differences between deaf pedophiles and hearing pedophiles (Miller & Vernon, 2003). Deaf pedophiles had what is called a *primitive personality disorder*. Therefore, their competence to stand trial has been called into question. Also noted in studies with deaf pedophiles was a high rate of neurological impairment, illiteracy, poor communication skills, and other psychiatric illnesses (Miller & Vernon, 2003). Of these males, 17 were functionally illiterate, meaning that they read at the 2.9 reading grade level or below. Most of the individuals in the two studies also had criminal records involving offenses such as assault, burglary, arson, and car theft (Miller & Vernon, 2003; Vernon & Rich, 1997).

Other deviant sexual behaviors found in Deaf sex offenders include downloading child pornography and using the Internet and cell phones to exchange pornography and solicit sexual meetings. In unpublished data on three clinical studies, conducted by Andrews (2013), involving three deaf men who had no past criminal history but who were apprehended by the FBI for downloading child pornography or soliciting sex from a minor on the Internet, it was noted that these cases presented challenges to the courts because, by all appearances, the Deaf defendants appear to have had sufficient education history and had the language skills to use the Internet for child pornography or for texting to find partners despite their low reading levels. One case involved a young man with Usher syndrome who had enough functional vision to attend computer maintenance classes in a community college but read at the 2.8 reading grade level. The other deaf man, who was in his fifties, had mild cognitive disabilities, lived semi-independently with the help of a sister, and was employed as a janitor for 30 years at a city court. He had a 2nd-grade reading level. The third deaf man also had a 2nd-grade reading level and mild cognitive disabilities. All three men were physically and sexually abused as children. None were drug users. All three were social isolates who spent most of their time on the computer, had few friends, and depended on their families economically and socially. The court dismissed two of the cases because of linguistic incompetence, and the third individual was sentenced to prison.

These three cases pose challenges for the courts because on one hand these deaf adults may be linguistically incompetent to answer questions from the arresting officer or detective, to understand the Miranda Warnings, to work effectively with an attorney, and to stand trial. When charged with a sex offense, they may not understand the consequences of pleading guilty and having to register as a sex offender. They do not understand how the repercussions of being a registered sex offender will impact their living arrangements and job prospects. To complicate matters, there are psychosocial as well as linguistic factors that must be considered if they are to receive a fair hearing or trial. Most attorneys and judges often assume if the Deaf person graduated from a deaf school, they are literate. They most likely graduated with a certificate of completion, meaning they did not meet the requirements for a diploma. Texting and chat room conversations do not require high levels of literacy. This type of discourse is radically different from the discourse Deaf individuals face in the courtroom. The picture gets even more complex if the deaf person is sent to a treatment program. There are few facilities in the country that specialize in treating the Deaf sexual offender. These facilities are designed for the hearing offender with staff that has no knowledge of Deaf culture or ways of visual teaching and learning. While they may provide qualified interpreters, this accommodation is not enough for low language level Deaf offenders (Glickman, Lemere, & Smith, 2013).

Deaf Juvenile Offenders and Their Crimes

There are increasing numbers of older deaf youth with mental health issues brought on by early childhood/familial sexual abuse and neglect. When committing felonies, they are removed from school and sent to alternative schools or juvenile correctional facilities (Andrews, Shaw, & Lomas, 2011). Their crimes include drug and alcohol abuse, sexual abuse of minors, and violent offenses such as assault and murder. In effect, they become the victim and the victimizer because they suffered from many of these abuses when they were young children (Andrews et al., 2011; Jernigan, 2010). Etiologies also play a role as they may have associated impulse control disorders, attention deficit disorders, and language and learning disabilities. They also may have poor ASL skills and are unable to use sign language interpreters effectively. Due to their limited reading and writing skills, they cannot read court documents or fully comprehend the charges and the consequences of their charges against them (Jernigan, 2010). Data from nine case studies show the relationship between etiologies, low reading levels, low sign language skills, and criminal activity. Six out of the nine were physically or sexually abused as children. Seven out of nine had etiologies such as rubella and meningitis that are often accompanied by neurological sequelae (Andrews et al., 2011; Vernon & Andrews, 1990).

In another study of 20 deaf juvenile male felons, 35 felony offenses were committed over a 4-year time frame (Jernigan, 2010). Out of their offenses, 13 were for the illegal sale of drugs or alcohol, 6 were for illegal substance possession, 6 for hazing, 2 for threats to use weapons, 1 for a bomb threat, 3 for illegal possession of weapons, 2 for assault and battery, and 2 for rapes (Jernigan, 2010). Ten of the youths had a DMS-IV diagnosis, of which 70 percent were ADHD. The majority of the youth had a nonverbal IQ of 90 or above, with only four having a nonverbal IQ that was less than 90. Sixty percent of the youth were reading at the 1st to the 3rd grade levels, with 40 percent reading from 4th to 9th grade levels. Many of the families expressed frustration and difficulty in finding treatment programs that were accessible to these Deaf youths in their communities (Jernigan, 2010).

Within this small sample of Deaf youth, there are clear patterns of biological, cognitive, communication, and language factors that contribute to their delinquency. Many have average or below average IQ and have conceptual and background knowledge deficits. Most of them were not exposed to signing in the home, with many arriving at school at age 5 with little or no language. There is an increased risk for childhood abuse as the parents are stressed with having a difficult child to manage with whom they cannot communicate with (Andrews et al., 2011; Vernon & Vernon, 2010). These youth and young adults pose a challenge to the system because of their lack of communication, reading, and writing skills. When they are incarcerated in juvenile justice programs, they have difficulty participating in group discussions on sexual offending or violent offending and drug rehabilitation programs in the same way that hearing offenders can. Deaf juvenile offenders often languish in the courts because the system does not know where to place them. The young deaf offenders do not understand bond and parole issues; thus they often find themselves back in jail or prison for parole violations. Many go on to adult prisons, thus continuing the cycle of school to juvenile detention to prison pipeline (Andrews et al., 2011).

Cognition, Communication, and Language

Cognitive Functioning

In police and court proceedings, the lay public and legal officials often incorrectly associate hearing loss with an intellectual disability or mental illness (Vernon & Andrews, 1990). However, as discussed in Chapter 1, intelligence is normally distributed in the deaf population. Another factor in cognitive functioning is the presence of additional disabilities as many of the viral and genetic etiologies of deafness have medical and neuropsycholocial correlates, including various forms of brain involvement (Vernon & Raifman, 1997; Vernon & Vernon, 2010).

Diagnostic Issues

Some Deaf offenders have been diagnosed with a condition termed *primitive personality disorder* (PPD) or *surdophrenia* (Basilier, 1964; Miller & Vernon, 2002; Altshuler & Rainer, 1966). First described by Basilier (1964). PPD consists of psychological and personality traits that include a severely restricted or minimal language functioning with huge information gaps and little awareness of social norms or mores (Miller & Vernon, 2002).

The diagnostic criteria for PPD require three out of the five following conditions: 1) little or no knowledge of sign language, the primary spoken language in local use, or some other spoken language; 2) functional illiteracy of a reading grade level of 2.9 or lower as measured by a standardized reading achievement test, preferably the appropriate battery of the Stanford Achievement Test (SAT-10); 3) a history of little or no formal education; 4) pervasive cognitive deprivation involving little or no knowledge of such basics as what the U.S. Constitution and Social Security are or how to make change, pay taxes, follow recipes, plan a budget, or function on a job; and 5) a performance IQ of 70 or higher (Miller, 2004; Miller & Vernon, 2001). These criteria relate to how these deaf individuals diagnosed with PPD would have difficulty understanding legal documents, being able to work with an attorney, and understanding the language in the courtroom.

While PPD is controversial among some psychiatrists, as it does not appear in the DSM-V, it has been used for diagnostic purposes with Deaf defendants because it provides a set of conditions that can be identified by an observer. PPD and other psychiatric diagnoses are best diagnosed based on in-depth interviews by a psychologist who is fluent in ASL (Miller, 2004; Vernon & Raifman, 1997). The courts have recognized PPD as a valid psychiatric disorder (*People v. Lang*, 1979) even though few forensic psychologists, psychiatrists, attorneys, and judges are aware of how it relates to prelingual deafness and how it is applied when the deaf defendant is incompetent to stand trial based on linguistic grounds (Vernon et al., 1999). However, as Glickman (2009) notes, PPD seems to be a pejorative label as it further stigmatizes this group of people and obscures the developmental and linguistic issues of this diagnosis. While PPD is a useful diagnosis in order to obtain mental health and allied services for this population, Glickman prefers the term *language deprivation with deficiencies in behavioral, emotional, and social adjustment* and provides a comprehensive list of diagnostic criteria that mirror the PPD criteria, albeit with more details.

Adjudicative and Linguistic Incompetence

Many police, criminal justice staff, judges, and prosecuting attorneys are not familiar with the terms *linguistic incompetence* and *adjudicative incompetence* and how they relate to a deaf defendant's case (Miller, 2004). They are familiar with the term, *mental incompetence*. Mental incompetence is defined as the inability of a person to make or carry out important decisions or as being psychotic or having an unsound mind, either consistently or sporadically, by reason of mental disabilities such as cognitive disabilities, schizophrenia, and dementia (LaVigne & Vernon, 2003).

Adjudicative competency is a term that is currently used for the legal standard to refer to a person to be mentally fit to participate in court proceedings (Dawes, Palmer, & Jeste, 2008). This construct was defined by the United States Supreme Court in the decision in *Dusky v. the U.S.* (362 U.S. 402) case where the court determined the key test of competency was whether the defendant could communicate with his lawyers to understand the charges against him (Dawes, Plamer, & Jeste, 2008).

Many Deaf defendants are mentally competent and even *communicatively competent* in their ASL for social reasons. However, they are often *linguistically incompetent* in that they cannot understand the police officer during the arrest, the jail and prison staff during booking, nor the legal proceedings around them in court situations. Competency to stand trial is an important consideration because of the constitutional requirement that the defendant must be able to work with his or her attorney (*Dusky v. United States*, 362 U.S. 402, 402 [1960]).

While it appears that a hearing illiterate person can simply ask questions when he or she does not understand, oftentimes he or she has a language impairment and does not know how to ask questions that would be helpful in the defense (LaVigne & Van Rybroek, 2014). A Deaf person will need an interpreter, but even with an interpreter, there are no guarantees, similar to the hearing language impaired person (LaVigne & Van Rybroek, 2014), that the Deaf person will understand legal concepts (LaVigne & Vernon, 2003).

LaVigne and Vernon (2003) present six factors that contribute to linguistic incompetence. The first factor is the lack of early, consistent, and fluent sign language. One example is that of Victor, the Wild Child of Averyon, a teenager with no language who was found in the French woods in 1797 (Lane, 1976). In another example, Genie was locked in a closet until she was rescued in later childhood (Fromkin et al., 1974). Both Victor and Genie were not able to learn much language even after years of training. Similar to Victor and Genie, there are deaf persons who are physically isolated from daily communication and language and learn a smattering of language later in childhood, well after the critical period for language acquisition (see Chapter 4). A second factor is that many deaf children leave school with an inferior education and limited linguistic skills in ASL or English. A third factor stems from the isolation that is imposed by well-intentioned albeit overprotective families who keep their deaf adult offspring at home, use their Supplemental Security Income (SSI), and create an even more isolated environment where the deaf adults live without language and have no opportunity to develop job skills or become independent. A fourth factor is the 2.9 or below reading grade level, related to lack of language, type of instruction, and motivation. This inability to read creates major obstacles during the arrest, booking, trial, and rehabilitation. The presence of a language and learning disability in addition to the deafness is the fifth factor. Some of the deaf adults could very well have an undiagnosed sign language disability in addition to their low reading levels. Most have average nonverbal intelligence abilities, but some do not, meaning they have low overall cognitive skills. Finally, the sixth factor is poor, underdeveloped ASL skills that make it difficult to effectively use a sign language interpreter or even a Certified Deaf Interpreter (CDI). Understanding the deaf defendant and the concept of linguistic incompetence will provide the court system with some understanding of the obstacles that deaf defendants face. Judges may order the Deaf defendant to achieve linguistic competence prior to a legal proceeding, but this is an almost impossible goal to accomplish because of the experiential, conceptual, and language deficits the Deaf person may have.

The police, court, prison, and legal system do not understand the language deprivation of Deaf defendants, its roots in early childhood, and how lack of exposure may result in severe deficits in spoken language. For example, by age 5, even with cochlear implants, speech training, and high levels of maternal education, many deaf children have less than 100 spoken words and also have difficulty placing two to three words together (Cupples et al., 2014). In comparison, by age 18 months, the hearing child has an expressive vocabulary of 150 to 200 words, and by age 6, the hearing child has an average vocabulary of 8,000 to 14,000 words and knows most of the basic grammar structures of English (Andrews, Logan, & Phelan, 2008).

Misunderstandings often arise with police and criminal justice officials when a deaf suspect or offender can talk using speech for common phrases such as *thank you, yes,* or *no,* but cannot understand or use spoken language to sustain longer conversations, especially during police questioning, booking, and subsequent interrogations. When the deaf person talks and nods, legal officials may construe this to mean that the deaf person understands what is going on. In effect, the "deaf nod" simply signals that the deaf person wants to cooperate, not that he/she fully comprehends the proceedings (LaVigne & Vernon, 2003).

Police, criminal justice, and legal officials often assume that deaf people compensate for not being able to hear by being able to lipread, read, and write. A very small number of deaf adults may speechread far less than the average 30 to 40 percent of sounds that are visible on the lips, as many speech sounds appear the same on the lips, though for better speechreaders the context of the sentence will help the person understand what is being said (Ross, 1998; Vernon &

Andrews, 1990). Even if the deaf person wears a hearing aid or cochlear implant, during such a stressful time of arrest, interrogation, and incarceration, speechreading may not be an effective means of communication in situations requiring clear communication with new, complex, or abstract concepts.

For those with weak language foundations, English reading and writing notes are not effective means of communication. Deaf suspects may appear literate in the eyes of legal officials if they own a cell phone to send and receive text messages and a computer to send e-mail and surf the Internet. Deaf suspects may also have passed a driver's license exam with the aid of an interpreter, filled out job applications (with assistance) on a computer, or ordered food at a restaurant by pointing to pictures on the menus. All of these English-based activities suggest levels of functional literacy. In actuality, the Deaf suspect may be unable to use English to access the information surrounding them. Indeed, most are completely unaware about what is going on around them during an arrest, booking, and incarceration in a jail or prison. While aspects of the booking process are easy to understand, such as the fingerprinting, being handed a set of clothes, and the correctional officer pointing to a room to change, Deaf prisoners will not understand the whole process. The frustrated correctional officer may resort to writing or texting but the prisoner without a sign language interpreter or with a low reading level will not understand (Vernon, 2009a, 2009b).

As part of the booking process, the Deaf prisoners meet with a medical officer or counselor who will request information about medical and psychological conditions using an intake form. Deaf prisoners may not be able to provide information regarding medication, suicide risk, and necessary accommodations or assistive devices. Again, using written communication with a deaf person who is reading at the 3rd-grade level or below is dangerous when discussing topics such as heart issues, allergies needing medication, diabetes, and mental health issues like depression and suicide (Andrews, 2011; LaVigne & Vernon, 2003). The next example is further expanded in the case study of Gerald P. in the case study section of this book.

A Deaf man was booked into jail and the medical intake form was filled out without a sign language interpreter so his medical and psychological data were not obtained. ASL was his primary language. To ensure his safety from other hearing prisoners, the jail officials made the decision to put him in an isolated cell. The Deaf man committed suicide a few days later. A wrongful death suit was filed, and the family was awarded a settlement. This case and others point to the importance of providing interpreters at critical junctures in the booking process in jail or prison (*Ulibarri v. City & County of Denver*, 2012).

In another case, a Deaf suspect was not provided with an interpreter during the medical booking and could not communicate his back pain to the medical staff. He could not read the medical form so he refused to sign it. Later he was provided with other medical interventions (i.e., vaccinations) without his permission (*Zemedagegehu v. Arthur*, 2015). Such occurrences are frequent (National Association of the Deaf, 2015) and could be avoided if police, sheriff, and jail officials provided sign language interpreters for Deaf suspects during booking and medical intake procedures.

Deaf prisoners suffer in jail because of lack of communication and access to services (Vernon & Vernon, 2010). A jail or prison is an auditory environment filled with bells, buzzers, and announcements over the public address system, as well as orders from the correctional staff that Deaf prisoners will miss, including this one who missed many meals because he did not hear the buzzer for breakfast (*Zemedagegehu v. Arthur*, 2015). Visual or vibrating alarms would solve this problem but are not available at many correctional facilities.

Deaf prisoners are routinely physically and sexually assaulted and punished for using sign language to communicate, failure to obey spoken commands, failure to follow rules and procedures that were never communicated to them, missing prisoner counts that they were unaware of, missing meals, and for filing grievances about injustices and inequities. They may be beat up, assaulted, or even raped by other prisoners if the prison does not establish adequate protections or if correctional officers do not follow appropriate communication access protocols. Deaf prisoners who are assaulted cannot explain their side of the story and frequently are punished for fights they did not instigate. Further, Deaf prisoners do not have access to prison hotlines to report sexual and physical abuses that are available to hearing prisoners (HEARD, 2016; Vernon, 2009a, 2009b). The National Association of the Deaf has published a position paper to provide guidance for police and criminal justice officials on the rights of Deaf prisoners in correctional facilities (https://nad.org/issues/justice/fails-and-prisons/rights-deaf-prisoners).

For deaf prisoners, a jail or prison sentence means countless hours with nothing to do and with no services to access (Vernon, 2009b). Since many read at the 3rd-grade level or below, they cannot read books and magazines (Andrews, 2011; LaVigne & Vernon, 2003). They may not be able to understand the captioning on the television if it is available at all. Jails and prisons often prohibit DVDs and other digital signed information from entering onsite. If there are vocational or educational programs available, most require a 7th-grade or above reading level. If no interpreters are provided, these programs are inaccessible even though the ADA and Section 504 mandate that prisons must provide access to deaf and other prisoners with disabilities in the same capacity as hearing prisoners (Vernon, 2009a). Many deaf prisoners may feel isolated and confused by what is happening around them because no sign language interpreter was present to explain the routines and rules (*Pierce v. District of Columbia*, 2015).

ASL and Sign Language Interpreters in Police, Criminal, and Court Proceedings

When a deaf individual gets arrested, police should provide interpreter services for the arrest and the booking, at arraignment, and when bail is posted. The court provides interpreter services while in court. When the deaf person meets the lawyer, the lawyer should provide the interpreter. The court provides interpreter services for communication with the court, witnesses, and so on but not necessarily between the lawyer and the client (Andrews, Vernon, & LaVigne, 2007; LaVigne & Vernon, 2003). Interpreters for Deaf people interpret from English into ASL and from the Deaf person's ASL into English. For words that lack a sign equivalent, the ASL interpreter must fingerspell these words letter-by-letter or else mime them, draw a picture of what they stand for, give examples, and/or use gestures or other ways to try to convey the words that can come up in court proceedings. Coupled with fingerspelling, they use a bilingual strategy called *expansion* (LaVigne & Vernon, 2003) (see Chapter 5). Fingerspelling has little value in court for individuals with low literacy (2.9 reading level), who may also not understand the expansions. This is because the reading level of discourse in court proceedings ranges from grade 5.7 in a typical jury trial to 9.2 in an average plea and sentencing hearing with other court proceedings falling in between (Andrews, Vernon, & LaVigne, 2007). See Table 10.1 for specifics.

Attorney-Client Relationship and Communication

Due process happens when the attorney and the Deaf defendant have a qualified ASL interpreter during their meetings (LaVigne & Van Rybroek, 2014). Many hearing defendants, particularly juveniles, have difficulty communicating with their attorneys, but Deaf defendants have even more challenges because of the effects of hearing loss on language development, severe language deprivation, and poor education (LaVigne & Vernon, 2003). The Deaf defendant may face challenges such as asking questions, telling a story, sequencing the events, and making rational and informed decisions on how to handle the defense issues. As the attorney-client relationship is of vital importance to our criminal justice system, LaVigne and Van Rybroek (2014) write that we cannot avoid the challenges defendants who are language impaired have to deal with.

Table 10.1 Reading Levels of Court Proceedings

Type of Proceeding	Average Readability Level by Grade
Plea and sentence hearing	9.2
Motion for suppression hearing	8.4
Jury trials	7.4
Jury Trial (1) Volume I	6.6
Volume II	7.9
Jury trial (2)	7.8
Jury trial (3)	5.7
Jury trial (4)	6.1
Average	M = 7.4

Source: Vernon & Miller, 2001.

Average readability levels were based on eight different readability calculations: the Dale-Chall formula, the Flesch reading ease formula, the Flesch grade-level formula, the FOG formula, the Powers-Summer-Keurl formula, the SMOG grade-level formula, the FORCAST grade-level formula, and the Fry formula (Micro Power & Light, Co., 1995).

Professional Training of Sign Language Interpreters

It is unethical to use family and friends as interpreters in situations involving the police and criminal justice system (Mather, 2007). ASL interpretation skills are the result of years of professional training which entails the acquisition of cultural, cognitive, and linguistic knowledge as well as highly technical skills in producing and comprehending signing. In addition, trained and certified interpreters follow a code of ethics that includes confidentiality and are cognizant of state laws regarding sign language interpretation (Mather, 2007). While it is generally understood by the legal system that sign language interpreters are required in courtroom proceedings, interpreters are frequently not provided at pretrial detention hearings in police stations and correctional settings though interpreters are just as necessary during these preliminary court hearings (Miller, 2001).

Providing ASL interpreters around-the-clock in jails would make the costs unreasonable. However, it is reasonable to expect that interpreters be provided when communication takes place, such as during intake. It is also important to provide ASL interpreters during the prison orientation so that Deaf prisoners can learn and ask about the rules. ASL interpreters are also necessary during any GED classes and other educational classes or religious services that the prison provides. In addition, if the deaf prisoners face disciplinary charges, then calling in an ASL interpreter is necessary (Andrews, 2011; Vernon, 2009b).

Factors of Speed in Simultaneous and Consecutive Interpreting

During courtroom proceedings, for many Deaf defendants who are language deficient, the voice-to-sign interpreting process takes longer due to the need for extensive expansion, mime, gesture, etc., in order to convey the meaning of words. Deaf defendants often will not know the meaning of many legal terms. Rarely will a Deaf defendant learn the basic necessary concepts in order to be linguistically competent to stand trial. As mentioned earlier, many can never become linguistically competent (LaVigne & Vernon, 2003).

Because of the complexities involved in sign language interpreting, even deaf college students do not get as much information from lectures interpreted into sign language as matched hearing college students get from the same lectures in spoken English (Marschark et al., 2005). If this is true of deaf college students, it is true many times over for a Deaf defendant with low literacy.

Simultaneous interpreting, with the interpreter keeping up with the speaker who is using legal words or concepts, will be difficult for some language-deficient Deaf defendants to follow. Since it may take longer to sign something, as contrasted to expressing the same material through speech, the court ASL interpreter may have to eliminate some of what is said. When this kind of distortion of the discourse occurs in a court procedure, the Deaf defendant loses the right of equal access. Therefore, simultaneous interpreting should not be used in any but the simplest of cases, such as those involving misdemeanors or when the defendant is highly literate. Instead, consecutive interpreting should be required in the overwhelming percent of trials in which the defendant is deaf. In this procedure, attorneys, judges, and witnesses speak a sentence or several sentences and stop. Then the interpreter signs what was said, taking as long as necessary to ensure that the defendant understands the concepts just spoken. If they are not understood, the interpreter or defendant informs the court. It is a simple procedure to carry out but can be a slow process. However, it goes a long way toward ensuring the deaf defendant's due process rights if the defendant needs this type of interpreting. Nonetheless, judges may decline the use of consecutive interpreting because it extends trial time.

In a small minority of cases, the deaf defendant has such a meager knowledge of English and ASL that even consecutive interpreting is inadequate to convey due process rights. Such cases represent linguistic incompetence to stand trial (Vernon & Miller, 2001) (see earlier in this chapter).

Use of CDI Interpreters

For Deaf defendants with low language levels, the use of a Certified Deaf Interpreter (CDI) is an option to gain access to courtroom information. CDIs are Deaf individuals, often children of deaf parents, who have grown up with ASL and have been certified by the Registry of Interpreters of the Deaf. These deaf interpreters are required to have special linguistic skills in ASL idioms and usages understood by deaf people who have very limited English and ASL competency. Their skills allow them to transmit information from the hearing interpreter into language the deaf defendant can comprehend. They serve as a double-checking system regarding the deaf defendant's understanding of what is said in court. CDIs also provide a grace period for processing the information. They act as a monitor for effect and neutrality. CDIs protect the right of the defendant to understand what is said in court and can increase the comfort level of the Deaf defendant (National Association of the Deaf, 2015).

Literacy and Telecommunication Accessibility Considerations

Literacy, or the ability to read and write, is a skill that the general public assumes most deaf people have because they cannot hear (Chapters 5 and 6). To be able to read the captions of a real-time court reporter, the waivers, and the documents that suspects are expected to read and place their signature on (e.g., Miranda Waiver, Guilty Plea questionnaire) require high reading levels, as do other legal documents and jail and prisoner handbooks. Most deaf suspects and prisoners do not have the reading and writing skills to accomplish these tasks.

Real-Time Captioning in Court

During hearings or jury trials, with the best of intentions, the courts may provide real-time captioning versions of what is being said. Judges may perceive this accommodation as providing Deaf defendants with all the information they cannot hear and need access to. However, the court transcriptions may be impossible for Deaf defendants who read at the 3rd grade or below. As Table 10.1 showed earlier, the readability analyses show that jury trial transcriptions are written at the 6.9 reading level. Other courtroom proceedings that are provided with real-time captioning such as the hearings for plea bargaining, sentence hearings, and motions for suppression of evidence hearings are also written at high reading levels that a Deaf defendant with a 3rd-grade reading level will not comprehend.

Document Literacy

Deaf suspects and defendants are frequently asked to read and sign legal documents to indicate they understand the information in the documents. Document literacy is difficult for many hearing suspects, but hearing individuals have the advantage of asking jail officials or fellow prisoners for clarification, not so for a Deaf person without a sign language interpreter.

The National Center for Educational Statistics (NCES) defines document literacy as "the knowledge and skills needed to perform document tasks (i.e., to search, comprehend, and use noncontinuous texts in various formats). Examples include job applications, payroll forms, transportation schedules, maps, tables, and drug or food labels" (https://nces.ed.gov/naal/literacytypes.asp). Also included are written legal documents such as the Miranda Warning, the Search and Seizure Waiver, the Guilty Plea Waiver, and prisoners' handbooks for those in correctional facilities (Andrews, 2011).

To ascertain the difficulty level or reading grade level of documents, readability assessments can be carried out. Readability assessments are objective standardized assessments that apply a mathematical formula to a reading passage. Such analyses provide information on the surface feature of the text, such as the number of syllables in words, the average number of words per sentence, and the different words on lists of commonly used words. Computerized readability assessments were used to analyze the reading grade levels of the Miranda and a number of other documents, including the prison handbook (Micro Power & Light, 1995).

Miranda Warning and Waiver

The Miranda Warning and Waiver is a short written document that police must recite before questioning a suspect taken into custody. Each state has its own version of the Miranda, but the concepts are the same. A confession cannot be admitted into evidence in court unless the person waived his or her right in a *knowing, intelligent,* and *voluntary* fashion. For Deaf persons who have problems comprehending the Miranda Warning, it is critical to have a sign language interpreter. If an interpreter is not provided and the police officer continues with the questioning, the evidence gathered by the police officer could be suppressed. This remains a distant possibility considering that many judges do not grant these motions to suppress (Talilia Lewis, personal communication, February 28, 2016). Table 10.2 lists cases involving the suppression of evidence because a qualified interpreter was not provided.

While the language in the Miranda Warning and Waiver appears straightforward, it poses complex legal and linguistic concepts. The reading levels required to read it range from grade levels 5.2 to 9.9 depending on which readability formula was used.

To determine comprehension of the Miranda Warning and Waiver, 34 Deaf college students viewed a videotape of a legal interpreter signing a version of the Miranda Warning and Waiver. After viewing each of the six segments in ASL, they read it in English. Following the ASL viewing and English reading of the Miranda, the participants were asked to retell what they understood. Using a back-translation technique, their retellings were transcribed by independent interpreters. The subjects differed on reading grade level and number of years using ASL. Results indicated that participants who read at the 8th-grade level and below could not comprehend the Miranda or some of its segments (Seaborn, Andrews, & Martin, 2010). One student interpreted "the right to remain silent" as "If I tell them, I wouldn't get as bad

Table 10.2 Cases Involving the Miranda Warning and Waiver and Deaf Clients

Case Name and Number	Place and Date	Crime	Findings
State of Maryland v. Baker (1977), Cases #17,995 and #19,580	Criminal Maryland Circuit Court, December 8, 1977	First-Degree Murder	An interpreter signed the Miranda Warning to the defendant. Motion to suppress statement to the police by the defendant was based on defendant's insufficient understanding of the Miranda Warning.
State of Oregon v. Mason (1980), Criminal Case #80-03-30821	Multnomah County Circuit Court, May 27, 1980	First-Degree Murder	Motion to suppress statement to police by the defendant. One of several issues was the competence of the interpreters to interpret in legal settings.
State of Wisconsin v. Robert Rewolinski (1987), Criminal Case #87CR155	Pierce County Circuit Court, 1987	First-Degree Intentional Homicide	Motion to suppress evidence from the defendant based on insufficient understanding of the Miranda Warning was granted. At issue was the lack of accuracy in the interpretation.
State of Minnesota v. Gary Lester Goehring, Case #K5-9302466	Ancka County District Criminal Court, 1993	Murder in the First Degree	Motion to suppress the confession of the defendant was granted in the District Court for Anoka County. At issue was the defendant's lack of understanding of the Miranda Warning and therefore the lack of knowledge waiver of rights.
State of Wisconsin v. George W. Hindsley, Criminal Case #99-1374-CR	Pierce County Circuit Court, 1999	First-Degree Intentional Homicide	Motion to withdraw guilty plea and motion to suppress evidence from the defendant based on insufficient understanding of the Miranda Warning was granted by the trial court. At issue was the fact that the interpreter used transliteration versus interpretation. The defendant's language was established as being ASL.
State of Tennessee v. Chester Lee Jenkins, Case #C-12430, 31	Blount County Circuit Court, 2001	Second-Degree Murder	Motion to suppress the confession of the defendant was granted in the Circuit Court for Blount County. The two issues that emerged were whether the defendant had adequate language competence to understand the Miranda Warning as it was interpreted and whether the interpreter had executed an accurate interpretation.

Source: Adapted from Witter-Merithew, 2003.

punishment, but if I wouldn't talk, it would be worse punishment." And another student was asked in ASL, "Do you agree to the question?" and the student answered with his interpretation: "I prefer to tell them [police] everything. Forget lawyers. Who needs them? If I honestly admit and answer, then I make it easier on myself. I get less jail time" (Seaborn et al., 2010). With such misconceptions, a defense lawyer can make a case that the Deaf defendant did not understand the Miranda, and thus this evidence can be suppressed in a court hearing or trial (see Table 10.2 earlier). Obviously, even with a sign language interpreter, the comprehension of the Miranda Warning and Waiver is not guaranteed because the legal concepts are not understood.

After the Miranda Warning and Waiver is administered, police interrogations typically begin. Mandy deaf suspects have memory problems and will experience difficulty. This can lead to false confessions, especially if the attorney and an ASL interpreter are not present (LaVigne & Vernon, 2003; Vernon & Andrews, 2012). In one case, a police interrogator asked the Deaf individual, "Are you guilty?" and the Deaf person answered in sign, "I FEEL GUILTY." Later, when asked to explain, the Deaf person said was that he felt guilty that the victim was hurt, not that he himself committed the crime (Marc Charmatz, personal communication, November 8, 2015).

False confessions are common and involve not only deaf individuals, but also the uneducated, those with low intelligence, and those with cognitive and learning disabilities. It is strongly suggested that video recordings be taken of all police interrogations with Deaf defendants in order to ensure that they receive their constitutional rights and that interpretation was accurate (Vernon & Andrews, 2012).

Other Legal Documents

Besides the Miranda Warning and Waiver, Deaf defendants are often asked to sign their names on other legal documents (based on various amendments) containing highly specialized vocabulary that is complex linguistically to comprehend. Table 10.3 provides a description of five legal documents: the Miranda Warning and Waiver (5th and 6th Amendments), the Waiver of Search (4th Amendment), the Blood and Breath Test (4th Amendment), the Guilty Plea Questionnaire (5th Amendment), and the Polygraph Exam (5th Amendment). Given a deaf defendant's low reading level of 3rd grade or below, these documents are written at much higher reading levels than the Miranda Warning (average reading grade level of 7.0) to the Waiver of Search written at the 13.6 reading grade levels. Also, documents such as regulations for sex offenders, orders to appear in court, conditions of bond, and notice of suspension of driving licenses, among others, are written at the 9th-grade level or higher. These documents are intimately related to due process as guaranteed by the 14th Amendment (Vernon & Andrews, 2011).

Another document that is impossible to read for Deaf prisoners who are linguistically incompetent is the jail or prison handbook. Provided for each prisoner during orientation, this 30- to 40-page manual provides detailed information about the facility rules and regulations for daily life in jail or prison. It also outlines information about the prisoners' rights for services and rights to present and resolve grievances. A list of the types and consequences of misbehaviors while incarcerated is also given. There are sections that describe emergency medical care, dental, dietary, optometry, and medical services and the procedures for getting these services, how to pay for these, and the jail and prison rules for using medications, as well as information on the kinds of items (e.g., food, clothing, razors, reading materials, toiletries, stamps) that are allowed in the cell. It also has information on types of religious, educational, and visitation programs that are available.

Table 10.4 presents information on the readability of these inmate handbooks. The reading grade levels range from 11.6 to 14.8, clearly impossible for language-challenged deaf inmates

Table 10.3 Legal Documents, Protecting Amendments, Reading Levels, and Difficult Vocabulary of Five Legal Documents

Legal Document and Description	Amendment Providing Legal Rights	Reading Level Required	Vocabulary Difficult to Read for a 5th Grader or Below (Micropower & Light, 1995)
The *Waiver of Search* states that an individual gives up his constitutional right not to be searched.	4th Amendment (rights of people to be safe from unreasonable searches and seizures, including arrests or taking of belongs)	13.6	Aforemention, authorized, conduct, consent, constitutional, evidence, hereby, hereinafter, located, mentioned, otherwise, permission, police, premises, promises, property, search, signature, states, thorough, threats, understanding, violation, voluntarily, waiver, warrant, witness, written
The *Blood and Breath Test* is given to a suspect when under arrest for an offense arising out of acts alleged to have been committed while he/she was operating a motor vehicle or watercraft in public place when intoxicated.	4th Amendment	13.5	Admissible, alcoholic, alleged, beverage, certify, denial, detectable, approximately, offense, penalties, presumed, prosecuted, refusal, statutory, subsequent, suspension, consequences, hearing, inform, operating, permit, specimen provided, severe, whether
The *Guilty Plea Questionnaire* involves the right to a trial and the requirement that a guilty plea must be made knowingly, intelligently, and voluntarily.	5th Amendment (applies to the right to remain silent, the right against self-incrimination)	9.7	Plea, penalty, defendant, attorney, convicted, testify, felony, waiver, signature, restitution, questionnaire, probation, mandatory, constitutional, voluntary, subpoenas, revoked, prosecution, presumptive, plaintiff, firearm, exclusion, cross-examine, confront, complaint, deportation, diploma, disorder
The *Miranda Warning* reminds suspects of right to remain silent; the suspect cannot be forced to self-incriminate; the right to an attorney.	5th and 6th Amendments	7.0	Right, remain, silent, anything, against, attorney, afford, proceed, lawyer, request, understand, questioning
Polygraph Exam involves rights against self-incrimination.	5th Amendment	13.2	Hereby, submit, witness, coercion, contemporaneously, deception, detection, duress, examiners, harmless, interview, liability, polygraph, recordation, sexual, signature, submit, voluntary

Source: Andrews, Vernon, & LaVigne, 2007.

Table 10.4 Readability and Difficult Vocabulary of Five Jail/Prison Handbooks

	Handbook 1	Handbook 2	Handbook 3	Handbook 4	Handbook 5
Average readability/ reading grade level	11.6	13.9	11.6	14.1	14.8
Difficult vocabulary and phrases	complaint, media, incident, occurred, deputies, witnesses, discharge, accrued	commissary, counseling, delivered, probated, sanctions	book in, ensure, jailee, unimpeded, disposition, emergencies	unauthorized, horseplay, verbal, self-discipline, intoxicants, herein, blackmail, assaulting	confinement, specified, separation, inmate, designee, corrective, recreating, reprimand

Source: Andrews, 2011.

(Andrews, 2011). There are also multisyllabic vocabulary and phrases representing difficult concepts with multiple meanings at the 5th-grade level or higher (Andrews, 2011).

Prisoners who are hearing and illiterate can ask their fellow prisoners or the criminal justice officers questions about the handbook content. Because ASL translations of the handbooks via video are not provided, Deaf prisoners may find themselves incarcerated without knowing the rules and routines to the same extent that hearing prisoners do, thus creating anxiety and frustration (Vernon, 2009b). While most Deaf prisoners have to figure out the rules on their own by watching other prisoners' behaviors, this can be confusing as there are many rules that need explicit directions. It can also result in the Deaf prisoners being punished for infractions they were not aware of as "inappropriate" or "illegal," sometimes leading to privileges being removed and time being added onto their sentences.

The prisoners' handbook can be read in sections, but at the sentence and discourse levels, the handbooks contain features of legal language that are difficult to comprehend such as technical vocabulary or jargon (e.g., detainee, pretrial); archaic or unusual words (e.g., prisoners shall be deemed to have violated . . .); impersonal constructions (e.g., if this prerequisite is met, a prisoner may fill out . . .); overuse of nominalization; and passive modal verbs, multiple negations, and complex sentences (Andrews, 2011; Tiersma, 1999).

Some Deaf prisoners without ASL proficiency may need a CDI to fully comprehend the rules and regulations. ASL translation via video may remove the barrier to accessing information in the prisoners' handbook for some deaf prisoners but does not allow the prisoners to ask questions when sections arise that they do not understand (www.chron.com/news/houston-texas/article/Deaf-Harris-County-prisonerss-seek-more-assistance-1641695.php). Thus, these video translations are not adequate for every prisoner.

Availability of Telecommunication Technology

Studies show that, if incarcerated persons can maintain contact with family members and the community, they have fewer infractions in prison and increased possibility of success when they return to the community (HEARD, March 25, 2013). All prisoners, deaf and hearing, have rights to access communication through the telephone or visual telecommunication equipment (e.g., TTY, videophone) with family, friends, advocates, and attorneys outside of the prison as well as toll-free prison abuse hotlines for protection.

The most commonly used technology in prisons is the TTY, which allows the phone to be connected to a device or coupler that allows a conversation to be typed out between the caller and the receiver. It necessitates a teletypewriter device (TDD) or use of the computer on both ends. Today, TDD devices are antiquated, outmoded, and becoming obsolete while videophones allow Deaf prisoners to use their native language rather than type words. Since English is not the first language for many Deaf prisoners and many have low English reading levels, TDD technology is inadequate and not an effective communication device. In contrast, videophones allow Deaf prisoners ease of communication using their ASL. Video relay services (VRS) provide access to sign language interpreters who can relay conversations between the signing Deaf person and hearing telephone users. Videophones require Internet access for transmission purposes (e.g., www.fcc.gov/consumers/guides/video-relay-services and https://apply.sorensonvrs.com/secured_ntouch_apply_form). TTY relay services are also available but are much more time-consuming due to the need to type back and forth between the relay operator and the Deaf prisoner; the relay operator reads the dialog to the hearing phone user and types the hearing user's words back to the Deaf prisoner.

Within the prison system, making a call on a TTY or by videophone, or using TTY relay services or VRS, requires much more time compared to hearing prisoners making voice telephone calls. Many Deaf prisoners with hearing attorneys, advocates, or family members who do not know sign language use TTY or VRS relay interpreters during their videophone calls; this makes the communication take even longer. Further, some Deaf prisoners have family members who speak Spanish so they require access to Spanish relay services. All this means excessive phone call bills for family members and Deaf prisoners as explained in the next section. Consequently, phone justice for Deaf, DeafBlind, Deaf-disabled, and hard-of-hearing prisoners continues to be inequitable. Additional factors that contribute to inequity include high cost factors, lack of equipment availability, Internet access issues, and lack of access to what technology is available. But positive changes have been undertaken by the Federal Communications Commission (FCC), which has issued measures for reform and cost regulation.[5]

FCC Rulings and Cost Regulation

On August 9, 2013, the Federal Communication Commission (FCC) limited the high costs charged by the Inmate Calling Services (ICS) providers to family members of all prisoners, including deaf prisoners. For years, ICS has charged excessive rates for calls through TTY technology that requires more time to make and that families have to pay for due to the need to use collect calls. As for videophone or VRS calls, while there is no charge for the service per se, the need for Internet access, specialized equipment, and the time consumed with explaining legal aspects among other things add to the cost factor for Deaf prisoners. To build on the reform initiated by the FCC in 2013, on October 22, 2015, the FCC added further steps to curtail excessive rates paid by all prisoners by capping costs that previously could skyrocket up to $14 to $17 per minute for hearing and deaf individuals and their loved ones or their attorneys. The FCC also banned add-on fees imposed by Inmate Calling Service (ICS) providers (FCC News, October, 22, 2015). In the case of deaf prisoners, flat rates were being charged in addition to these already excessive rates.

In a letter from a female prisoner in Texas who explained that she got help composing her letter to HEARD, she compellingly wrote,

> Videophones are the only way I can effectively communicate with my family. The unit I am on is equipped with TTY phones; however, calls are limited to 15 minutes. By the time the connection is made added to the length of time it would take me to type and receive messages, using a TTY phone is counterproductive. The possibility of miscommunication is high. The cost of the phone call is too high for such limited communication.
> (Letter to HEARD, February, 11, 2013)

A male prisoner in Maryland wrote along a similar vein:

> The TDD conversation takes significantly longer because I have to read rather than listen to what's being said. It's also a financial burden to my family and loved ones because the institution uses a private service company to provide relay services. Inmates at this institution are required to make collect calls when using the TDDs and are charged an 8 dollar connection fee as well as 30 cents a minute. I cannot use a prepaid system, which the hearing inmates use, so there goes my telephone rights again.
>
> (Letter to HEARD, February 10, 2013)

Lack of Availability of Equipment

Even before the prohibitive cost factors kick in, availability of equipment is sporadic or even nonexistent. In many jails and prisons, the telephones are located in a room that is accessible to all of the prisoners, but the videophone and TTYs are often in separate locked rooms for security. Thus, the deaf prisoner must make scheduling arrangements to use this equipment, and security guards are often not always available when the deaf prisoner has been scheduled to use the equipment. Another problem is that TTYs or videophones may be locked in a closet with no one knowing how to connect them or remembering where they are located. An additional consideration is that the prison or jail needs a high-speed broadband connection for videophone use.

Availability is often curtailed by lack of accessibility of prison officials to monitor the use of the technology. When they are available, oftentimes the prisoner loses privacy in making the calls. As one prisoner wrote,

> While they DO have a TTY machine here, but it doesn't work properly—AND the only time we are able to use that machine is when someone is available to "monitor" it. What that means is my "counselor" has to take time of her work to sit beside me and read our conversation.
>
> (E-mail to HEARD, January 10, 2013)

And still another prisoner complained there was no power outlet near the phone for the TTY to continue working (Letter to HEARD, January 10, 2013).

Families also present barriers. Too often they own cell phones that cannot connect to prison/jail TDD equipment. A text telephone would solve this problem, but many prisons and jails do not have them. Even with the TDD technology, many Deaf prisoners have poor English skills, and it takes them longer to read and write messages.

Many organizations have supported the FCC's movement to reform the ICS providers by submitting hundreds of letters written by Deaf prisoners, various civil rights and disability organizations, churches, public defender offices, and the National Technical Institute for the Deaf among others.[6]

Parole and Life after Prison

The parole process is complex and involves many communication and language barriers for Deaf prisoners. There are forms to be filled out and appointments made with the parole officer. Many prisoners find these rules and forms confusing. After release, deaf prisoners frequently have difficulty returning to society, finding housing and a job, and attending court-mandated substance abuse and sex offender programs. Many Deaf parolees are rejected by their families and the Deaf community (LaVigne & Vernon, 2003).

Communication, Language, and Culture Assessment

Because deafness presents its major challenge in the area of communication and language, a comprehensive evaluation should include an assessment of communication skills, including speech, speechreading, reading, and expressive and receptive abilities of sign language competence. A person with expertise in deaf education or a related field (e.g., psychology, counseling, or social work) who has experience working with culturally Deaf persons should conduct the evaluations for communication, language, and reading. Formal speech and audiology assessments should be undertaken by a certified speech/language pathologist and audiologist. The components of a communication and language evaluation are found in Table 10.5.

Data gathered in these evaluations can be used to educate attorneys, prosecutors, judges, and juries about the communication and language issues in cases with Deaf clients. This information will more than likely come out in the trial or hearing setting and may or may not influence the judge or jury's decisions.

The communication and language evaluation for Deaf defendants consists of three sections (Vernon & Andrews, 2011). In the first part, the focus is on gathering the deaf person's communication, language, and school history. This information can be obtained partially from interviewing the client and supplemented with school records if available. The second part involves language testing in both English and ASL. One reading test most commonly used to measure reading achievement with deaf students is the Stanford Achievement Test (SAT-10). This test is normed on the deaf student population and has vocabulary and reading comprehension subtests. Informal tests that evaluate responses after the defendant reads a short magazine or newspaper article can be used. Written syntax tests have been developed for deaf people such as the Test of Syntactic Abilities (TSA) (Quigley, Steinkamp, Power, & Jones, 1978). The TSA has a screening test that assesses the deaf person's ability to comprehend nine basic

Table 10.5 Components of a Communication/Language Evaluation

I.   Communication, Language, and Education Background History

a.   Conduct an interview with the deaf person in sign language to gather information on communication, language, and educational history (age of onset, etiology, use of hearing aids, use of cochlear implants, use of videoconferencing, type of school placement, communication/language used at home, attained educational level, reading level, use of pager/text, parents/sibling sign skills).
b.   Interview parents, siblings, and spouses if available.
c.   Review any educational files, including any testing on academic level over time, speech, psychological, psychiatric, psychodiagnostic, IEPs, etc.
d.   Review any medical examination, audiological evaluation, and psychological or psychiatric evaluations.

II.   Tests of English

a.   NTID Speechreading test: CID Everyday Sentences Test (Simms, 2009).
b.   Stanford Reading Achievement Test: screening battery, vocabulary and reading comprehension.
c.   Test of Syntactic Abilities (TSA, Quigley et al., 1978).
d.   Read and sign a newspaper article.
e.   Free writing sample.

III.   Test of American Sign Language

a.   No standardized test available, 15-minute interview about favorite hobbies, etc.
b.   This data will be analyzed using a 6-point scale (Black & Glickman, 2006).

IV.   Linguistic Document Analysis: Using computerized readability formulas, analyze any documents the deaf suspect was asked to read such as the Miranda Warning, the Guilty Plea, prison/jail handbook, etc.).

Source: Vernon & Andrews, 2011.

English sentences: negation, conjunction, determiners, question formation, verb processes, pronominalization, relativization, complementation, and nominalization. Another method is to have the deaf client write about a topic of interest. This language sample can be analyzed for vocabulary, sentence, and discourse features. Speech and speechreading are other key aspects to be evaluated because it is commonly believed among hearing people that if deaf people have some speech for social purposes, they can "get by" in the jail, prison, or courtroom setting. It is important to determine the functional hearing level of the Deaf individual in normal communicative contexts. Deaf suspects with residual hearing and speech skills may still not be able to follow the conversation during a police interrogation or during the jail intake process because of the seriousness of the content and the consequences if misunderstandings occur.

It is also important to obtain a measure of the client's ASL skills. Currently, there is no commercial instrument available for adults as most of the instruments have been developed for children or for research purposes. A rating scale can be used in this case by videotaping a 15-minute segment of a signed conversation. Such an assessment is highly indicative of factors such as basic linguistic competence, affectivity, acceptance of a deaf person, and basic capacities to interact with others (Vernon & Andrews, 1990).

Another approach is to conduct readability analyses of any documents the deaf person must sign (Andrews et al., 2006; 2007). Comparing the reading levels of the documents to the Deaf defendant's reading level is one clear way to determine if the Deaf person could understand these documents. And still another approach is to videotape all interactions between police and the Deaf person, including, for example, the booking process, medical intake and so on. Also, all court proceedings involving a Deaf person should be videotaped (Vernon & Andrews, 2011).

Final Thoughts and Directions for Future Research

Barbara Raimondo, attorney, advocate, and parent of a Deaf child, cogently summed up the challenge of providing due process to Deaf defendants who are linguistically incompetent (www.barbararaimondo.com). She traces the problem back to early childhood and language deprivation. In one case, she reports that a Deaf youth who found himself in the legal system after having raped two women and murdering one could not defend himself because of linguistic incompetence. Prior to his conviction, the state of Ohio spent 7 years trying to teach him sign language so he could understand the charges against him. Raimondo questions the Deaf youth's early language history and comments that, if the youth had been taught sign language by the school system in early years, the language incompetence issue would not be a barrier. Of course, early language acquisition is but one factor, albeit a critical one that needs to be highlighted in deaf education. By not providing early access to language, we are in essence creating barriers down the road for Deaf individuals in obtaining their due process and constitutional rights.

Education about the situation of Deaf suspects and defendants can occur through blogs such as David Greenberg's Deaf in Prison (www.deafinprison.com), through online ASL videos, and advocacy by organizations such as the NAD, HEARD, and the American Civil Liberties Union's National Prison Project (ACLU, 2016). Information about constitutional rights and the reading of legal documents can be presented to Deaf high school students in civics and history classes. Related to research, case studies of Deaf prisoners who can describe their experiences in jail and prison and their interactions with the prison and legal system are needed in order to improve accommodations and services and reduce recidivism. Research directed at analyzing cost factors such as the cost benefit of grouping Deaf prisoners in jails and prisons, not only for social reasons, but also to centralize interpreting services for educational and rehabilitative programming could possibly ameliorate current access issues.

Suggested Readings

Burch, S., & Joyner, H. (2007). *Unspeakable: The story of Junius Wilson*. Chapel Hill, NC: University of North Carolina Press.
    Born deaf in Wilmington, North Carolina, Junius Wilson (1908–2001) was an African American man who lived for 76 years in a psychiatric hospital, including 6 years in a criminal ward. Wilson was never found guilty of any crime, nor was he declared legally insane by a medical professional. His biographers show how race, disability, language, and community impacted his life.

Lewis, T. (2015, May/June). Deaf inmates: Communication strategies and legal considerations. *Corrections Today*, 44–49.
    Written by attorney, advocate, and president and founder of HEARD, a nonprofit advocacy organization for Deaf prisoners, this article provides a concise summary of the challenges and needs of a misunderstood prison population—Deaf, DeafBlind, hard-of-hearing, and Deaf-disabled individuals.

National Association of the Deaf. (2015). *Legal rights: The guide for deaf and hard of hearing people*. Washington, DC: Gallaudet University Press.
    This book describes current legislation that prohibits discrimination against deaf and hard-of-hearing people. Also included is information on health care and social services, fair housing regulations, employment, and the use of sign language interpreters in legal situations.

Vernon, M., & Vernon, M. (2010). *Deadly charm: A biography of a deaf serial killer*. Washington, DC: Gallaudet University Press.
    Patrick Colin McCullough (1960–2001) was a deaf serial killer who was born in Maryland 2 months premature. Using police and court reports; witness reports; newspaper accounts; and interviews with family, friends, counselors, and teachers, the authors describe his history of theft, robbery, three murders, and suicide. McCullough posed a challenge to the courts because of his poor communication and language skills.

Notes

1   The term "semilingual" has been considered to be derogatory as it views the language learner through a deficit lens that blames the learner rather than focusing on the impoverished language environment (MacSwan, 2000).
2   Helping Educate to Advance the Rights of the Deaf (HEARD) is an all-volunteer nonprofit organization that uses education, research, and advocacy to promote equal access to justice for deaf defendants, prisoners, and returning citizens nationwide. HEARD's advocacy is aligned to the ADA, Section 504, and other federal and state laws that protect the rights of people with disabilities (HEARD, January 19, 2016).
3   TTYs are text telephones that were used by deaf people to communicate with each other and with hearing people. Today, videophones are more commonly used.
4   To protect privacy, a pseudonym has been used.
5   The Federal Communications Commission (FCC) is an independent agency of the United States government, created by congressional statute (see 47 U.S.C. § 151 and 47 U.S.C. § 154) to regulate interstate communications by radio, television, wire, satellite, and cable in all 50 states, the District of Columbia, and U.S. territories (https://en.wikipedia.org/wiki/Federal_Communications_Commission).
6   This letter was provided by Talila Lewis, founder and CEO of HEARD (Helping Educate to Advance Rights of the Deaf), to Jean F. Andrews on December 1, 2015.

11 Deaf-Hearing Relationships in Context

Deaf futures hinge not only upon the recognition that stereotyped beliefs, values, and attitudes are the scourge of minority communities, but upon an understanding that a restriction of diversity prevents growth and adaptability.

Corker (1996, p. 202)

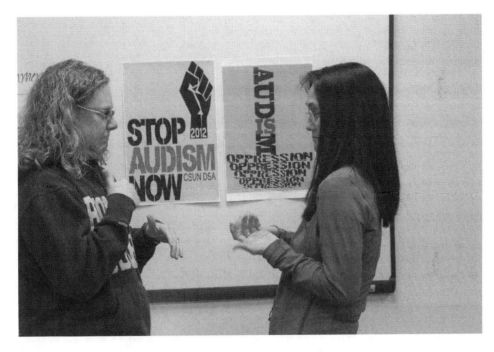

Figure 11.1 Photo of two females in front of audism posters
Source: Used with permission.

When Brenda Jo Brueggemann (1999), who is hard of hearing, arrived at the Gallaudet University campus in 1991, every day she was asked, "Are you Deaf or hearing?" Daily she struggled with the answer.

The salience of this identity question is a powerful one, implying as it does that, if you are one, you are not the other. For deaf persons firm in their Deaf identity, the answer is clear. For persons on the margin of the deaf community who are struggling to define their identity, this question may force them to navigate the unchartered territory of Deaf-hearing community dynamics. For naïve hearing persons, the "Deaf or hearing" question is outside the realm of their experience, since "hearing" tends to be an unconscious status taken for granted. Hearing people don't know that they are hearing until they encounter deaf people, and they do not know what "hearing" represents for deaf persons. For example, Dirksen Bauman (2008b) reports that, growing up, he had absolutely no idea that he was a hearing person until at age 21 when he took a job as dormitory supervisor at a school for the deaf and was bluntly informed that he was hearing. He interprets that to mean he was on the other side of the border between Deaf and hearing. During a lecture on Deaf culture for psychology interns provided by Irene W. Leigh, one of the authors, she asked them how culturally Deaf people labeled them. Not one was aware that they were *hearing*. Complicating matters, those who are hard of hearing may struggle with where they belong and decide that they are neither and/or even both, depending on the situation, as Brueggemann (1999) finally decided. To say that one is "both" is to take a "bicultural" stance, which acknowledges a comfortable attitude toward both worlds. For hearing children of Deaf parents, the "hearing or Deaf" question can reflect a minefield of confused answers. On the one hand, they are the true inheritors of Deaf culture, having been born into the culture; on the other hand, they hear as hearing people do (Hoffmeister, 2008).

Whatever the choice, the decision carries with it not only the issue of Deaf-hearing identity but also the assumption, either explicit or implicit, of how the relationship with the "other" culture is to be played out and how one is to behave with the "other." In this chapter, we now consider the issue of hearing-deaf relationships and attitudes.

Chapter Objectives

This chapter explores the power of stereotyped reactions to deaf persons, based on typical perceptions, values, and attitudes of hearing society, exceptions notwithstanding. It also explores how deaf persons react to hearing persons. These typical responses can have an impact on hearing and deaf communities, interactions at school, and work relationships. Professionals bear a heavy responsibility as shapers of how these relationships are constructed. The chapter also discusses the nature and influence of attitudes conveyed by professionals. Healthy deaf-hearing relationships are described. We note that these relationships are heavily influenced in part by sign language interpreters. We examine their influence as conduits between deaf persons and the larger hearing society. We then take a look at attitudes within the deaf community before concluding with the belief that through greater positive exposure to each other, attitudinal barriers between deaf and hearing people could possibly crumble.

A Look at Attitudes

- During a job interview for an administrative position, the coauthor of this book, Irene W. Leigh, who is deaf and happens to be well versed in both spoken and written English in addition to ASL, was asked about her proficiency in written English because, as the interviewer put it, deaf people had serious problems with writing, and there was concern about how the written English requirements of this position would be handled. This was in spite of the fact that Leigh already had her doctorate, her resume included listings of professional publications, and she had never needed editing on daily writings at work. This was not a question asked of hearing applicants.
- Kellye Nelson, an African American nurse clinician at Johns Hopkins Hospital in Baltimore, Maryland, and also a clinical instructor at the Johns Hopkins University School of Nursing, still has people assuming she cannot do anything once they see her hearing aids. She has to assure them that she is up to the task (Task Force on Health Care Careers for the Deaf and Hard-of-Hearing Community, 2012).

- Despite the fact that Trish Nolan, a Deaf medical records technician, had been in her employment site longer than anyone else and had seniority, she was turned down each time she applied for promotion to supervisor even though she had the full qualifications and ability to do the job (Task Force on Health Care Careers for the Deaf and Hard-of-Hearing Community, 2012).
- When highly qualified Christen Szymanski applied for a psychology doctoral internship, she included the fact she was deaf in half of her applications and left that information out of the other half. She received no offers for interviews from sites that knew she was deaf, and 100 percent offers for interviews from sites that did not know she was deaf (Szymanski, 2010). This type of incident buttresses the findings of a research project that involved sending resumes and cover letters on behalf of fictitious candidates with disabilities for thousands of accounting jobs (Scheiber, 2015). Results indicated that employers followed up on letters that disclosed a disability about 26 percent less frequently compared to letters that did not disclose, a percentage that researchers did not expect to be that large. Further analysis showed that small businesses were less interested in applicants with disabilities compared to larger companies and firms with federal contracts, both of which may be more sensitive to Americans with Disabilities Act regulations that ban discrimination for employment settings with 15 or more employees. Interestingly, employers were less interested in experienced workers than in novice applicants, perhaps because of the potentially higher salaries and costs for experienced applicants. This study illuminates the presence of discrimination as personified by the overall reluctance to hire people with disabilities, with only 34 percent employed as of 2013 compared to 74 percent of those individuals without disabilities (Scheiber, 2015).
- During one episode of ABC News' *What Would You Do?* with John Quinones, hidden cameras were used to depict the efforts of two female deaf actresses to "apply" for a job at a small coffee shop (Yee, 2011, as cited in Gournaris & Aubrecht, 2013). The coffee shop manager, also an actor, was instructed to provide increasingly provocative comments that revealed blatant discrimination, such as: "I'm not going to hire a deaf person. I'll let you know right now, I'm not going to waste your time." Actual customer witnesses rolled their eyes and for the most part did not get involved with the exception of a few, including two human resources professionals who offered advice on how to "legally" discriminate to minimize litigation. In contrast, during other equally provocative segments involving Hispanics and waitresses, Caucasians protested strongly against racial profiling and restaurant patrons protested strongly against the actor/patron who "stole" the waitress's tips. We need to ask why the reaction was so muted for the deaf scenario compared to the Hispanic and waitress scenarios.
- The National Association of the Deaf (NAD) (2014b) found sufficient evidence that apartment complexes treated potential deaf and hearing renters differently. Evidence cited included the following: 86 percent gave less information to deaf persons, 56 percent informed deaf individuals of the need for further background and financial checks to determine qualifications, and 40 percent hung up on deaf callers. The NAD also notes the lack of accessible low-income housing for deaf individuals and has repeatedly met with the U.S. Department of Housing and Urban Development to ensure that national housing policy addresses this lack.
- In stories of mainstream experiences, even those students who are successful academically or very "hearing" oriented acknowledge experiencing different levels of rejection (Oliva, 2004; Oliva & Lytle, 2014). Although deaf students with good speech and speechreading skills can easily interact with hearing peers, relationships are often not perceived to be as close as they would have liked.
- As a hearing son of deaf parents, Lennard Davis (1995) wanted to escape "deafness" but eventually discovered that he really sought to flee the deafness constructed by hearing

society. This was built on experiences of discrimination to which his deaf parents typically reacted by stating that they were as good as anyone else. In other words, they "knew" they had to prove they were equal to their hearing peers.

Yes, deaf people have come a long way. They have achieved far more than hearing persons ever thought possible, as witnessed by the number of deaf people in different prestigious occupations (see Chapter 9). The public is much more familiar with deaf people than they were in the years before the Deaf President Now movement, thanks to mass media reports of the event (Christiansen & Barnartt, 1995) plus increased social media. Deaf financial advisors are now working with both deaf and hearing clientele, thanks to technology such as e-mail and other Internet venues that reduce communication barriers. Patients who hear are comfortable about requesting advice from deaf physicians such as Phillip Zazove, M.D., and Michael McKee, M.D., among others (https://amphl.org). Deaf religious leaders minister to both deaf and hearing individuals; see, for example, Father Joe Bruce, Rabbi Rebecca Dubowe, Rabbi Darby Leigh, and Reverend Tom Hudspeth. The rehabilitation field led the move toward hearing staff working together with deaf supervisors and deaf administrators. The fields of education and mental health have increasingly followed suit, and now there are more opportunities for deaf teachers and deaf administrators.

The Influence of Perceptions

Unfortunately, despite these advances, experiences such as those reported in these vignettes have not disappeared from the scene. They emanate from typical perceptions by hearing persons that, because deaf persons cannot hear, that suffices to classify them as having a disability since communication using spoken language is blocked or limited and therefore subtly implies a disadvantage. Despite the fact that deaf people through the centuries have found different ways to communicate and have created lively communities, those different ways do not fit the parameters of spoken language to which hearing society is accustomed. Even if deaf people use speech, they are not always easily understood. Because they frequently cannot follow hearing discourse, they are often seen as living in a world of silence and as being limited in the ability to handle what their hearing peers can. As Teresa Blankmeyer Burke (2014) notes, "I am often struck by the divide between accounts of what it is to be a Deaf person and what hearing people think it must be like to be a deaf person" (p. 3).

Mass media has continued to extol the miracle of any device that supposedly restores hearing and brings the world of sound to deaf persons (Christiansen & Leigh, 2002/2005). The arts have also been guilty of reinforcing negative stereotypical perceptions of deaf people or of ignoring deaf people. For example, Davis (1995) examined written literature and drama from the nineteenth century onward that included descriptions of deaf people. He found that these descriptions typically depicted deaf characters as ones who are ostracized from mainstream society, often ending up as "the butt of many 'eh what?' jokes" (p. 114) or as melancholy characters in a world of silence. Esmail (2013) analyzes the lack of deaf characters in Victorian literature with the exception of Charles Dickens's *Dr. Marigold* and Wilkie Collins's *Hide and Seek*. The entertainment industry's portrayals of deaf people have historically been ones that often do not resemble real-life deaf people, thereby perpetuating society's misunderstanding of deaf people and reinforcing discriminatory attitudes (Krentz, 2014; Schuchman, 1988). For example, films reinforced the stereotypes of deaf people as "dummy characters"; as perfect speechreaders and speakers; or as solitary, unhappy figures. Thankfully, that has changed considerably with TV shows such as *Switched at Birth* and *America's Next Top Model*, both of which highlight deaf individuals and portray intelligent deaf people confronting issues and challenges just like anyone else. As a matter of fact, the winner of *Dancing with the Stars* was Nyle

DiMarco, a culturally Deaf actor and Gallaudet University graduate who grew up in a culturally Deaf family and whose first language is ASL. Krentz (2014) highlights how what he labels "the hearing line" contributes to a literary perspective of deaf people that differs from how deaf writers and filmmakers might present deaf people themselves, with the latter possibly portraying a relatively greater richness of character descriptions. He recommends further study of the hearing line in the interest of acknowledging the diversity and achievement that deaf people have demonstrated.

Meanings of Disability and Deaf

Because deaf people do not hear physiologically, they become part of the construct of disability. In this regard, they have all too often been categorized as living on the margins of society, a categorization many deny because they view themselves as part of a community with a common language. When people talk about diversity, disability tends to be mentioned as an afterthought. This is ironic because when people think about the largest minority group in the U.S., the Latinx/Hispanic category comes to mind, even though disability is certifiably the largest minority group in the U.S. and in the world (Invisible Disabilities Association, 2011; United Nations, 2006).

What does disability really mean? To literally translate *disability* is to say that one is not able. This logically leads to a response set that encourages thoughts about disability as a state of being that is not "normal," that reflects loss, weaknesses, helplessness, or heroism in the face of adversity. This frame of reference is bound to encourage ambivalence toward disability, involving both compassion and callousness.

This ambivalence extends to deaf persons. Just like people with disabilities, they may feel oppressed, become objects of pity, or are treated as individuals who don't quite make the grade because they don't fit what society expects of hearing individuals. If they achieve in the world of work, they are regarded with admiration as having overcome a disability. In the book, *Damned for their Difference: The Cultural Construction of Deaf People as Disabled*, Branson and Miller (2002) illustrate the irony of a society that declares all people are created equal and yet creates structured inequalities based on social class, gender, age, race, ethnicity, and ability/disability. Even though many culturally Deaf persons do not make much of having a disability and maintain some distance from the disability rights movement despite the presence of a common history of oppression (the Deaf President Now movement was not a disability rights movement; rather, it was a civil rights movement), the vignettes earlier in this chapter show that hearing society does not readily distinguish between disability and Deaf. Nor is hearing society sensitive to the fact that hearing people with physical or invisible disabilities are not the same as people with hearing disabilities who are dealing specifically with communication access. All of these have reinforced the uneasy coexistence that defines the disability/deaf relationship (Burch & Kafer, 2010).

What hearing society tends to overlook is that disability is not static. When a community makes a commitment to remove barriers, the disability is redefined. If a wheelchair user enters an accessible movie theater and is watching the movie in the same seated position as theater patrons are, who is then disabled in the audience? If there are open captions on the screen, so that deaf theater attendees have visual access to the spoken dialogue, who is then disabled in the audience? If voice dialogue is deleted and the hearing audience coming to watch a play sees actors communicating in ASL, who is then disabled in the audience?

Despite the fact that disability is to some extent defined by the environment, leveling the playing field is often hampered by, for example, cost factors that become a prime argument against the widening of every door for wheelchairs or installing elevators in school systems (N. Stewart, 2015) or producing captions for every feature film (https://nad.org/issues/technology/

movie-captioning/cases). Not recognized is the irony that sound systems are far more costly than captions and that video relay services do not incur up-front costs for users. In any case, this point essentially reflects a facet of discrimination that society does not own up to. To put it bluntly, society continues to reinforce the disability rather than create an equal playing field. In a society that runs on economic rules, the equal access of persons with disabilities is often seen as too costly. It took legislation in the guise of the Americans with Disabilities Act of 1990 (ADA, amended in 2008, see Chapter 1) to require accommodations that can benefit all, deaf persons included. Considering that lawsuits to enforce the ADA are still entering the legal system (see Chapter 9), it is clear that all too often society does not accommodate disabilities gladly and that prejudiced attitudes toward deaf people continue to influence their daily lives.

With the ADA in place, and in the face of increasing tolerance accompanied by the recognition that society is as responsible for those with disabilities as it is for all its able-bodied citizens, subtle discrimination against persons with disabilities has gradually begun to replace overt discrimination (as is evident from some of the earlier vignettes). This is a more insidious form of discrimination, one that is difficult to prove and fight. When deaf persons in the workplace are not privy to information that may be critical for job performance, when it is insinuated that deaf people are less capable than their hearing peers, when deaf children are rarely called on to be team members by their hearing peers in mainstream or inclusion educational settings, or when deaf callers get hung up on when using video relay services (see Chapter 9), such incidents are frequently dismissed as oversights, even when the argument that these are examples of subtle discrimination could be made.

Professional Attitudes

Considering the lingering reluctance of hearing society to accommodate the needs of deaf people, or even in some situations, the tendency to ignore deaf people, the task of defining how hearing-deaf biculturalism can be implemented in a sociologically healthy manner continues unabated. For example, the Internet has multiple examples of how deaf individuals are left in the dark when crisis situations such as tornados, hurricanes, or shootings occur; this speaks to the lack of attention that emergency management teams have paid to potential deaf victims. The reluctance to place sign language interpreters on center stage next to the podium of the person conveying critical information via television or video streaming is a disservice to deaf people who urgently need to be in the know during crisis situations. Take a look at the Deaf in Government website (www.deafingov.org). Its mission statement, listed on the home page, is that of empowering "Deaf and hard-of-hearing federal employees to overcome communication barriers, resolve accessibility issues, and promote a fully inclusive work environment through networking and fostering professional growth." This speaks to the ongoing barriers and issues such employees face in the workforce.

Neglect is not the answer. Professionals with responsibility for those they are protecting, leading, working with, or educating must endeavor to maintain a mindset or attitude that incorporates awareness of and respect for the needs of these deaf individuals. This requires attention to cross-cultural issues between hearing and Deaf workers (Glickman, 2009; Gournaris & Albrecht, 2013) in order to create mutually beneficial work environments.

Despite documented changes for the better, the majority of individuals in charge of organizations, agencies, schools, and businesses serving deaf individuals continue to be hearing, to network within themselves and not with deaf professionals, and to feel that they have the best interest of deaf people at heart (Benedict & Sass-Lehrer, 2007; Gertz, 2008; Gournaris & Aubrecht, 2013). Deaf people continue to protest when hearing superintendents are selected to fill positions at schools for the deaf (e.g., Stevenson, 2015). Go to most major deaf education conferences, and more often than not, you will see deaf professionals communicating amongst themselves and hearing professionals communicating amongst themselves, with the latter typically running the conferences. Access is not always guaranteed. For example, the International Congress on the Education of the Deaf, which took place in Athens, Greece, in July 2015 had only hearing keynote speakers and did not allow for universal language access for professional Deaf attendees (Tucker, 2015).

This is what Lane (1992) means when he uses the term *mask of benevolence* (the title of his book) as a guise for oppressing deaf people and exploiting them for financial gain. He claims the presence of "a hearing way of dominating, restructuring, and exercising authority over the deaf community" (p. 43) that does not take Deaf perspectives or input into account. To describe this phenomenon, he uses the word *audism*, which was coined by Tom Humphries. Eckert and Rowley (2013) further clarify this word to reflect social relationships constructed by the hearing-speaking majority, whether overt or covert, on the basis of assumed superiority over deaf people. This in turn engenders oppressive stances toward this minority group. In any case, Lane (1992) does provide a disclaimer in his preface that some of the hearing professionals are unjustly accused of audism since they are in the business of empowering deaf persons. Nonetheless, the book proper is a powerful indictment of these hearing professionals who are audist.

In a devastating critique of *The Mask of Benevolence*, Moores (1993) accused Lane of audism as well. As a prime example, Moores uses Lane's narrative to illustrate how Lane himself made decisions regarding deaf education in Burundi without consulting deaf professionals, either White or African, or deaf organizations with expertise in African educational systems for deaf children. Clearly, however well-intentioned professionals may be, sensitivity to one's own potential audist tendencies requires being open to criticism and addressing blind spots.

Lane (1992) emphasizes the financial incentives for hearing professionals. This does not consistently play out on the individual level, since motives for working with deaf people are not always based on money but rather on complex factors and good intentions (Benedict & Sass-Lehrer, 2007; Vernon & Andrews, 1990). In moving from denunciations of hearing professionals to more individual scrutiny, Hoffmeister and Harvey (1996) recognize that people choose to work in the field for a variety of reasons. Some have deaf family members or have encountered deaf people, some are intrigued by sign languages, some see the field as a challenge, and some will show a "missionary zeal" in that they feel deaf persons need their guidance. They could be altruistic, identify with the oppressed, or religiously inspired. What is important in the long term is how they relate with deaf persons in the course of their work. Do they immerse themselves in the Deaf community and then become disillusioned because they can never be Deaf? Do they intervene to help those who are "less fortunate than hearing people" or become so jaded that they see deaf "victims" as ungrateful? Do they experience frustration because, contrary to their opinions, the deaf people they want to help have different notions of how to get things done? As members of the dominant hearing society, do they in some manner continue to oppress the deaf people they work with by imposing their perspectives or value systems on deaf persons who might "see otherwise"?

Hoffmeister and Harvey (1996) describe several relational postures or patterns of behavior that hearing people may enact in relating to deaf people. One is the *freedom fighter posture*, in which individuals "fight" to correct past wrongs imposed on deaf people. Another posture, the *pathological posture*, reflects a belief that the deaf person cannot function optimally without the assistance of a hearing person who knows best, while in the *blame the victim posture*, the hearing person views the deaf person as someone who simply cannot make it because of the inability to hear rather than because of extenuating circumstances such as limited communication in the environment. In the *idealization and betrayal posture*, the hearing person heaps accolades on the deaf person, who eventually is seen as less than perfect, thus engendering feelings of betrayal on the part of the hearing person. Lastly, the hearing person who overidentifies with deaf people and integrates into the Deaf community is labeled as having a *confusion of boundaries posture* that can lead the hearing person to the point of exaggerating their importance to deaf people.

Hoffmeister and Harvey (1996) warn that these hearing relational postures, or perceptions of deaf people, if not worked through, will interfere with potentially healthy hearing-deaf collaboration. According to Gournaris and Aubrecht (2013), these types of hearing relational postures are what create cross-cultural conflicts between hearing and deaf people that may happen in the workplace. "Hearing privilege," which reflects advantages or entitlements accruing to hearing people that place deaf people at some disadvantage, may explain some of the responses made by hearing individuals. Deaf-related experiences of discrimination, communication problems, and prejudicial attitudes factor into these conflicts, with hearing people not always aware of what they are perpetuating.

The Other Side

So, in turn, how do Deaf people perceive hearing people? Their question, "Are you Deaf or hearing?" is a powerful one. It asks, "Are you with us or with the other?" It highlights the issue of belongingness and the issue of cultural values as well as potential cross-cultural conflicts. If the answer is "hearing," what does this signify? According to Padden and Humphries (1988), "hearing" is not the central point of reference; rather, it represents the greatest deviation from "Deaf" and as such can be less than complimentary or as representing the external world outside of the Deaf-World. This makes sense when acknowledging the resentment deaf people feel when they are defined by perceived inabilities or limitations, when their hearing loss is equated with presumed deficits, or when their strengths are minimized (Gournaris & Aubrecht, 2013).

As a qualifier, it goes without saying that deaf people's lifelong experiences with hearing people are subject to wide variation, ranging from supportive to dismissive or outright rejection. Much depends on their background and the extent and nature of their exposure to hearing people, as indicated in previous chapters of this book. As Gournaris and Aubrecht (2013) indicate, these experiences or social context will form the foundation of their attitudes, responses, and behavioral patterns toward hearing people. The authors have categorized some common deaf relational postures, which are not meant to be exhaustive. First, they discuss the *submissive posture*, which reflects internalized audism. What this means is that the deaf person either consciously or unconsciously internalizes hearing people as authorities who can validate or affirm their responses or behavior instead of using an internal locus of control that is more affirmative in terms of strengths related to being deaf. The submissive posture can be interpreted as reflecting a state of inferiority or powerlessness, to the point that such individuals question their own ability.

In contrast, the *militant posture* reflects what Glickman (1996) labels as the immersion stage in Deaf identity development (see Chapter 8). The militant individual is quick to denigrate anything and everything related to hearing people, putting this into the framework of "us" versus "them." Their attacks on hearing people do not allow for compromise or the perspective of differing viewpoints, thus rendering them "difficult" in the eyes of others who do not subscribe to their viewpoints. Then we have the *activist posture*. Imagine a deaf person continually alert to any intimidation of oppression and quick to challenge these, particularly if these come from hearing people. They make efforts to work within the system in conjunction with hearing colleagues, their goal being to effectively change the status quo. At times, they may appear to be militant.

The *native posture* describes individuals who live their lives within the Deaf community. They do not necessarily inveigh against hearing people; rather, they see hearing people as "outsiders" and deal with them as part of the necessity of doing business. They believe that the Deaf person is the expert on anything related to being deaf. Lastly, there is the *objectifier posture.* This is a relatively more complex posture that covers deaf individuals who use their Deaf identity personally and professionally but yet subtly affiliate with hearing people depending on the power dynamics centered on how being deaf and hearing are used as strategic assets. Their stance may give rise to perceptions that they are hypocritical, particularly in situations such as, for example, when hearing people are preferred for critical assignments despite the availability of qualified deaf individuals.

These postures can lead to predictability in how these deaf individuals will relate with hearing people and how cross-cultural dynamics are influenced. These postures also need to be understood within the context of how recent decades have impacted the "voices" of Deaf people. As these voices have grown stronger in recent decades, emboldened by the support of a Deaf culture frame of reference (Humphries, 2008), Deaf people are articulating more than ever their needs for self-definition and equality with hearing peers. To accomplish this, they have at times told hearing people to "back off," to let Deaf people assume more of a say in their destinies. This could be viewed as an articulation of prejudice against hearing people. Neil Glickman (1996) captured this sentiment when he described the immersion stage in Deaf identity development as one in which Deaf culture values reign strong and the hearing world is disparaged. At some level, it really reflects efforts to gain some transfer of power, considering that hearing people have long been in the role of policy and implementation decision-maker in areas that affect the lives of Deaf people (Benedict & Sass-Lehrer, 2007; Gournaris & Aubrecht, 2013).

When Deaf people assert themselves, they often confront bewildered hearing participants, who may react with "What is it with you deaf people? . . . What is it about Deaf culture that makes you have a chip on your shoulder when the hearing world is trying to help you?" (Drolsbaugh, 2000, p. 12). These stereotyped responses reinforce the feelings of being misunderstood or maligned that many Deaf people have. At the same time, it reveals the difficulty hearing people have in seeing their own paternalistic attitudes and in recognizing that deaf people are trying to help themselves and be independent. For example, film studios will often claim that the best solution is to hire a hearing actor who may need to learn some signs for the role, even when deaf actors are available who could attempt the role and who would not need to learn sign language (Callis, 2015; Frank, 2015). When the hearing establishment claims that deaf actors cannot fulfill role expectations, they appear to be taking on an audist or paternalistic stance. For this reason, deaf organizations have banded together to rally for the hiring of deaf actors as opposed to hearing actors for deaf roles in films. This exemplifies how the Deaf community does take its own counsel and express its opinion, most often through deaf organizations.

When deaf people identify more closely with an integrated or bicultural stance, the focus shifts toward that of supporting Deaf people rather than attacking hearing people (Glickman, 1996). People in this stage are able to recognize that the "Hearing" category does not necessarily have to be one of denigration. Rather than simplistically reflecting a paternalistic force, Deaf people can also see "hearing" to mean a person with a different set of experiences based on hearing or who may be judged as a trustworthy peer or colleague.

The boundaries between deaf and hearing individuals have become increasingly porous in recent decades due in great part to increased communication using visual technology such as e-mail, the Internet, and video relay services; greater use of mainstream settings for education; and the lowering (note: not removal, unfortunately) of barriers to employment opportunities. Therefore, deaf people who "behave as hearing people do" are less often criticized as not being Deaf enough. In concrete terms, biculturalism has become increasingly acceptable. This is reflected by the greater number of hearing and deaf teams working together more or less as equal partners in various venues, including education, mental health, politics, policymaking, and so on. That deaf people can be the "boss" in organizations with hearing employees is personified by Jim Macfadden, a Deaf businessman and Gallaudet University graduate who founded his information technologies company and grew it to a large entity before selling it to his employees (see www.macf.com/about-us/our-history-vision.html for a brief history).

Oppression

In education as well as mental health, it is common knowledge that deaf people have long been excluded from decisions about the education of deaf children (Benedict & Sass-Lehrer, 2007; Moores, 1993) or mental health service delivery for deaf people (Gournaris & Aubrecht, 2013). For too long, Gallaudet University existed without a deaf president (Christiansen & Barnartt, 1995). While it is now more common than ever for deaf people to become superintendents of schools for the deaf, assume faculty positions at community colleges and universities, or run agencies such as those for abused deaf women, for example, it is still an uphill battle to get hearing professionals in decision-making positions to acknowledge the capabilities of deaf colleagues. We now turn to a consideration of how this reflects oppression.

The word *oppression* has become a popular cliché to define the behavior of many hearing professionals. People who enter the helping professions tend to perceive themselves as enablers who want to empower those they help. For many of them, being told they are *oppressors* is mind-boggling. Why does the term *oppressors* keep appearing in the literature even with growing evidence of the greater willingness of Deaf people to take on the mantle of biculturalism and display comfort with hearing people?

The process of oppression takes place in the guise of social, political, and economic relationships with marginalized groups, including people with disabilities and people who are deaf (Corker, 1998; Haualand, 2008). Oppression happens when hearing persons control decision-making processes involving deaf people instead of working with them to enact accommodations that benefit all. The concepts of hearing privilege and audism both contribute to oppression, whether overt or covert.

In industrialized societies, for example, jobs are power. When economic opportunities are limited because one is "deaf" despite the fact that there are ways to reconstruct jobs in order to focus on abilities instead of "disabilities," this reinforces the expectations of "inability" (Corker, 1998). When deaf people are repeatedly stymied in their efforts to make advances—whether in school, in training opportunities, on the job, or in the political arena—they may see society as unwilling to work with them and therefore oppressing them. When they attempt to criticize the advice of hearing persons, their points may not be seen as valid, and they can be perceived as being ungrateful.

Deaf people can respond in different and complex ways to situations they perceive as oppressive, as indicated earlier. They may uncritically accommodate to hearing society, withdraw into Deaf culture where their attributes are seen as positive, or work with hearing society to change oppressive tendencies (Corker, 1998; Ostrove & Oliva, 2010). Their responses may vary depending on the situation in which oppression takes place and their individual attributes and past experiences. In looking at the larger picture, Corker emphasizes the need to look at not only the oppressors and the oppressed but also the process of oppression, specifically the dynamics of the power relationship between these two groups. The Deaf President Now movement required consciousness-raising to illustrate the dynamics of this power relationship and to upend the balance of power so that it did not remain fully in the hands of hearing decision-makers (Jankowski, 1997).

Although perceptions of oppression do predominate, a counteracting perspective claims that hearing people do not necessarily oppress deaf people. Larry Stewart, a deceased deaf professional, ASL user, and prolific as well as outspoken author, ridiculed the paradigm of deaf people as being oppressed or framed as victims of hearing society (L. Stewart, 1992). He claimed that, although some hearing people do treat deaf people badly at times, they also treat other hearing people badly. He has explained that, compared to other parts of the world, deaf people have been supported to a far greater degree in the United States and do have many opportunities to achieve. He even went so far as to suggest that getting a taste of life in, for example, Iraq or Cuba, would teach people a new definition of the word *oppression*.

Stewart acknowledged that, compared to hearing counterparts, deaf people have had to struggle that much harder to overcome "ignorance, prejudice, and at times cruelty" (p. 141) and to achieve comparable linguistic, educational, and occupational achievement and equal community participation. He has reminded us that many groups of hearing people—of varied ethnic origins size, and shape, disabilities, religious, or whatever—have had to struggle against oppression by other hearing groups as well and that deaf people are no different. According to Stewart, many deaf people are satisfied with the quality of their lives, so defining them as oppressed does not make inherent sense. And finally, he made a case for avoiding the needless splintering between deaf and hearing people, for which he laid blame on Deaf culture because of its "rejection" of those who differ in their perspectives. Incidentally, research findings indicate that quality of life for deaf participants tends to be comparable to hearing comparison groups in social relationships (not so for physical and psychological domains) (Fellinger et al., 2005), while other research indicates that those deaf individuals with solid psychological resources appear to demonstrate satisfaction with life (e.g., Hintermair, 2008; Kushalnagar et al., 2014).

The fact that deaf people in the United States do have it good in comparison to other places in the world, particularly when it comes to educational and job opportunities as well as access to services, does not obviate the need to examine the tensions between groups whenever that happens. All in all, for diverse groups, whatever their group affiliation, there is a critical need to work together in coalitions that respect the value of difference in order to advance opportunities for *all* people. Society needs techniques to minimize the continual discrimination and splintering among groups. At the same time, it is important to learn about the unique traits and the diversity within each group. Many hearing and deaf professionals are working toward that end.

Healthy Ways of Relating

In order to establish trustworthiness in the eyes of deaf people, it is recommended that professionals undergo the admittedly difficult process of honest self-analysis in trying to understand why mistrust may exist and how they can ensure healthy relationships with "the other" (Benedict & Sass-Lehrer, 2007; Gournaris & Aubrecht, 2013; Hoffmeister & Harvey, 1996; Ostrove & Oliva, 2010). In describing this process, Ostrove (hearing) and Oliva (deaf) write:

> True alliance means that the traditional power dynamic would shift, and dominant group members not only would take responsibility for their own identities and related privileges but also would acknowledge their own struggles and behaviors in response to cross-identity issues or predicaments.
>
> (2010, p. 109)

By way of example, this speaks to how willing hearing participants are to modify their behavior to communicate with deaf people, for example, instead of expecting deaf people to accommodate the hearing person's communication. This also speaks to the question of who needs the interpreter—the deaf person, or rather the hearing person who does not know ASL, or both. The hearing person does not always understand this and frames the interpreter as something the deaf person needs rather than that interpreting is a need mutually beneficial to both. The issue of communication is repeatedly cited as playing a critical role in hearing-deaf relationships (Gournaris & Aubrecht, 2013; Ostrove & Oliva, 2010). Hearing professionals, who are sensitive to hearing privilege, recognize how that privilege affords them higher status and greater privileges than might have otherwise happened. Trying to become fully integrated into Deaf culture is not necessarily the answer. What works better is to examine one's own attitudes intensively, be sensitive to deaf-hearing relations in any arena, work toward a status of mutual respect, and understand that hearing professionals do not always have all the answers. Deaf professionals do not, either.

Gournaris and Aubrecht (2013) take the stance that cross-cultural conflicts are normal and common and provide vignettes illustrating how these conflicts play out. Resolving such conflicts requires mutual teaching. Hearing and Deaf people need to be open to understanding and working with each other's perspectives as part of an ongoing educational dialogue. They also need to be open to how they are embedded in their own cultures. They need to be willing to examine both personal and cultural biases in a nondefensive way. Respectful dialogues coming out of these interactions can focus on cultural exchanges to increase understanding of each other's perspectives, thus facilitating resolution of conflicts that may come up (Benedict & Sass-Lehrer, 2007). When communication procedures within bilingual settings are clearly outlined, and when the environment is perceived as safe enough to allow frank, respectful feedback, the potential for improved relationships between hearing and Deaf people or professionals significantly increases (Gournaris & Albrecht, 2013; Sheridan, White, & Mounty, 2010). Sheridan, White, and Mounty (2010) also address the need for deaf-hearing collaboration, with focus on barriers and strategies in the field of social work.

In cases of perceived discrimination, misunderstandings need to be discussed in safe places where neither the hearing nor the deaf person feels threatened. Efforts to create mutual accommodation and compromise go much farther in terms of helping hearing and deaf people understand each other and working together in mutually beneficial ways. Lawsuits should be seen only as a last recourse, since these set up either-or situations and engender bitter feelings in the process, even though the end result may mean permanent changes for the better.

Many examples of positive deaf-hearing working relationships can be found in various contexts. Take a look at the book *A New Civil Right* (Peltz Strauss, 2006), and you will note how closely the hearing author, a lawyer who initially held positions at Gallaudet University and the National Association of the Deaf and learned ASL in the process, collaborated with multiple deaf individuals to achieve legislative advances for functional equivalence (equal access) in the use of telecommunications. Benedict (Deaf) and Sass-Lehrer (hearing) (2007) point to their own collaborative experiences in organizing presentations for educational conferences where the focus is hearing-oriented and Deaf perspectives are not highlighted, and also recognize organizations such as the Conference of Educational Administrators of Schools and Programs for the Deaf (CEASD) that have a long tradition of supporting deaf perspectives and providing communication access for both deaf and hearing administrators. When Deaf professionals in the Association of College Educators for the Deaf and Hard of Hearing (ACEDHH) established a bilingual special interest group (SIG), Deaf attendance and participation quadrupled. The authors of this book (one hearing and one deaf) are illustrative of the numerous examples of deaf and hearing collaborative projects where both deaf and hearing authors and researchers share their diverse opinions and beliefs. Such hearing-deaf collaborative research and teaching relationships are crucial in forging attitudinal changes and leveling the playing field for everyone as well as providing positive bicultural modeling for the next generation of Deaf children and youth.

Another way to promote healthy deaf-hearing relationships is to forge alliances between hearing and deaf groups, whether in the professional, political, or social arenas (Lane, Hoffmeister, & Bahan, 1996). This increases "cross-pollination," creates the potential of producing a more relevant research agenda, and encourages changes in attitudes when mutual respect is maintained. This is not always an easy process, considering that the issue of sharing and control will always be present. Such alliances are what enabled passage of the ADA of 1990 and the Universal Newborn and Infant Hearing Screening and Intervention Act of 1999 by Congress, which saw an united front composed of diverse constituents passionately supporting both bills.

If both hearing and deaf professionals go about their work in a collegial and collaborative manner, giving careful consideration to each other's perspectives, this encourages healthy deaf-hearing relationships (Benedict & Sass-Lehrer, 2007). It is up to these professionals to set examples and train future generations to recognize this as status quo. This is exemplified by programs such as the training program for deaf and hearing interns who are fluent ASL users in psychology, social work, and medicine set up at the University of Rochester Medical Center Department of Psychiatry via the Deaf Wellness Center (www.urmc.rochester.edu/deaf-wellness-center.aspx). In this program, deaf trainees are not cordoned off into work with deaf patients only but also are exposed to training experiences throughout the department alongside hearing faculty and hearing patients as well, thereby permeating the culture of the institution in positive ways.

In recent years, agency, organization, and educational boards with responsibility to deaf constituents, for example, have drastically increased deaf membership in the interest of parity, setting a precedent for others to follow. Examples include the Gallaudet University Board of Trustees, the Lexington School/Center for the Deaf Board in New York City, and the board of the Alexander Graham Bell Association for the Deaf and Hard of Hearing, which had its first deaf president back in 1976. However, boards of other prominent organizations have been slow in following suit. For example, few if any deaf adults have been invited to serve on selected otolaryngology, audiology, or speech and language boards to offer advice to professionals, hearing aid manufacturers, and researchers on various issues that involve policy, product, and service provision for deaf people. For a significant period of time, Beth Benedict, Ph.D., was the only Deaf member of the Joint Committee on Infant Hearing, a professional committee that includes representatives from 11 educational, audiological, and medical organizations involved with infant hearing, early identification of hearing loss, and early intervention (Benedict & Sass-Lehrer, 2007; www.jcih.org/members.htm). In her role, Benedict was instrumental in focusing the committee's attention to issues that tend to be overlooked, including the need for more deaf professionals in early intervention programs. However, her stand was a lonely one with no other deaf colleagues on the committee. At present, due to her efforts, there are two deaf members on this committee who represent one organization (www.jcih.org/members.htm).

There are more deaf teachers and social workers today, even though barriers in the guise of examinations make it difficult to obtain certification in some locations (Mason & Mounty, 2005; Singletary, 2005). Some examination sections might cover material unrelated to classroom practices or that make it difficult for deaf test-takers to pass because of complexities inherent in the language used for test items. Professionals today are scrutinizing this practice in the interest of ensuring that potential deaf teachers are not discouraged from entering fields requiring examinations for licensure or certification and can join hearing peers in providing collaborative models for their students.

The fact that day programs for the deaf rarely feature deaf adults as administrators makes it that much harder to enhance deaf-hearing professional relationships in such settings. Individuals such as Kathleen Treni, principal of the Hearing Impaired Program at the Midland Park Schools district in New Jersey (http://bcss.bergen.org/index.php/hip-mp-home), have broken through this barrier and held on to their administrative positions by virtue of good deaf-hearing collaborative approaches. Another example is that of Connie Ferguson, the only deaf supervisor in the Texas Regional Day School, a position she held for many years until her recent retirement. Under her leadership, a bilingual-bicultural program was implemented in Bryan, Texas, and numerous Deaf teachers were hired at all levels of instruction from elementary to high school to work with hearing peers.

In the field of audiology, Gallaudet University has enrolled deaf students in its audiology doctoral program. Deaf audiologists such as Samuel Atcherson, Ph.D., director of the Auditory Electrophysiology and (Re)habilitation Laboratory and Interim Director of Audiology at the University of Arkansas for Medical Sciences, have clearly succeeded in a hearing-dominated environment (www.ualr.edu/sratcherson/people.html). Atcherson also enjoys teaching ASL. Such individuals are able to work with hearing colleagues and help their respective fields incorporate different perspectives about "hearing" in the course of evaluating the needs of deaf and hard-of-hearing children and adults and providing amplification or education information.

Ostrove and Oliva (2010) mention that Deaf and hearing individuals in formal settings tend to use sign language interpreters for communication access in the interest of maximizing interactivity, and we address the role of sign language interpreters in the next section.

Interpreter Issues

The development of healthy deaf-hearing relationships is very often contingent on how sign language interpreter issues are resolved. Most hearing professionals and hearing peers or colleagues do not develop sign language proficiency, and not all deaf persons develop proficiency in spoken English. Some will use the text feature on their smartphones for communication, but such conversations do not necessarily flow easily. When sign language interpreters are used during face-to-face interactions, they serve as bridges for the facilitation of interactive dialogue.

Sign language interpreting, traditionally seen as a service for deaf adults, developed out of the need for deaf people to communicate in depth with hearing people. Early interpreters were family members who could sign, particularly hearing children of deaf parents, friends, and other local resources (Cokely, 2005; Hoffmeister, 2008). Although their social intentions were often above reproach, hearing people stepping in to interpret could intrude themselves into the dialogue, provide options, and without being aware, inadvertently influence not only the outcome of such interactions but also reinforce how hearing people might perceive deaf people as dependent or in a powerless capacity (Kushalnagar & Rashid, 2008). And deaf people themselves at that time might have found it difficult to complain because of their dependency on these volunteer interpreters.

Sign language interpreting evolved into a professional field because of an increasing demand for interpreters by deaf adults and the inability of informal volunteers to meet this demand, aligned with a shift towards enhancing professionalization of the individuals doing the interpreting (Cokely, 2005). The establishment of the Registry of Interpreters for the Deaf (RID, www.rid.org) was the outcome of the professionalization of the field. Because of ethical issues related to confidentiality and interpreter exploitation of information obtained through interpreted situations among other things, the RID developed a stringent code of ethics that covers the use of sign language interpreters. This ensures confidentiality and accurate reflection of ongoing dialogue, whether it is voice to sign or sign to voice.

Clearly, it is best to use certified interpreters who are fully qualified to handle many interpreter situations both linguistically and ethically Throughout the United States, there are interpreter agencies that are a valuable resource for providing sign language interpreters as well as oral interpreters and CART (Communication Access Realtime Translation, using computers for those who prefer to use typed English) services. The National Consortium of Interpreter Education Centers focuses on collaboration between interpreter education programs to enhance the quality of sign language interpreter education. While this reflects professionalism, the preponderance of hearing professionals (Winston, 2005) has led Cokely (2005) to view such efforts as a diminishing of the control the Deaf community has as stakeholders in the interpreting realm.

As noted throughout this book, there has been an upsurge in the number of deaf professionals who are in the position of having a larger degree of power and authority vis-à-vis the use of sign language interpreters (Kushalnagar & Rashid, 2008). Due to their professional needs and their knowledge of the linguistic demands of their occupations, such as, for example, scientific or legal terminology, these individuals are managing how they use interpreters to a greater extent compared to historical use. In turn, interpreters need to be aware of their own attitudes, particularly as these relate to the possibility of audism, so as to ensure a positive collaboration with the individuals they serve.

Why is this so important? Many deaf people are acutely aware that their ability to develop positive relationships with hearing peers, whatever the context—the workplace, the social setting, the classroom, the conference, etc.—depends to a significant degree on the quality of the interpreters being used and their skills in formulating accurate translations. Deaf people see interpreting as a valued and cherished service. For many, this has provided entry into job opportunities that might have otherwise been unavailable or into social, educational, and recreational situations that maximize the potential for participating in hearing society activities. However, there are ongoing issues that need to be acknowledged and dealt with in order to enhance deaf-hearing relationships.

Sign language interpreters regularly deal with a variety of demands, including linguistic, environmental (e.g., court, see Chapter 10; classroom, see Chapter 5, business conference, etc.), interpersonal, and extrapersonal (role expectations, knowledge of specialized language relevant to the setting, such as medical or statistical terminology) demands. In addition, research reveals that they are at risk for chronic physical disability such as carpal tunnel syndrome and tendonitis as well as increased mental and cognitive stress (Rochester Institute of Technology, 2008). Interpreters must constantly judge appropriate responses, oftentimes in difficult situations. Recurrent frustrations include, for example, situations when deaf persons are unfamiliar with interpreter roles or when hearing people start talking to interpreters instead of focusing on the process of communicating with deaf persons through these interpreters. Unfortunately, some deaf persons are not particularly sensitive to interpreter stress, considering their dependency on interpreters and their expectations of how interpreters perform their duties. For both hearing and deaf parties, training will facilitate the comfort of interpreting situations and sensitivity to the role of the interpreter.

Admittedly, sign-to-voice interpreting is more difficult than voice-to-sign interpretation. Adequate translation requires a true understanding of linguistic nuances in whatever way the deaf person chooses to express herself or himself, especially in individual facial nuances, gestures, and signs. When the interpreter's first language is spoken English and not ASL, there can be considerable stress in working through the translation process, particularly when interpreters at least hopefully understand that they are responsible for how the deaf person is represented to the hearing public.

In turn, what is extremely frustrating for deaf persons themselves are situations when they recognize that they are not being accurately interpreted. Interpreters are *not* neutral conduits. Instead, they significantly affect interchanges through their ability to understand, their knowledge of terminology, and their translation selection (Turner, 2005). These issues are manifestations of how interpreters potentially control situations, often unconsciously, and affect hearing perceptions of deaf people.

For example, speeches by deaf presenters may sound less than excellent when poorly interpreted. Hearing listeners will then develop poor opinions of the presenters. When professional terminology is translated incorrectly, this can negatively affect perceptions about the sophistication level of deaf professionals. During a professional meeting, a deaf sociolinguist used the term *language acquisition* in the course of his lecture (S. Nover, personal communication, January 15, 2002). The interpreter interpreted this term as *language pick-up*. By selecting this phrase, the interpreter unwittingly created false impressions that put the deaf sociolinguist at a disadvantage in the minds of hearing scholars at this academic conference.

Multiplied many times over, such situations leave ASL users at the mercy of interpreters. They do have the means of evaluating whether they have been accurately interpreted, but unfortunately, that is typically after the fact—that is, after they have completed their presentations. Deaf professionals who have presented have conveyed to the authors their concerns about being accurately interpreted after having read transcriptions of their presentations as conveyed by interpreters that revealed significant misinterpretations.

Clearly, what is needed is to have interpreters who are familiar with the professional language being used and who can work with deaf professionals in advance, using PowerPoint slides and the like, to ensure as accurate a translation as possible. To rectify mistakes, deaf people need to become extra-sensitive to hearing respondent dialogue, correct misunderstandings as these emerge, and obtain feedback from trusted hearing colleagues, particularly when there are no transcripts. If real-time captioning is available, deaf people can verify interpreter translations by checking text as they go along. These tactics demand a level of sophisticated awareness that the typical deaf person may not always possess, and training efforts in this direction will help.

In addition to questions of interpretation, some deaf professionals may be wary of the hidden ambitions of some sign language interpreters. Based on on-the-job informal networking and exposure to job duties, hearing coworkers and supervisors may feel that interpreters understand both the subject matter and the roles of the deaf persons for whom they are interpreting. People, deaf or hearing, are more comfortable in situations that involve direct communication. Thus, having to work through an interpreter requires some adjustment. There have been stories of job openings being filled by the interpreter instead of qualified deaf applicants. Deaf professionals who rely on sign language see this as a thorny issue, reflecting ongoing oppression. Training of hearing personnel about interpreter roles and boundaries may help rectify this situation. Other than that, there is no clear resolution apart from recourse to the ADA. People who might think of suing have to deal with concerns about their professional reputations as potential troublemakers with negative implications for future job possibilities.

It is important to remember that many sign language interpreters embrace interpreting as a lifelong career and establish excellent reputations. Some use their interpreter training and interpreting work to obtain in-depth understanding of what it means to be deaf and related issues. Others pursue higher education to improve their qualifications for working in different capacities with and for deaf people. Their abilities to form positive relationships with deaf colleagues is a key factor in their being accepted by deaf people and deaf professionals in particular (Hauser, Finch, & Hauser, 2008).

Are sign language interpreters adequately sensitized to the perceptions of deaf consumers in the course of whatever training they receive? Considering the lack of consistency in criteria for interpreter training programs (Winston, 2005) and the fact that the term *qualified* has yet to be specified throughout the country, training and subsequent experiences should involve ongoing feedback regarding performance, particularly from deaf consumers themselves.

One overriding issue regarding interpreters is cost. Many administrators may be willing to accommodate deaf people on the job, but they are concerned about this ancillary expense. This is a valid concern that needs to be addressed, as noted, for example, in the Task Force on Health Care Careers for the Deaf and Hard-of-Hearing Community Final Report (2012), which offers suggestions about innovative approaches to deal with cost. Medical providers and hospitals continue to deny communication access or interpreters for patients and claim that writing is sufficient, based solely on economic or profit considerations. Even today, you can use Google and find out about lawsuits against hospitals for not providing sign language interpreters. These lawsuits generally are settled in favor of the plaintiffs. In any case, such situations are blatant examples of oppression in which hearing perspectives about the communication needs of deaf people are superimposed over the perspectives of deaf consumers. What is overlooked is that, in the medical setting, cost effectiveness as part of the greater picture can be argued when deaf people in most typical situations fully understand their medical issues, take care of themselves, and reduce their need for medical attention and in turn for medical insurance payment. It is heartening to hear reports of medical offices inquiring about communication preferences when deaf patients call to schedule appointments so that interpreters can be on site if needed. While medical settings have started to install video remote interpreting systems as a cost-cutting approach, there are problems with video transmission, and medical situations do not always permit patients to position themselves to watch a computer screen (National Association of the Deaf, 2008b).

To look at the cost issue from a different perspective, a hearing organization may automatically include sound systems that enhance communication for hearing people as part of operating costs but will question whether to enhance communication access for deaf persons as an integral part of operating costs. Admittedly, this is an expensive proposition. Some effort to consider creative financial solutions will go a long way in conveying the message that accessibility is important for *both* deaf and hearing people. Not making this effort does deaf people an enormous disservice and perpetuates discrimination. The ADA of 1990 has provisions that apply to both privately and publicly funded settings as well as an undue hardship provision that covers settings having 15 employees or more. If settings claim undue hardship, both the program or subdivision resources and the resources of the entire institution or agency are examined in order to ascertain whether operating costs for interpreting services do justify denying accessibility because of undue hardship.

Attitudes within the Deaf Community

Although this chapter focuses on deaf-hearing relationships, we cannot leave the topic of attitudes without very briefly touching on attitudes within the deaf community. Yes, the deaf community is diverse, and one can find a multitude of deaf members of various ethnic and racial groups, members who are gay, lesbian, bisexual, transgendered, DeafBlind, affiliated with various religious groups, and so on, mingling amicably at large deaf community events. The commonality of being deaf does facilitate cohesiveness in these diverse groups of deaf people, even to a greater extent than may be found in hearing gatherings.

However, the deaf community is also a microcosm of the larger hearing community. It has factions that do not always coexist in full harmony or that exhibit bigotry (Lane, Hoffmeister, & Bahan, 1996; Leigh & Lewis, 2010). And sadly, some deaf people absorb the discriminatory values of the societies in which they develop and perpetuate the ongoing oppression of deaf peers on the basis of religion, race or ethnicity, sexual orientation, language preference, and disability.

Take the case of DeafBlind persons, arguably among the most isolated of all people. Many deaf people understandably harbor some fear of vision loss, and seeing DeafBlind persons will ignite that fear (Bailey & Miner, 2010). Even more, there is the stigma of additional disability. To deal with this, some sighted deaf persons will minimize social contact with DeafBlind people, thus perpetuating their isolation. Openly gay deaf people still confront varying types of rejection, ranging from snide remarks to overt rejection by heterosexual deaf people (Gutman & Zangas, 2010). The African American and White deaf communities have historically gone their separate ways because of institutionalized racism (Corbett, 2010; Jankowski, 1997), although today there are increased efforts to intermingle. Deaf people who object to spoken language values have ostracized deaf people who prefer spoken English, even if they can sign (Leigh, 2009). The history of deaf women approaching parity with deaf men in running deaf organizations is relatively recent (Lane, Hoffmeister, & Bahan, 1996; Robinson, 2006).

In coming to terms with the fact that we are a diverse society, we can turn to models of deaf people who reject such behavior and who strive for common causes that bring deaf people together. These causes include civil rights and empowerment, employment equity, and access to communication, whether face-to-face or via technology. Just as society struggles with discrimination as an ongoing process, the deaf community is engaged in a parallel struggle to learn about respect for diversity in the face of an increasingly multicultural deaf component. It is the schools, ranging from preschool through postsecondary settings, which bear most of the burden for increasing sensitivity to diversity. Many have responded to this call by instituting multicultural programs that teach about respect for diversity.

Even though deaf people have worked hard to ensure their places in society, it has taken them a long time to learn that if they are not seen as a united front, they will fail to achieve desired political agendas. The number of organizations in the deaf community is large in proportion to the small size of the community (Van Cleve & Crouch, 1989). All of these organizations have their own mission and objectives, and historically they were seldom united on issues related to the lives of deaf people (Christiansen & Barnartt, 1995). This often sabotaged political possibilities.

The Deaf President Now movement showed that the deaf community was capable of media manipulation, a united front, and political savvy. Since then, national organizations of deaf people have banded together to form the Deaf and Hard of Hearing Consumer Advocacy Network (DHHCAN, Lucas, 2012). Organizations composed of hearing people who work to serve the interests of deaf people can be associate members but do not have voting rights. The network engages regularly in the political process and advocates for different legislative initiatives that affect the educational, rehabilitation, mental health, occupational, social, and political lives of deaf people. In doing so, DHHCAN not only informs hearing society of the perspectives and goals of deaf people, but it also draws deaf organizations together and limits the potential for infighting.

Conclusions

When deaf and hearing administrators of schools and programs for deaf and hearing children are seen as equally desirable, when no eyebrows are raised at the announcement of deaf professionals heading major institutions and corporations, when the expectation is that deaf people from diverse backgrounds can contribute as much to society as hearing people, and when subtle discriminatory biases that reinforce the perception that deaf people are limited in some way because of their inability to hear are eliminated, then one may say that the potential for healthy relationships between deaf and hearing peers or colleagues has been fully achieved. The possibility of that happening today is far greater than it was decades ago, but as indicated throughout the book, there continues to be room for improvement.

We believe that through recurrent positive exposure to each other, deaf and hearing people will endeavor to work together in dismantling attitudinal barriers that hamper healthy coexistence. This requires ongoing education and sensitivity in view of the fact that society at large is still engaged in the process of breaking free of lingering stereotypical perceptions of deaf people.

Suggested Readings

Burch, S., & Kafer, A. (Eds.). (2010). *Deaf and disability studies: Interdisciplinary perspectives*. Washington, DC: Gallaudet University Press.
    This book consists of 14 essays covering the nature of the Deaf/Disability coexistence, highlighting the tensions and common parameters of both constituents while also noting the influence of economics, race, location, and culture.

Hauser, P., Finch, C., & Hauser, A. (Eds.). (2008). *Deaf professionals and designated interpreters*. Washington, DC: Gallaudet University Press.

If you are interested in learning how Deaf professionals take charge of the interpreting situation and how this collaborative relationship can be mutually beneficial, this is the book for you.

Stoffel, S. (2012). *Deaf-blind reality*. Washington, DC: Gallaudet University Press.

How do DeafBlind people communicate with hearing-sighted people? This book provides a sense of what works for this unique group of individuals.

Torres, A. (2009). *Signing in Puerto Rican: A hearing son and his Deaf family*. Washington, DC: Gallaudet University Press.

Get a glimpse into what a Deaf Puerto Rican family with a hearing son is like by reading this book. You will get a sense of the frustrations, misunderstandings, and love expressed in this minority cultural family with Deaf and hearing members interacting with each other.

12 From Now to the Future

Life can only be understood backwards; but it must be lived forwards.

Søren Kierkegaard (1843)

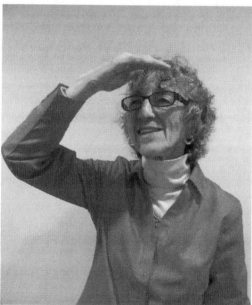

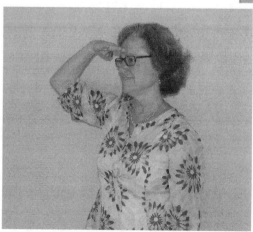

Figure 12.1 Irene W. Leigh (top right) and Jean F. Andrews (lower left), two authors looking towards the future

Nationwide, approximately 45 million people have hearing differences ranging from mild to profound. This can affect language comprehension and communication to varying degrees. Some causes of hearing loss can be treated medically, but the majority of profoundly deaf persons have a sensorineural hearing level that is currently not amenable to medical treatment aside from cochlear implantation (Chapter 3). In this book, our primary focus has been on this population, although we have briefly covered those individuals who have confronted issues related to changing hearing levels over the course of their lives.

In the Preface, we introduced questions about deaf people. Throughout the book, we have attempted to answer these questions, starting in the first chapter with an exploration of the field of psychology and deaf people. The issues discussed in that chapter—including intellectual testing, mental health services, changes in standards of care, professional training, and the effects of Deaf culture—illustrate how the field has evolved. Chapters 2 through 11 provided additional information, expanding on these issues and more. This chapter briefly reviews critical points and uses these as stepping-stones to envision what the future may bring in terms of research, development, educational practices, and life changes.

Changes in the Deaf Community

Hearing people not intimately acquainted with deaf people have traditionally seen the deaf community as a ghetto apart from the "real world," hence the urge to "bring deaf children into the hearing world." But deaf people are full participants in their communities, just like hearing people are participants in their own communities. This reinforces the drift away from the sole focus on the medical model of how deaf people should function and encourages different perspectives on the lives of deaf people within their communities.

In addition to the sociocultural model that is predicated on a dynamic community rooted in American Sign Language (ASL), we have Deaf Studies scholars creating different lens for understanding Deaf people, thereby encouraging a more nuanced and diverse picture of what Deaf people are and what their communities are like. We now have Deaf ethnicity, Deafnicity, Deafhood, People of the Eye, and Deaf Gain (see Chapter 1 for details). These frames of reference have emerged only in the last 20 years or so, encouraged primarily by Deaf scholars who are creating new paradigms of what it means to be deaf. Carrying this development further, research into these areas is generating different perspectives of what being deaf entails in ways that have never previously been framed. Thanks to these contributions, we see a maturing of the Deaf Studies discipline. This phenomenon is one recognized by Tom Humphries (2008, p. 3), who views this maturation as part of "the reorganization of DEAF" thanks to the narrative shift away from medical aspects towards a more expansive discourse of language and culture. Because of the dynamism of Deaf Studies, we can expect ongoing productions of "new forms, explanations, representations, and identities" (Humphries, 2008, p. 17).

Of critical note is that, parallel with the demographic shifts currently taking place in the United States, the face of the deaf community is changing significantly (Chapters 2 and 9). Historically, the deaf community has been portrayed with a White face. Growing up on the north side of Chicago, Illinois, Irene W. Leigh never knew there were Black Deaf students in Chicago's South Side. Moving on to New York City, she slowly became aware of a large Russian Deaf contingent in Brooklyn, the Orthodox Jewish Deaf community also in Brooklyn, the Puerto Rican Deaf individuals in the Bronx, a thriving Black Deaf organization representing individuals from the various boroughs, and so on. These Deaf religious and ethnic groups are what give the deaf community its vibrancy and its diversity.

To expand on the diversity issue, while we recognize the bonds bringing groups of deaf people together, we need to also acknowledge the unique nature of each deaf group, of which there are many as indicated in Chapters 2 and 9. A sobering note is that research of diverse Deaf groups is still in its infancy, with the exception of studies such as those on African American Deaf persons done by McCaskill, Lucas, Bailey, and Hill (2011) and Williamson (2007). The good news is that there has been an explosion of publications describing the different groups that form deaf communities worldwide, such as *A Lens on Deaf Identities* (Leigh, 2009); *Many Ways to be Deaf* (Monaghan, Schmaling, Nakamura, & Turner, 2003); *Deaf People around the World* (Moores & Miller, 2009); and *Citizenship, Politics, Differences* (Cooper & Rashid, 2015), as well as diverse groups within the United States (e.g., *Psychotherapy with Deaf Clients from Diverse Groups* [Leigh, 2010]). As we move into the future, we can anticipate more scrutiny on the lives of these diverse deaf groups.

Deaf culture serves to draw all these diverse deaf people together with a set of shared experiences and worldwide social and educational networks (Chapters 2 and 9). It is a vibrant culture vividly expressed at the many Deaf cultural festivals occurring in cities, and through Deaf art, ASL storytelling, and Deaf theater and literature. For Deaf people, such artistic expressions provide an opportunity to share the "Deaf perspective." In particular, these cultural expressions serve as a forum to vividly illustrate their experiences at the hands of hearing society, in particular their feelings of oppression (as outlined in Chapter 11). This is a form of empowerment. One end result of these expressions has been to provide hearing viewers with new perspectives that counteract their natural and traditional urges toward ethnocentric and egocentric behaviors when it comes to Deaf people. In essence, these cultural expressions serve to reinforce the fact that Deaf people want to be understood. In turn, we also want to emphasize that not only culturally Deaf people but also deaf people who have different types of affiliations with the deaf community, and outside the deaf community, want their views and opinions considered as well in the larger hearing society.

Historically, the community of deaf people expanded as graduates of residential schools for the deaf entered its ranks. That has changed. Today, the vast majority of deaf children are being educated in the public schools, whether cordoned off in day classes or placed with hearing peers. Many of these deaf children will not form social networks with deaf people until a much later age, if at all. This clearly influences psychosocial development in general and the development of deaf identities in particular (Chapters 7 and 8). Furthermore, this new development is now changing the face of the deaf community to one that is more diverse in terms of experience.

Additional factors impacting changes in the deaf community include the fact that the ways in which deaf people socialize has moved beyond the traditional structure of Deaf clubs. These clubs have declined due to home entertainment captioning and the Internet, as well as the emergence of a deaf professional middle class less reliant on old forms of socializing (Padden, 2008; Chapter 9).

The concept of Deaf space used to bring to mind deaf clubs. No longer. Deaf space is now increasingly fluid and less permanent. Murray (2008, p. 103) describes the major features of "the new Deaf cultural landscape" as one that consists of gatherings in various public spaces as well as virtually, through such sites as www.deafzone.com that provide information on where international deaf gatherings are planned to take place. More to the point, the Internet provides opportunities for Deaf people to establish and maintain national and international digital Deaf spaces or communities, and smartphones are now Deaf spaces in the midst of hearing chaos (Kurz & Cuculick, 2015). Murray (2008) cautions that such spaces are not just because of technology, considering that even before the Internet, there were national and transnational connections between nineteenth-century deaf people. Physical Deaf space is increasingly transient, with Deaf expos, world congresses, national conventions, and so on taking over hearing spaces such as hotels or convention centers for a few days at a time. Nonetheless, nontransient Deaf spaces exist, now known as DeafSpaces, one noteworthy example being that of the Sorenson Language and Communication Center at Gallaudet University, which serves as a model for future Deaf space creations (Bauman, 2014). The focus is on architecture that expresses connections rather than barriers and visual openness rather than closed-off spaces.

When people enter the deaf community, they will find that this involvement fosters strong interdependence among its members. This continues from early childhood into old age. Elderly deaf persons from residential schools typically maintain lifelong friendships developed in childhood. Those who enter the deaf community during adolescence and adulthood also develop close bonds within the community. Their social networks sustain them, even after they have retired. The number of deaf retirees has greatly increased, with many joining Deaf Seniors of America (Chapter 9). A good number of deaf retirees are clustering in areas such as Las Vegas, Nevada; Surprise, Arizona; and the Villages and Boynton Beach, Florida. There are some retirement settings throughout the United States that have been set up for deaf senior citizens. Additionally, there has been an increase in the number of ethnic-based deaf organizations and gay/lesbian/bisexual/transgender/questioning groups, to name a few, each of which encourages group bonding and community involvement.

The issue of tolerance in the face of increasing diversity within the deaf community is one that demands attention. Although the community has traditionally been known to welcome this diversity, tolerating different types of people still continues to be an issue at the local level, as witnessed in bullying situations and conscious or unconscious racism and microaggression towards others who are viewed as different. Research into effective ways of fostering tolerance, particularly in the schools, will ameliorate the insidious effects of discrimination. Leadership training, such as those provided by various deaf organizations as mentioned in Chapter 9, will encourage development of effective leaders that will model tolerance for a widely diverse deaf population.

Historically, in their choice of occupations, many deaf persons were limited to blue-collar jobs such as printing, shoe repair, factory work, peddling, and barbering. With today's proliferation of interpreter services, wireless and digital technologies, relay services, increasing positive media representations, free and appropriate education, and legal protections from discrimination, deaf people intermingle in the broader society as never before. They increasingly benefit from the larger society's offerings in education, employment, and recreation. Gallaudet University continues to have deaf presidents, the most recent one being the first female Deaf president (Roberta "Bobbi" Cordano), and RIT/NTID has continued also to have deaf vice presidents/deans who hold that rank under the umbrella of RIT and its president (currently Gerard Buckley). Deaf academicians now number in the 300+ range, and their roles in higher education have the potential to influence both hearing and deaf college-age students in a proactive and positive fashion. The number of deaf teachers working in schools for young deaf students has increased exponentially. Thousands of deaf adults are now studying and have studied for graduate degrees and teacher certifications at various universities in the country. With postsecondary and graduate education accessibility enhanced by the use of interpreters, voice-to-text software, video relay services, real-time captioning, and distance learning and tutoring, many deaf adults are succeeding in higher education and in various professions and trades. Today, even more occupations are accessible to deaf people (Chapters 2 and 9). Many are employed as computer programmers and software developers, educational researchers, scientists, inventors, physicians, religious leaders, lawyers, teachers, administrators, CEOs of companies, stockbrokers, chefs, auto mechanics, ad infinitum. Limits continue to be tested. For example, there is even a push to allow deaf people into the military, via a potential pilot program, the Keith Nolan Air Force Deaf Demonstration Act of 2015 (www.congress.gov/bill/114th-congress/house-bill/1722), which President Obama signed in November 2015. The Department of Defense did a feasibility study report that was released to Congress in April 2016. As of May, 2016, Congress was considering the findings of this report (Keith Nolan, personal communication, May 17, 2016). Although automation continues to hinder the deaf unskilled worker, job opportunities in an increasing number of fields are open to them. Overall, again, the deaf community's exposure to hearing communities is greater than ever previously.

There is a dark side, too. The deaf community is plagued by illiteracy, underemployment, and underachievement. Too many deaf persons get caught in the criminal justice system and need special services (Chapter 10). Some refuse to work and abuse the Social Security system. Some cannot get work or are unable to work. Learning to read and write continues to be difficult for many (Chapter 6). The gap between many deaf persons' intelligence levels as indicated on intelligence tests and their low academic performance remains. All of this is quite discouraging. But looking at the big picture, it is not difficult to see how many hearing Americans are struggling with the same issues. Like many Deaf Americans, African American, Latinx, Asian American, Native American, and immigrant communities struggle daily to survive economically, get a good education, enjoy all the freedoms and benefits the United States has to offer, and acclimatize into U.S. society without sacrificing their cultural identities.

The media continually reflect ongoing debate about the best ways to resolve these complex issues. But solutions can be effective only when the strengths of the people involved are utilized. With deaf people, their problems can more readily be addressed when instructional programs are culturally sensitive and are built on their sensory, cognitive, and survival strengths rather than on their limitations. Framed in this way, there is hope that future research can alleviate the problems that continue to plague deaf people. In addition to the need for educational research, mentioned in Chapters 5 and 6, and later in this chapter, cross-cultural studies of ethnic communities and deaf communities that focus on the skills they use to succeed may be one way to address these issues. With the inclusion of more deaf professionals on research teams, different perspectives and creative solutions have the opportunity to emerge.

There is also a need to reinforce the perception, both professionally and on the lay level, that there are psychologically healthy deaf adults who choose the hearing world or the deaf world or, most commonly, who gravitate between both worlds. We repeat this observation yet again because too many tend to forget that these adults, who are able to confront life and to fashion satisfactory adjustments for themselves, are more the norm than the rarity. Studying these psychologically healthy deaf adults will help develop parameters of normalcy within the deaf population and clarify more who the deaf community members are, as contrasted with those who struggle with mental illnesses and other significant difficulties.

American Sign Language

ASL is now firmly entrenched as a bona fide language, not only as the language that Deaf people use, but also as a language worthy of research. The use of ASL has been explored, and is continuing to be explored, through research into its role in psychological functioning, best practices in education, bilingualism and second language learning, psycholinguistics, neurolinguistics, and literacy learning, as has been reported throughout this book. The study of cognitive processing and learning styles in deaf children with the addition of ASL as an investigative tool now boasts a growing corpus of studies, some of which are briefly reviewed in Chapter 4. In mental health, measures delivered in computerized ASL format have begun to be developed and researched for reliability and validity (Chapter 8). Analyzing the ASL expressions of Deaf people who are psychotic will facilitate accurate diagnosis of deaf persons, particularly in terms of differentiating them from those deaf individuals who are language and learning challenged and who may thus appear to be psychotic when in fact they are not.

The use of ASL has enabled neuroscientists to explore the frontiers of the brain in order to understand where sign language is processed and to develop increasingly accurate data about how the brain is organized for and processes language. Today's noninvasive brain imaging techniques, including magnetic resonance imaging (MRI), functional magnetic resonance imaging (fMRI), positron-emission tomography (PET), and functional near infrared spectroscopy (fNIRS), among others, have allowed neuroscientists to successfully explore the brains of Deaf individuals who communicate in sign language with the goal of probing further for the neural roots of signed languages. It is now confirmed that, even though signed languages have visual-spatial organizational features that relate to right-hemisphere functioning, the neural organization of signed languages have more in common with that of spoken languages than previously thought. This of course has generated and is generating more research into how signed languages are processed in both left and right hemispheres.

There have been significant advances in the development of the first generation of standardized cognitive and language screening tests that contribute to the diagnosis of acquired neurological impairments in British sign language users (University College London, 2015). Used in conjunction with brain scans, it is now possible to confidently diagnose dementia and other neurological impairments at an early stage, thus allowing for potentially timely services and better health outcomes. Hauser et al. (2016) have developed an American Sign Language Comprehension Test with acceptable reliability and validity results, a development long awaited.

Taking into account the fact that many deaf persons are delayed in their exposure to language (Chapter 4), research into how deaf children and adults process language can provide insights regarding the nature of the so-called sensitive or critical period for language acquisition, which has fueled the expansion of cochlear implant use to ensure maximum language acquisition early. Interestingly, anecdotal evidence points to some who have been able to internalize a language after age 6, with exposure to ASL. One of the authors (Andrews) routinely asks Deaf graduate students at what age they acquired language. Many of them reported that they did not acquire a full language until after age 6 when they entered school and did not fully acquire sign language until well into their elementary school years. Their language learning experiences challenges past thinking about the critical periods for first and second language acquisition. A seminal paper by Hakuta, Bialystok, and Wiley (2003) argued against this critical period hypothesis for second language learning based on their study of immigrants who developed the ability to learn a second language that gradually decreased over the life span, rather than the expected discontinuity earlier in life. A review of the evidence for this hypothesis by Qingzin (2012) suggests a more nuanced view, specifically the possibility that there are different critical periods for different aspects of second language acquisition, rather than a single one, as based on the premise that language is not a unitary phenomenon. This has implications for those attempting to learn ASL or English as a second language. The sensitive or critical period hypothesis appears to be more germane for first-language acquisition, but how long it lasts appears to be due to numerous complex factors that are difficult to weed out. Ongoing study of how deaf children acquire their first and second languages can provide further data in evaluating this theory of sensitive or critical periods.

Research into Total Communication and other sign systems failed to note significant gains in language and literacy achievement test scores despite better face-to-face communication skills compared with spoken communication alone for many deaf children and their families. Interest in bimodalism has resurfaced due to the advent of the cochlear implant and research results indicating that literacy skills, while improved, are still not increasing to the levels that we want for deaf children. Consequently, within the context of bimodalism and bilingualism, researchers have increasingly turned to an examination of the links between the acquisition and use of ASL and English reading and writing abilities with the goal of evaluating the applicability of these findings to the language and learning needs of deaf students (Marschark, Tang, & Knoors, 2014). Language and literacy teaching approaches are increasingly incorporating the use of ASL (Allen, 2015; Allen, Letteri, Choi, & Dang, 2014; Freel, Clark, Anderson, Gilbert, Musyoka, & Hauser, 2011; Hoffmeister & Caldwell-Harris, 2014; Kuntze, Golos, & Enns, 2014; McQuarrie & Parrila, 2014; see also Chapters 5 and 6).

It is important to note that research into the extent to which bilingual (sign and spoken languages) deaf education is associated with cognitive development is still in its early stages and evidence continues to be mixed due to a multiplicity of complex factors (Marschark, Knoors, & Tang, 2014; see Chapters 3, 4, 5, and 6). The authors conclude that there are deaf and hard-of-hearing children with cochlear implants who succeed with sign language (see also Davidson, Lillo-Martin, & Pichler, 2014; Mitchener, 2015), as well as those who succeed with spoken language (see also Geers & Sedey, 2011; Ruffin et al., 2013) and who succeed with both (see also Hassanzadeh, 2012; Rinaldi & Caselli, 2014), with no one route to be expected for all such children. Today, researchers have available new tools to measure ASL in babies, toddlers, and young school children (Enns et al., 2013; Simms, Baker, & Clark, 2013). Results from these assessments will enhance knowledge regarding how deaf children develop linguistically in ASL.

Education Issues

Since the enactment of Public Law 94–142 and subsequently the Individuals with Disabilities Education Act (IDEA), parents legally have had access to a continuum of school placements for their deaf children. These placements cover public schools that provide inclusion experiences, mainstream settings, self-contained classrooms, day schools for deaf children, co-enrollment, and state residential schools or center schools for deaf children. Each type of placement has its advantages and disadvantages (Chapter 5). The bottom line is that each deaf child deserves a quality and communication-driven program that is also sensitive to their cultural needs. To this day, parents continue to request hearings to evaluate the appropriateness of school district placement decisions for their deaf child, since parent perspectives and school district perspectives do not always align with each other.

With IDEA, the trend toward educating all children with disabilities in schools with their nondisabled peers has significantly accelerated. While educating deaf children in these settings has typically been viewed as inclusive and therefore preferred to segregated education, this may in fact be an exclusion setting for far too many deaf children (Siegel, 2008; Tucker, 2010/2011). Although well-intentioned, this law has created a situation where too many deaf children are now in hearing classrooms without access or with limited access to the support services that are essential for effective communication, language development, or academic learning. Consequently, many are deprived of an appropriate visual and linguistic classroom that is culturally friendly for deaf children. These children are at risk for experiencing academic failure and feelings of isolation, rejection, and negative self-worth (Oliva & Lytle, 2014). Unquestionably, with appropriate services in place, whatever the setting, the chances for academic success and optimal psychosocial development are far greater.

Deaf children need a setting where they can develop age-level language skills in their first language, whether it is spoken English, the non-English spoken language of the home, or ASL, together with corresponding skills in English literacy. In addition, deaf children benefit most from a critical mass of communication, age, and cognitive peers in order to develop healthy self-perceptions and resilience (Tucker, 2010/2011; Zand & Pierce, 2011). It remains to be determined what a critical mass consists of, but being the only deaf child in the entire school brings with it its own set of challenges, including the feeling one is the only deaf child in the world (Oliva & Lytle, 2014). It is important to ask these children how they feel and how they are doing, so that appropriate supports such as, for example, summer camp programs with other deaf children, can be implemented. Parents have reported benefiting most from deaf or hard-of-hearing role models, and having these models in early intervention programs is now considered best practice (Pittman et al., 2016).

Teachers and staff should be able to communicate directly with deaf students. Interpreters, note-takers, captioning, tutoring, opportunities for inclusion in extracurricular activities, and speech and audiology services, as well as school counseling and school psychology services with appropriate training in working with deaf children, are services that can improve the performance of deaf children in public schools. Administrators in public school settings often are not aware of, but do need to understand, the unique needs of deaf children. These children often lack exposure to adult deaf and hard-of-hearing role models as too few of these role models can be found within the public school system. Parents who are knowledgeable about what services and opportunities their deaf child needs can legally demand appropriate support services when canvassing school programs.

Oliva and Lytle (2014) have several systemic recommendations, some of which are as follows: If organizations serving deaf people collaborate with school systems, common concerns about how deaf children develop can be addressed. A new profession—the educational specialist for deaf and hard-of-hearing children—could be developed to better support deaf children dispersed through mainstream schools. This should minimize the fragmentation of services that currently exists in the public school system. The United States Department of Education (DOE) needs to do a better job of gathering and reporting data by disability group, including deaf and hard-of-hearing students.

Taking this further, for example, DOE could set up a system to track deaf children from birth throughout their school careers. Oftentimes, the education trajectory of deaf children is bumpy and full of change. They start out in speech and hearing centers and then move into public schools. Those who fail to develop sufficient language are transferred to center or special schools in later childhood or adolescence (see later). After these children needing more services are moved out, studies show the public school placement is superior when in fact, the low achievers have been removed, thus showing a selection bias in studies favoring general education placement. By tracking the children from infancy forward, more rigorous research can be conducted to provide the services that individual deaf children need, rather than promulgating the notion that "one size fits all" and that all deaf children should be educated with their nondeaf peers. This will provide a far better and richer picture of how these students are doing compared to what we have now and guide the profession towards focusing more on needed academic enhancements.

Self-contained classrooms can be a boon in that these bring deaf children together within mainstream settings because they receive the support they may need. However, especially in rural areas where the number of deaf students is low, teaching becomes more complicated. For example, a teacher may have several children in the classroom, each one of different ages and having different language backgrounds and communication needs. Even though children benefit from interacting with each other during group teaching situations (Rogoff, 2003; Vygotsky, 1978; Wenger, 1999), such instructional practices in this case may be less than ideal, even nonexistent. For instance, what does the teacher do when the class contains children who have cochlear implants and require speech and auditory training, a hard-of-hearing child who uses a Total Communication or simultaneous (speech and sign) approach, and a profoundly deaf child who benefits from an ASL/English bilingual approach? These are just some of the myriad of issues teachers of the deaf in the mainstream face.

In 1975, when Jean F. Andrews entered the field as a teacher at the Maryland School for the Deaf in Frederick, Maryland, she noticed a trickle of deaf and hard-of-hearing junior high students who transferred to the center school because of low reading levels and behavior issues. After working in more than ten center schools as a researcher and supervisor of student teachers and serving on the governing board at one school, she has observed a flood of deaf transfer students to center schools. Center school administrators and teachers are put in the position of "picking up the pieces" of these language-deprived children who were neglected or not provided with appropriate services in clinics and public schools where professionals expect deaf children to function as "hearing" in regular classrooms. From "last resort" to "centers of deaf education expertise," these center schools play an important role in addressing the language and literacy needs of these children by providing outreach, parent training, summer camps, professional training for interpreters and teachers with a staff of deaf education experts who can provide expertise to public schools who educate deaf children. Their atmosphere is that of a Deaf culture-friendly atmosphere with full linguistic access. But even within these strong cultural and linguistic school communities, there is room for reflection. For example, based on an ethnographic case study of a state residential school for the deaf, there continues to be competing discourses of deaf as a disability and Deaf culture (O'Brien & Placier, 2015). Recommendations include changing teacher/administrator hiring practices, improving professional development options, and distributing power more evenly between Deaf and hearing educators.

While the Common Core Standards (CCS) provide teachers with language arts and mathematics benchmarks, currently there are no standards for providing educational and support services that apply to teachers and administrators in public schools, day programs, and residential settings for deaf children and youth. These standards might minimize some of the difficulties teachers currently face. Such standards need to be developed and evaluated for effectiveness by sophisticated educational researchers. Additionally, there is a need for more research that examines the effectiveness of using state or county curricula in residential schools for the deaf to improve academic quality. The Maryland School for the Deaf has implemented Maryland State Department of Education's State Curriculum and participates in the Maryland Assessment Program (www.msd.edu/academics/vsc.html). Results of these assessments as well as those of other state schools should be evaluated for effectiveness in teaching approaches and academic achievement.

With the emergence of new language approaches for teaching deaf children, it is extremely important to accurately reflect the level of success for each approach in facilitating language development and focus on the unique needs of individual students rather than the communication method. With the current controversy over the extent to which high-stakes testing has gone, the benefits of frequent testing of deaf children has to be assessed against time taken from classroom teaching. This may change with the recent passing of the Every Student Succeeds Act (ESSA, 2015), which gives states more control in student testing and teacher preparation.

Today, more than 50 percent of deaf school-age children are from nonwhite homes with almost 30 percent Latinx (from homes where most often Spanish is spoken), 5 percent Asian American, and 15 percent African American in addition to those who are Native American and biracial (Gallaudet Research Institute, 2013). These deaf children of color are under-represented in getting services, and the education system is often remiss in not tackling their psychological, social, and education needs head on due in part to racism. This needs to be confronted to give equity and justice to this underrepresented population.

There is also an influx of deaf immigrants from Mexico, South and Central America, and Southeast Asia. Many of these individuals arrive in late childhood or during the adolescent years without having had much formal education in their home country. These deaf immigrants pose a unique educational challenge for schools in the United States. They need sign language immersion and job training programs, and educational institutions have been working to address this issue. What these institutions need and continue to need are trained educational researchers, teachers, and administrators who are deaf and persons of color who can facilitate the ability of educational institutions to meet this critical challenge.

Major research centers, including the three described later, are generating projects that likely will have a profound impact on the education of deaf children and will provide direction on how deaf education evolves in the future. Theirs is a daunting task due to the complex issues and multiple factors, including significant variability within a small population, that impact how deaf children learn, but an important one nonetheless.

The Center for Education Research Partnerships (CERP, www.rit.edu/ntid/cerp/) focuses on research partnerships that are involved in researching development and learning among deaf and hard-of-hearing students in various national and international educational settings. The goal is that of optimizing educational opportunities and success for these students. CERP's publications have incorporated an extensive synthesis of global research data that have the potential to influence educational approaches for years to come.

Visual Language and Visual Learning (VL2, http://vl2.gallaudet.edu), an NSF Science of Learning Center at Gallaudet University (also mentioned later), has as its goal the advancement of the science of learning, specifically involving how higher cognitive functioning is enacted through vision. The focus is on how visual processes, visual language, and social experiences relate to the development of cognition, language, reading, and literacy. Studying the learning processes of monolinguals and bilinguals is being done in order to promote optimal practices in education and provide new insights into language.

The Center for Research in Language (CRT, http://crl.ucsd.edu/paddenlab/) carries out research on sign language structure, the role of gesture in sign and speech, and cultural transmission of language. The goal is to understand the role of the visual-manual modality in learning.

Mental Health Developments

Historically, deaf people were perceived as less than mentally competent. In the past half century, society has learned that deaf people have similar ranges of intellectual abilities as hearing persons do. This discovery was accomplished by professionals who recognized that intelligence can be defined in a variety of ways. It was not necessary to rely solely on verbal testing to measure intellectual functioning. Using performance tests to assess cognitive and intellectual abilities facilitated professional recognition of the strengths and abilities of deaf people. This was a significant advance in that the professional community began to perceive deaf people, not as deficient human beings, but as persons with different types of capabilities. Professionals now know that with optimal innate factors and environmental stimulation, deaf people can maximize their potential. This means that services are necessary to facilitate that process. This also means that professionals need to internalize the expectation that deaf people can benefit from mental health services (Chapters 1, 7, and 8).

In their work with deaf individuals, psychotherapy providers can take advantage of the wide range of therapy approaches that have been developed. In the general population, outcome results for an increasing number of approaches have been investigated relative to various mental health problems in the interest of developing proven evidence-based practices. This has not happened with the deaf and hard-of-hearing population, in large part because of small sample sizes available for research (Wilson, Guthmann, Embree, & Fraker, 2015); the significant variability within potential samples (due to the heterogeneity of the deaf population); and limited funding. The National Association of the Deaf Mental Health Subcommittee of the Public Policy Committee (2008) has cautioned that the evidence-based practices endorsed by the Substance Abuse and Mental Health Services Administration have not been adequately researched for deaf individuals and other linguistic minorities due to the lack of focus on these groups in study samples, thus leading to questions about validity and reliability. The Colorado Daylight Project has developed standards of care for serving deaf and hard-of-hearing clients, including caution regarding evidence-based practice without adequate research (Spark Policy Institute, 2011). Consequently, the focus has to be on deducing what works based on clinician experience. There are some reports of efforts to explore efficacy, including, for example, the use of constructionist therapy with a reflecting team of hearing therapists seeing deaf clients

(Munro, Knox, & Lowe, 2008), but these are not evidence-based reports. Reliable and valid sign language-based outcome measures are sorely needed to evaluate therapy results, with one having been developed in Australia (Munro & Rodwell, 2009). An outcome study comparing substance abuse and residential treatment programs found similarities in outcomes, but results were questioned because of the unacceptably small sample size (Wilson et al., 2015).

There has been a significant decrease in the availability of specialized inpatient services for deaf children and adults due in part to the focus on community-based treatment. Deaf children with serious mental health issues have to be placed in hearing residential facilities. State departments of mental health with deaf components can collaborate with community-based facilities as well as state/center schools for the deaf to provide culturally affirmative services (Gournaris, Hamerdinger, & Williams, 2013). Such statewide specialized services with administrators who are experts in deaf-related issues are not present in every state, but should be.

We know that the availability of community-based services that is accessible for deaf clientele is extremely limited and that trained service providers are scarce in most parts of the country, thereby reinforcing the disparity in service delivery compared with the hearing population. One way to get around this is to enhance the use of telehealth services for clients in far-flung areas. Increasing numbers of locations have started to implement such services for the benefit of deaf clients, thereby making scarce resources such as bilingually trained psychiatrists, psychologists, and other mental health clinicians more readily available for increasing numbers of clients. However, the nonrecognition of professional licenses across state lines due to differing requirements for licensure in each state, limited reciprocity across states, and concerns as to liability issues across states creates unique difficulties for professionals attempting to serve a wider geographical range, and there is increasing recognition that states will need to collaborate on how to address these issues. The American Psychological Association has been in the vanguard of developing guidelines for telepsychology, including those to implement technical security in transmission of confidential information (Nordal, 2015). Bills have been introduced in Congress to increase the use of telehealth in federal systems. We can expect state regulatory entities to oversee telepractice. For example, in Maryland, the Board of Examiners of Psychologists has begun to consider what safeguards are necessary to ensure good telepsychology practice (as of this writing, Irene W. Leigh is a member of this Board). These and future developments can only enhance service delivery for deaf clients.

There has been an explosion of video remote interpreting services (VRI) due in part to the expectation that such services represent cost-cutting measures in multiple settings, including mental health settings that provide services to deaf clients but do not have sign-fluent clinicians. While deaf clients will consider working with nonsigning clinicians at agencies where interpreter services are available, no research project to date has investigated the efficacy of face-to-face interpreting compared with video remote interpreting. It is far easier to ensure whether on-site interpreters are competent in mental health interpreting in comparison to general VRI interpreters. VRI interpreting agencies need to have listings of such interpreters and technical ways of contacting mental health competent VRI interpreters; this would aid in strengthening quality assurance.

Psychologists have used a variety of psychological tests with deaf children and adults. Only a few measures have deaf sample population norms. The field continues to need rigorous evaluation of numerous existing measures to determine their validity and reliability for deaf test-takers. While ASL-based measures that can appropriately assess psychiatric symptoms are being developed (e.g., Eckhardt, Goldstein, Creamer, & Berry, 2013), more needs to be done in this endeavor. The use of sign language interpreters in test administration has not received sufficient attention in the research area despite ongoing use. It would be useful to compare such administration with administration provided by sign-fluent test administrators to gauge how each administration does accurately reflect the deaf person's functioning in the different domains being tested. Other areas ripe for study include, for example, how psychological evaluations should be conducted and/or altered, considering new knowledge about normal attentional development in deaf signers (Hirshorn, 2011). Finally, it is time to take a closer look at computerized and neuropsychological testing (see the ASL section on neuropsychological measures for dementia) and assess reliability and validity for deaf test-takers.

The move away from dealing with deaf people as a homogenous entity has resulted in the need to understand the unique influences of various factors that differentiate deaf people from each other. We now know that a more sophisticated understanding of these influences and using this knowledge to treat deaf people requires professional training. While there has been significant increase in the number of professionally trained mental health clinicians, this number continues to be insufficient for the deaf population in need of services. Additionally, such professionals must be cognizant of the interaction between communication issues and how these interact with differing cultural backgrounds. This need is critical, considering the significant lack of mental health service providers from different ethnic backgrounds despite training program efforts to recruit qualified applicants who are ethnically diverse and interested in working with deaf and hard-of-hearing populations. Those school psychologists without specialized training in assessing deaf children and who nonetheless provide assessment services for deaf children should be required to take continuing education in order to ensure that their assessments capitalize on the unique strengths of each deaf child.

Criminal Justice System Recommendations

It has become increasingly evident that there appears to be a positive correlation between being deaf or hard of hearing and being the victim or perpetrator of "challenging behaviors" (O'Rourke, Glickman, & Austen, 2013, p. 323). Deaf people are overrepresented in the criminal justice system, not only in the United States, but also in Great Britain. O'Rourke et al. (2013) have reason to believe that a paternalistic attitude that avoids holding deaf people accountable for their criminal activities until these become serious coexists with widespread violation of their rights, which potentially traumatizes them, as noted in Chapter 10. Their trauma is exacerbated by the lack of due process and the difficulties in getting communication accommodations during the arrest and jail booking process, in the courtroom, while in prison, and during the parole process. Authorities who typically lack knowledge about Deaf culture are often reluctant to comply with the rights of deaf defendants because of the extra work and costs that this entails.

Recommendations include the need to hold deaf people accountable for their behaviors, even when their criminal activity is mild, in order to avoid reinforcing their expectations that they can get away with anything, so to speak (O'Rourke et al., 2013). It is necessary to reiterate the need for culturally affirmative school, rehabilitation, and mental health programs to address such challenging behaviors as these occur. Personnel in criminal justice systems need to at the very least have a basic awareness of linguistic and cultural issues in dealing with deaf people. This could be provided as part of their mandatory training on diversity. Additionally, criminal justice personnel working with experts in deaf mental health could collaborate in developing court ordered and probation processes that work for deaf defendants and in holding these defendants accountable if their follow-up is inadequate.

Access to qualified interpreters and monitoring of communication in court proceedings needs to become a standard procedure to ensure that the rights of deaf defendants are not violated. The use of professional Deaf intermediaries to explain procedures to deaf defendants and alert the court to potential problems is also recommended, particularly for those deaf defendants who are linguistically challenged. If states have centralized prison sections or small specialized units at various levels of security devoted to deaf and hard-of-hearing inmates, with staff who know Deaf culture and linguistic issues and who can communicate with Deaf people, and with available appropriate communication devices such as videophones, this could alleviate the lack of understanding typically demonstrated by prison officials throughout the criminal justice system. In addition, these recommendations can also alleviate the frustrations, safety fears, and loneliness expressed by deaf inmates. Data on the number of deaf and hard-of-hearing people in the criminal justice system and the communication situations they encounter would buttress the need to develop procedures that do not deprive deaf defendants and inmates of their rights.

Developments in Cochlear Implantation, Genetics, Stem Cell Regeneration, and Neurology

The deaf community continues to face critical developments that have the potential for radically influencing the lives of its members and future generations of deaf people. These developments are related to advances in cochlear implantation, molecular genetics, stem cell regeneration, and neurology. The work in each of these areas raises profound and complex biological, ethical, and social issues, as mentioned in Chapter 3.

Cochlear implant technology continues to advance based on research demonstrating its effectiveness in speech recognition with intensive training. Researchers have been working on a new implant design that eliminates the need for external hardware (Paddock, 2014). The internal hardware could be wirelessly charged. Instead of the external microphone, sound can be picked up using the natural microphone chamber of the inner ear, which tends to be intact after surgery. Wolfe (2014) reports on various technological innovations related to the cochlear implant and includes an abbreviated summary of the following updates: Individuals who are deaf only on one side now qualify for cochlear implantation. While bilateral cochlear implantation has gained in popularity, there is a trend toward the provision of bimodal use, meaning a cochlear implant in one ear and a hearing aid in the other ear. The outcomes for this trend, together with bilateral implantation, appear to be superior compared to those of unilateral cochlear implant use. One of the biggest complaints has been cochlear implant performance in noise; this is being addressed by improved technology. The use of hybrid cochlear implants involves the use of shorter electrode arrays within the cochlea designed to preserve hearing and sound processors capable of providing low-frequency acoustic amplification and high-frequency electrical stimulation.

One study of the effects of pediatric cochlear implantation has found that genetic diagnosis and imaging results are two predominant factors in determining speech recognition scores, resulting in a recommendation that genetic examination and imaging studies be included in the battery of preoperative evaluations (Wu, Lee, Chen, & Hsu, 2008). Research is currently underway to evaluate the possibility of using cochlear implants to help the auditory nerve regenerate by delivering gene therapy that can regrow neurons subsequent to its being tested in guinea pigs (Bourzac, 2014). We can anticipate ongoing technical changes with the cochlear implant, considering what has been happening to date.

While the Food and Drug Administration has approved the use of cochlear implants for children aged 12 months or older, babies younger than 12 months have been implanted "off label" in the interest of minimizing the amount of time without sound, based on reports of improved outcomes in communication (Wolfe, 2014). Implanting infants poses a quandary for parents, who struggle with the implications and potential risks of elective surgery for such young individuals. The ethical argument for the pro side is that with cochlear implantation, the potential benefits of improved access to spoken language outweigh the risks, particularly surgical risks.

Regarding concerns related to surgical risks, there have been new developments in surgical techniques and electrode array design (electrode arrays are inserted in the cochlea) that should augur for improved results (Wolfe, 2014). Also, it is important to acknowledge that there are many other factors extraneous to the genetic basis of deafness, including individual variability and environmental input, which play significant roles in predicting whether individuals will benefit from using the cochlear implant. At this time, research data continues to indicate considerable variation in how well children learn to decipher and understand the information they receive through the cochlear implant. Some will have optimal access to information that can help them understand spoken language and speak intelligibly. Their numbers are growing. Others will only recognize environmental sounds. Researchers are still investigating reasons for this variability (e.g., Pisoni, Conway, Kronenberger, Henning, & Anaya, 2010). The risk is that of linguistic deprivation for those who do not progress with spoken language unless these cochlear implanted children are provided with the opportunity to access bimodal and bilingual education, as is being done at the Laurent Clerc National Deaf Education Center at Gallaudet University as well as at other settings (Gárate, 2011; Nussbaum & Scott, 2011, see also Chapters 5 and 6). Since the expectation that cochlear implants will re-create the deaf child as a "hearing" child has not died away, it continues to be an ethical imperative for professionals to prepare parents for the possibility of variability in results and the importance of modest expectations and hard work in providing language input.

The issues pertinent to genetics and deafness are not new. There is a history that is filled with controversy and tragedy (Chapter 3). The recognition of hereditary deaf families began in the late 1800s, when schools for the deaf noted large numbers of families with deaf siblings and relatives. The burgeoning eugenics movement (see Chapter 3) culminated in the policies of the Nazi Germany regime that ordered the sterilization and eventual extermination of deaf children and adults (Biesold, 1999; Friedlander, 2002; Proctor, 2002).

Current work in genetics has generated significant ethical concerns regarding how new information is to be used in altering specific population characteristics, including deafness. Scientists continue to make major strides in identifying and locating the genes involved in hereditary deafness. Recent listings of genes and their clinical manifestations can be found in Smith, Shearer, Hildebrand, & Van Camp (2014). It is known that genetic deafness occurs more often in hearing families than in deaf families. Overall, genetic information, when properly used, can offer many benefits to hearing and deaf people in terms of knowing what to expect.

But there are issues of concern. Those who view being deaf as a normal part of the diversity spectrum are not necessarily comfortable with the possibility of deafness being altered. Gene therapy is now viewed as a promising treatment option for a number of inherited conditions, some types of cancer, and specific viral infections, but it remains a risky alternative to be used only when there is no other cure (Genetics Home Reference, 2016). Extensive publicity about the unknown and potentially fatal consequences of gene therapy leads one to seriously consider the ethical issues of this procedure, but researchers continue to forge ahead. Should the goal be to prevent deafness altogether by using genetic engineering to modify the structures of specific genes through adding, replacing, or repairing the gene?

And could and should deafness be prevented with the use of fetal testing in the early months of pregnancy? This remains a controversial issue with the emergence of fertility legislation, a very sensitive issue for a number of deaf people (see Chapter 3). Concerns arise when self-determination and autonomy on the part of those most directly affected are not respected. This exemplifies how the medical desire to enhance the human condition by eliminating so-called genetically based pathology has an uneasy coexistence with the view that genetic diversity is an expected and acceptable part of the human condition (e.g., Valente, Bahan, & Bauman, 2008). How capable is hearing society of considering signing deaf individuals as an expected part of the diversity spectrum?

While genetic treatment for hereditary forms of deafness has yet to happen, the debate on its ethics will become heated once such treatment becomes possible. Whether it means the eradication of Deaf culture in the future is subject to conjecture. Who will decide whether gene therapy should be available—the medical community, the potential parents of deaf children, or deaf people themselves? The issue of cochlear implantation has also led to fears about the demise of Deaf culture. Christiansen and Leigh (2011) note that currently there is an ongoing core of ASL users that will continue in the near future. They predict that the Deaf community will continue to exist, probably more so in countries where cochlear implantation is not standard due to economic and social reasons compared with countries that have a high rate of pediatric cochlear implantation.

Researchers have started working on stem cell research in the hopes of finding a biological method to restore typical hearing by repairing the hair cell damage in the cochlea itself (https://hearinglosscure.stanford.edu/research/stem-cell-therapy/). One research team is working on producing human hair cells in a culture dish, with the hope of eventually being able to transplant such cells into the cochlea. Researchers are also studying the possibility of using embryonic stem cell-based approaches in developing new drugs to treat hearing loss rather than relying on animal testing. It will be a long time before such efforts yield results related to restoring hearing.

The study of the neurological underpinnings of language has significantly expanded with the addition of tools that can illuminate brain functioning (see ASL section earlier). The Brain and Language Lab, part of the Visual Language and Visual Learning Center at Gallaudet University (http://vl2.gallaudet.edu/labs/brain-and-language-lab/), is capable of conducting neuroimaging and behavioral studies capable of researching biological mechanisms and environmental factors that lead to language learning, particularly bimodal and bilingual language. With the increasing use of ASL-based neurology measures as mentioned in the ASL section, we can expect an era of brain explorations that will result in data with implications for language learning approaches and diagnostic pathways for neurological dysfunction.

Advances in Technology

The use of new technology for medical, research, educational, work, home, and social purposes is in high gear, with new developments constantly appearing on the scene. The earlier sections have touched upon evolving hearing and genetic technology, neuroimaging technology, Internet tools, and smartphones. Many deaf and hard-of-hearing people are taking advantage of auditory technology, including digital hearing aids, assistive listening devices, cochlear implants, and other implantable devices. There are assistive systems and devices to minimize background noise and room reverberations. Bluetooth technology now connects hearing aids or cochlear implants to computers, cell phones, and handheld devices. Visual technologies include real-time captioning, captioning software, and systems such as CAN (computer-assisted note-taking), CART (Communication Access Real-time Translation), and C-Print that can be used in classrooms, courtrooms, and professional meetings to provide verbatim or summary transcriptions of spoken communications. Communication technologies such as e-mail, smartphones with text and video capabilities, videophones, live video messaging such as the Glide app, video relay systems (now provided worldwide), videoconferencing, video remote interpreting, Internet chat rooms, live chat on company websites, Facebook, YouTube, Twitter, and so on—all provide access. Software apps are available to alert users to incoming calls. SmartBoards, LCD projectors, multimedia software with text graphics, animation and ASL movies, signing avatars, virtual reality adventure games, electronic books, digital cameras and camcorders, web-based courses, and computer software all can be used to present both ASL and English to deaf students. Wireless light signalers visually alert deaf people to doorbells ringing, babies crying, wake-up alarms, and smoke alarms going off. Vibrating alert devices are also available depending on preference. Video baby monitors bring peace of mind, not only to hearing, but also to deaf caretakers. Such technology, and new technology yet to be developed, are shaping and will continue to reshape deaf people's communication experiences.

While technology is ever-changing, human needs will continue to pose new challenges for technology. For example, voice recognition software such as Siri has come a long way in quality, but is not accompanied by ASL or text capabilities. MotionSavvy has a product called UNI, a device that allows translation of signing to speech or text (www.motionsavvy.com). Its accuracy is in the process of being improved. Group discussions continue to be inaccessible, but with emerging technology such as the Ava app (www.ava.me) that involves smartphones capable of showing each group member speaking with voice recognition technology converting speech to text, the future looks bright. While YouTube has the capability for video captioning, less than 3 percent are accessible (TDI World, 2015). There is a need to convince YouTube users to caption their videos.

Additionally, it has been necessary to enact laws such as the Twenty-First Century Communications and Video Accessibility Act of 2010 that required broadcasters to include captioning for cable TV programs that are shown again on the web and, again in 2012, to include closed captioning for programs delivered through the Internet (NCI, 2015). Closed captioning technology for movie theaters have tended to be awkward and variable in comfort for deaf and hard-of-hearing users, with open captioned films that everyone in the audience can see being resisted due to expectations that hearing viewers would find it intrusive despite the lack of research evidence to support this expectation (Boboltz, 2015).

DeafBlind people are also beneficiaries of improved technology, although developments for this population lag behind those for Deaf people due to the small size of this population. For example, DeafBlind video relay calling ability is now being tested with the use of specialized software that enables the user to contact the video relay center, sign to the video relay interpreter who voices to the hearing person and types back to the DeafBlind person who receives the information via Braille display (Laird, 2015). DeafBlind individuals can use Bluetooth to pair a HumanWare Braille device to an iPhone, iPod, or iPad to enable text-based conversation (www.humanware.com/en-usa/products/deafblind_communication_solutions/humanware_communicator).

Yes, increasingly sophisticated technologies have made communication access far easier for deaf and hard-of-hearing individuals. However, one must be cautious in expecting that such technology will totally eliminate the communication challenges deaf people confront when interacting with hearing people, as witness the ongoing need for applications to ensure the access of evolving technology. Additionally, we must recognize those deaf individuals who continue to face discrimination in the hiring and upward career mobility processes despite the availability of access technology. Hurdles include, for example, such aspects as reluctance to install videophones due to the need to ensure security measures for privacy purposes, which has a cost component to it, and the desire of hearing people to rely solely on spoken language, thereby putting sign language users at a disadvantage. Deaf people know what technology can be used on the job; it is up to hearing individuals to listen to them and work with them to find cost-effective approaches. The key to implementing changes and comfort with the use of technology lies in attitudes and attitude changes that will equate the playing field for both deaf and hearing participants.

Professional Issues

Many of the Deaf people who are graduates of the deaf education system and choose to come back to teach in the very schools they graduated from, and who can help us solve important education problems, are routinely kept out by testing that puts them at a disadvantage, by lower expectations, and by the lack of mentoring (Chapter 5). Audism and racism are subtle influences that need to be scrutinized. We have discussed professional issues throughout the book, particularly in Chapters 5, 9, and 11. Here we remind the reader of challenges in various fields.

To start with, in the field of deaf education, teacher certification for deaf teachers continues to be an issue. Teacher examinations need to be developed that fairly assesses their knowledge of academic content and teaching strategies. Teaching portfolios and classroom observations can assist in evaluating teacher competencies. With more deaf teachers, deaf children will have access to deaf role models and can hopefully be inspired to work up to their academic potential. Power issues between hearing and deaf educators and administrators continue to be an issue that needs to be addressed through changes in hiring practices as well as attitudinal changes (O'Brien & Placier, 2015). Deaf/hearing collaboration such as that reflected by the authors of this textbook should be standard practice in deaf education. Researchers—both deaf and hearing—should set up collaborative teams to jointly address education problems. Hearing researchers should share the presentation platform with deaf researchers instead of dominating conferences. There is something inherently uncomfortable about listening to hearing researchers at deaf education conferences lecture on the directions deaf education needs to take without deaf collaborators involved in their projects. This collaboration is a two-way street, with hearing collaborators who do not sign needing to learn how to work with Deaf researchers.

The increased popularity of ASL courses on college campuses (Murphy, 2013) has meant more teaching opportunities for deaf ASL instructors. Public schools need to open more positions for deaf ASL instructors so that deaf children can learn ASL and benefit more from their sign language interpreters in the classroom. There are increasing numbers of deaf academicians at colleges and universities across the nation, but access issues continue to be a problem mainly because of institutional concerns about sign language interpreter costs. This of course limits their ability to obtain teaching positions. However, the possibility of evolving technology access, particularly with online courses and technology enabling ASL to speech translation, and vice versa, should improve the opportunities for deaf academicians to obtain positions for which they are qualified.

While deaf people still have to go the extra mile in competing with hearing peers for positions in their chosen field, struggle with whether to disclose their being deaf on application forms because of ongoing discrimination, and/or deal with access issues depending on training site attitudes or job expectations, overall there has been significant improvements in terms of expanding career possibilities, access to career training opportunities, job accommodations, and legal resources when all else fails. Deaf professionals continue to forge ahead in making contributions within their chosen fields, and this momentum will continue into the future.

Final Words

In this book, our goal was to present many of the issues that deaf persons face in society at large. We focused on interactions with hearing families, at school, at work, and during recreation. We emphasized the critical need for professionals to utilize the experiences and expertise of deaf people themselves as a valuable resource, particularly in deaf/hearing collaborative teams. This will enhance professional insight into the needs of the deaf children, youth, and adults with whom they work. Using Deaf culture represents an additional resource for professionals. We reflect on the observation of Frederick Schreiber, former executive director of the National Association of the Deaf, that deaf adults are our deaf children grown up. Deaf adults know what worked for them during different periods in their lives. They see themselves for the most part as more abled than disabled. Many have demonstrated resilience and endurance while experiencing oppressive situations and incidences of audism. Professionals who listen to these deaf adults have the potential to be more successful in creating optimal interventions, whatever their area of specialization.

We began this book with questions. And we end this book with additional questions. How can society continue to improve mental health, social, education, and support services for families, deaf children, and deaf adults? In what ways will the expansion of genetic research, gene therapy, neurological research, and cochlear implants affect the Deaf community? With advances in technology, how will the nature of interactions in the deaf community change? Where do the empirical data showing the results of monolingual, bimodal, and ASL/English bilingual language approaches lead us in terms of educational approaches? What are the model literacy teaching methods that work? How will psychological research contribute to the well-being of deaf children and adults? Are researchers careful to eliminate bias when investigating the various approaches? How can more deaf/hearing partnerships be forged in education and research? Will the criminal justice system adjust to the presence of deaf defendants and deaf inmates? These questions and more will encourage ongoing debate and highlight areas that warrant further study. We invite you, the reader, to join us in this ongoing endeavor to expand our understanding in these areas.

Case Studies

Adoption and Deaf Parents

Dr Martha Sheridan

When Shondra and Daniel, both deaf and aged 31, began their search for a deaf child available for adoption, they were shocked at how long and frustrating the journey had proven to be. At that time, they had been married for 10 years. Shondra's parents and siblings were hearing and Daniel's family was deaf. Shondra was mainstreamed in public schools and began to learn American Sign Language (ASL) in high school where she met two other deaf students. Daniel attended a private Catholic residential school for the deaf. Shondra and Daniel met when they were sophomores at Gallaudet University in Washington, DC. Shondra was a social work major, and Daniel majored in education. Both of them went on to obtain their graduate degrees in their fields. At present, Shondra is a school social worker, and Daniel is a high school science teacher at a state residential school for deaf students.

Shondra and Daniel have dreams of starting a family but have been unsuccessful in their attempts to bear children. Shondra has had three emotionally devastating miscarriages, and this experience has led them to consider adoption. Because the two of them know ASL and have studied the developmental needs of deaf children, they believed they were extraordinarily qualified and could provide a loving home to a child who is deaf.

Daniel's parents were supportive of their decision to adopt a deaf child. Shondra's parents were ambivalent at first as they grieved for their daughter's experiences with miscarriages and hoped that she would have hearing children of her own, the hearing children that they never had. They looked back on the struggles they experienced as they searched for educational options and communication access for their daughter in a variety of situations throughout her childhood and adolescent years. These memories were painful for them, and they worried that she too would experience heartache at the discrimination her deaf child might face. Yet, they also remembered Shondra's many successes: her high school graduation and college acceptance, her success in athletics and as a dancer, her happiness upon discovering a community of peers in the deaf community, her graduations from college and graduate school, and her happiness in her marriage and career. They were proud of the young woman she had become and knew that she would make a wonderful mother to a deaf child.

When Shondra and Daniel first contacted a public adoption agency to inquire about the adoption process and express their interest in adopting a child, they requested an appointment and explained that they were deaf and would need an interpreter. They were told that the agency did not have interpreters on staff and ironically suggested that they should probably consider contacting the local residential school (where they were both employed) for information. Shondra and Daniel asked to speak with an agency administrator. On doing so, they explained the agency's obligation to provide sign language interpreters in compliance with the Americans with Disabilities Act. The agency administrator explained that they had never had such a request in the past, and Shondra and Daniel found themselves educating him on the law. He agreed to provide an interpreter and proceeded to refer them to an intake worker to discuss the application process and preservice training.

Shondra and Daniel arrived for their appointment only to find that an interpreter had not been scheduled. They rescheduled their appointment, and at the end of the intake interview, they were asked how they could parent a child if they were deaf. They were told that it was highly unlikely that they would be found eligible to adopt because the child's safety would need to come first. They were also told that other individuals with disabilities who had applied to adopt in the past were determined to be unsuitable. Recognizing that there was an information gap to overcome and not wanting their dreams to die, Daniel and Shondra began a process of self-advocacy by educating the intake worker about the potential fit of deaf parents to a deaf child. Daniel shared his life story about growing up with deaf parents and all of the ways in which his parents had been able to protect and provide for him and his deaf siblings. Shondra also shared her story and talked about how there were times when her hearing parents were not able to protect or provide opportunities for her because they were not proficient in ASL and were unaware of the resources, communication strategies, legal rights, and equipment that were available to her. She said that, as she found her way into a community of peers who were also deaf, she began to learn about all of this on her own and was able to provide that information to her parents in a way that allowed them to bridge their communication and information gap in her adult life and become closer than they had ever been. The intake worker listened, but when Shondra and Daniel left the agency, they were concerned that the agency would not be open to them as qualified parents for a deaf child. Shondra and Daniel obtained letters of recommendation from their employers and from hearing parents of deaf children who testified to their suitability for parenting a deaf child.

At the time of the home study, Shondra and Daniel proudly displayed how their home was accessible with telecommunication, door, safety, and educational features and resources that they would share with a child. They hoped to demonstrate that their home, their characters, qualifications, and education were suitable to the needs and best interests of a child who is deaf.

Four years passed, and Shondra and Daniel were becoming increasingly anxious as to whether or not the agency was discriminating against them. They were clearly aware that such discrimination does exist in the adoption system, and they had prepared themselves well for the self-advocacy they expected to undertake. While they maintained contact with the agency for updates, they also contacted a lawyer specializing in disability law for legal advice. They considered international adoption because they knew that many deaf children in developing countries do not have the educational opportunities that are available domestically and that this would be an alternative if they were denied the opportunity to adopt domestically. They also learned that international adoptions are often less stringent. At the age of 35, as they were beginning the international adoption application process, the local agency placed a 3-month-old deaf child with them.

Shondra and Daniel continue to work at the school where they were both employed. Their son Travis, who was a student at the school, graduated near the top of his class and is studying computer science in college. In high school, he was active in school activities including student council and basketball. He continues to be involved in student body government activities in college. He is well adjusted socially and works part-time on campus in the computer labs. Since the adoption, Shondra and Daniel have been involved with an organization that helps other deaf parents who wish to adopt.

Activities for Further Learning and Questions for Discussion

1.   Do an Internet search on adoption of deaf children and deaf-parented adoptions. From this, create a list of resources for deaf adoption support and describe the mission and services of each resource.

2.   Do a literature search on the adoption of deaf children and deaf-parented adoptions create an annotated bibliography.

3.   Identify and discuss parts of the Americans with Disabilities Act and other disability laws that apply to the protection and accessibility of deaf people in mental health and social service agencies. What legal resources (e.g., nonprofit advocacy organizations, private law firms) exist locally or nationally that could assist Shondra and Daniel if they lived in your state?

4.   Do an Internet search and create a resource list of sign language interpreting organizations in your state that you could make available to organizations or service providers that are required to provide them.

5.   Identify specific types of home telecommunication, structural, design, alerting, and safety features that deaf individuals have at home. Identify places where they can be obtained.

6.   Elaborate on what Daniel and Shondra might have been referring to when they discussed the potential fit of deaf parents to a deaf child related to language acquisition, cognitive development, and cultural role modeling. Give examples of how Daniel's deaf parents may have been able to provide a nurturing developmental environment for him and his deaf siblings. What specific things might Shondra's hearing parents have had to learn in order to provide opportunities and a nurturing developmental environment for her?

7.   Do a literature review on attachment theory and deaf children. What cultivates an optimal developmental environment for healthy parent-child attachment in families with deaf children?

Becoming Deaf in Childhood

Dr Martha Sheridan

Joshua had recurring ear infections when he was an infant. He was diagnosed with otitis media and had tubes placed in his ears at 10 months and again at ages 2 and 3. As a result, he developed moderate (50 dB) bilateral sensorineural hearing loss.

At first, Joshua's mother Carina, a single mom, wondered why this was happening to Joshua. In her concern, she asked many questions of the otolaryngologist and audiologist they worked with. She held onto the hope that this was a temporary situation as she sought medical solutions, but over time, she realized that this would be a permanent situation. She subsequently experienced a period of mourning and loss filtered with anger at herself and others. She wondered if she could have done more to prevent the infections he developed, if it would have made a difference if she got him in for medical appointments earlier, or if she had not sent him to day care where he was exposed to the illnesses of his peers. She was angry at her husband for leaving and not being there to contribute to Joshua's care. She was angry as she considered the impact Joshua's hearing loss would have on his language, education, relationships, career, and all that she had planned for their lives and wondered how she would manage with all these issues. She worried about whom she could talk to, how she would help him, and how she would communicate with him. She felt that no one understood what she was going through. She worried about giving her two older sons, ages 6 and 7, the attention they needed.

Joshua was fitted with hearing aids, and the audiologist told Carina about a preschool program for children with hearing loss that used an oral/aural communication philosophy. They indicated that, given his level of hearing loss, this would be the best approach. Carina was concerned about transportation to the program given that it was an hour away from where they lived. She also thought that since Joshua was "hard of hearing" and not "deaf," she didn't think he needed to be with other children who were deaf. Instead, she hired a speech and language therapist to meet with Joshua at their home twice a week for one-on-one speech and language development. Carina did some research on educational options and learned that deaf and hard-of-hearing children can be mainstreamed in public schools. She also began to meet other parents of children with hearing loss whose children were mainstreamed, and she thought this would be the best way to proceed. She inquired about cochlear implants but learned that since Joshua benefits from hearing aids he would not be a candidate for a cochlear implant at this time.

After educational and psychological testing, it was determined that Joshua was a good candidate for mainstream education. He started school in his local public school district and continued with his speech and language training. Although his speech and English-language skills were developing, he was not on par with his hearing peers. Some of the children made fun of his hearing aids and speech. Joshua was showing signs of difficulty fitting in.

Joshua's hearing continued to deteriorate, and by age 8, he had a 65 dB hearing loss. Carina had experienced an initial sense of relief when Joshua's educational program was established, and she was hopeful that he would do well. However, seeing that he was not achieving as she had hoped, her grief and concern set in all over again, and she switched back into her advocacy role as she looked to the school personnel to help her plan for his educational needs. It seemed to her that he was falling further behind rather than moving ahead. He was quiet and withdrawn in class and was assigned a resource teacher for language, reading, and math. During 1st grade, it was determined that Joshua had a learning disability in basic and applied mathematics. The resource teacher provided extra support to aid his math learning.

Outside of school, Joshua was involved in Little League baseball sponsored by his town's Boys and Girls club. He had excellent athletic skills and excelled on his team. He also participated on the local swim team during the summer and did well there. Despite his skills, he felt self-conscious around his hearing teammates and awkward when he did not understand what the coach and players were saying. He worried that they would not understand him and that his peers might make fun of him. Even while he was a part of the group, and he was one of the strongest and most accomplished athletes on both teams, he felt like an outsider and did not understand what to attribute this to. He did make a close friend on the team who stuck by him and helped him with communication. His mother and his brother, who was also on the swim team, helped with communication as needed. As Joshua moved toward his middle school years, he was becoming increasingly uncomfortable about relying on his mother to help out with communication, more aware of his "differentness," and saw that even his older brothers were pulling away and seemed to join their peers in laughing at him.

When Joshua was 11 years old, audiology testing indicated he had a 75 dB hearing loss. In the family, he and his mother and siblings were having more difficulty understanding each other. Carina had been dating a man, Cal, who was divorced with three children of his own. When the two families got together, Joshua felt resentful and more isolated. At first, Joshua coped with this by going to the basement playroom to play video games alone, by going outside to shoot hoops, or by going for a bike ride on his own. He started getting in more frequent fights with his brothers, pushed one of Cal's children, and purposely brushed into a teammate on the swim team, thereby knocking him down on the side of the pool. As a result, Joshua was suspended for a swim meet. Carina was worried about his self-destructive behavior and noticed he was becoming increasingly angry with her as well. She thought perhaps they should get counseling but didn't know if a counselor would be able to communicate with Joshua.

When Joshua entered middle school, he noticed there were six other deaf students at the school. Unlike him, these students used American Sign Language (ASL), had interpreters, and had some classes together. After some initial hesitation, and wondering if they could communicate, he eventually became acquainted with these students and began to learn some signs from them. At first, this group of students thought that Joshua was hearing. By 7th grade, he had become close friends with one of the boys in particular and started to develop some sense of commonality with this group even though he was not yet adept at signing. Inside he knew he was like them, and he wanted to learn more signs and explore that part of himself. He begged Carina to let him go to a summer camp for deaf kids with his new friends. Carina was reluctant because it would mean missing part of his summer swim team activities. She also didn't think he was deaf like his friends—she thought of him as hard of hearing and was afraid that if he learned to sign his speech and English skills might be affected. At the same time, she realized he was finally finding a place where he felt comfortable and happy, and he seemed to be discovering something about himself that was working for him. She discussed Joshua's desire to go to this camp for a week and how much he seemed to need it with his swim coach. When the coach agreed it was a good idea and that he would hold a place on the team for Joshua, she agreed to let Joshua give it a try.

When Joshua came home from camp, he told his mom it was the best summer camp experience he ever had and that he made a lot of friends and learned more signs. When she saw how happy he was she signed the family up for a sign language class with other parents and families with deaf members. Although some teachers, other professionals, and parents had suggested that she and the family take sign classes earlier, she had been concerned that this was not the right direction for Joshua. Now, however, she was willing to give it a try.

Joshua continued to experience social challenges with hearing kids at his middle school, and he also found that he did not necessarily fit perfectly with all the deaf kids either since they were as heterogeneous in their identities as hearing adolescents are. But his social, academic, and communication opportunities improved and expanded. By high school, he was using a sign language interpreter in some classes and was in language, math, and science classes with his peers. He joined his high school swim team and continued to excel in the sport. He also found his way to organize after-school and weekend activities with a growing group of deaf and hard-of-hearing peers, which he was excited about.

Carina eventually married her boyfriend Cal. While communication at home was not perfect, the family sign language classes improved the ease and depth of communication at home with Joshua's new blended family. In addition, his new deaf peer group and activities gave him a social space where he felt a sense of belonging and identification.

Activities for Further Learning and Questions for Discussion

1. Using this book, the Internet and additional literature, explain and critique various grief theories (e.g., Kübler-Ross, 1969; Neimeyer, 2001; Raporport, 1970; Schlossberg, 1981). Discuss how these theories relate to Carina's grief response. What events precipitated her grief reactions, and how did this play into the dynamics of her relationship with Joshua and decisions regarding approaches to his education, communication, and social activities? Was her experience typical of parents of deaf children? What resources might have helped to alleviate this process for her and provide support for the family?

2. How does Erikson's (1980) psychosocial theory apply to Joshua and Carina as depicted in this scenario?

3. From the perspective of social construction theory, what social construction frames of reference were implied at various points in Joshua's and Carina's lifeworld? What social forces were at work in shaping these perspectives, responses and decisions? How does Deaf gain factor into this vignette?

4. Read about symbolic interaction theory and consider how it relates to Joshua's perception of self as described in this scenario.

5. From the information provided in this text and from searching for additional literature, discuss how identity development theories relate to the developing deaf person. How do these theories apply to Joshua?

6. Review Chapters 11 and 12 of Sheridan's (2008) *Deaf Adolescents: Inner Lives and Lifeworld Development*. Consider the themes identified in Chapter 11 and the components of lifeworld development theory discussed in Chapter 12 as they relate to Joshua and his life situation.

7. Review information in the literature and on the Internet about the strengths perspective and resilience theory. What were Joshua and Carina's strengths? What internal and external protective factors were evident that supported their resilience?

8. What IEP goals might have been beneficial for Joshua at various points in his academic life?

9. Discuss factors related to the assessment and diagnosis of learning disability in children who are deaf.

10. What other educational, language, communication, social, and mental health resources might have been available to and beneficial for Carina and Joshua? Do an Internet search to identify such resources in your home community.

11. What is otitis media? Discuss its causes, treatment, and effects.

12. What is sensorineural deafness?

Hearing Children of Deaf Adults

Dr Martha Sheridan

Brian is a 5-year-old hearing child of deaf parents. His parents, Cheryl (age 40) and Patrick (age 42), also have a 3-year-old deaf daughter, Chelsea. Cheryl and Patrick both work outside the home. Cheryl has her master's degree in education and is a teacher of deaf students in a local elementary school. Patrick has a bachelor's degree in biology and works for a government agency. Because both parents worked, Brian and Chelsea attended a bilingual American Sign Language (ASL) and English preschool program offered by the residential school for the deaf, which is just a few miles from Patrick's place of work.

At home, the family communicates in ASL and English. Both Brian and Chelsea were native users of ASL. English is Cheryl's native language; she gradually became deaf beginning at age 9 and has good spoken English skills. She learned to sign in the middle school where she was mainstreamed along with other deaf students. Patrick, whose parents were deaf, is a native user of ASL and attended the local residential school for deaf students.

Cheryl and Patrick work hard to be sure they expose their children to early educational and language development opportunities. They make frequent trips to the library and read to the children every day. Brian, who just started kindergarten, is reading on his own and takes pride in reading to other children in his class when they ask him to. Both Cheryl and Patrick did well in school, and now Brian and Chelsea are also doing well. Preschool teachers told the parents that both Brian and Chelsea have advanced reading, language and math skills.

When it was time for Brian to start kindergarten, the parents worried about communication with Brian's teachers in the hearing public school he was to attend. They found a school that had a reputation of providing interpreters for parent-teacher conferences and school events and were pleased with the school's responsiveness to their requests for interpreters for the Open House and preadmissions testing. Brian did very well on the preadmissions testing, and the school was pleased to have him.

A couple of weeks into the school year, when Cheryl went to pick Brian up after school, she asked his teacher how Brian was doing. The teacher replied, "He doesn't pay attention in class and doesn't respond like the other kids do when I ask them to do something." Cheryl was puzzled. Brian had never had behavior problems, and none of his previous teachers had ever said he was disobedient. Cheryl asked for an appointment for a parent-teacher conference. When Patrick and Cheryl met with Brian's teacher, they saw that Brian was assigned a seat facing away from the teacher at a round table at the side of the classroom. Brian was making friends easily, but the teacher said that Brian often got out of the single file lines in the hall and went up to a friend in front of him or turned around to face the friend behind him to talk. He had been reprimanded for this on several occasions. The teacher also said that on two occasions, when she asked the students to put their books away and get out a different book, Brian did not do this. He continued to work on the previous task. She said she had given Brian three time-outs this week for those behaviors.

Cheryl and Patrick discussed this and realized that this situation was probably indicative of the adjustment Brian was making in his transition from bilingual visual communication environments at home and preschool to an auditory-based school environment. At home and at his preschool where he communicated with deaf and hearing people in ASL, it was necessary for two people to face each other and establish eye contact to communicate visually in ASL or English. His teachers, peers, and others at his new school came from a language culture that was auditory based. For this reason, the school personnel saw his behaviors as deviant. If Brian was seated facing away from the teacher and she vocally asked students to put their books away without getting Brian's visual attention, his language and communication norms indicated that she was not addressing him. His turning around to talk with someone behind him or stepping out of line to talk to someone in front of him to establish eye contact were also language and communication norms for him.

Prior to the parent-teacher conference, Cheryl and Patrick gathered information on hearing children of deaf parents (CODA) to share with Brian's teacher. They explained to her that Brian is bilingual and bicultural and that she and Brian were going to need some time to work together to adjust to their different language and communication norms. They asked that Brian be moved to a seat in the back of the classroom where he could see her and the rest of the class and also have eye contact with her while she was teaching. They also asked that she be sure to get his attention before speaking to him, such as by calling his name, tapping him on the shoulder, getting down to his eye level, or flicking the classroom lights to get the full class's attention. They asked her more about the lines in the halls and learned that the other children were talking with each other but were not stepping out of line. Cheryl and Patrick explained this was a cultural norm for Patrick and that it was going to take some time for him to adopt new cultural behaviors and asked for her patience (without punishment) during the process. The teacher reported that the meeting had been helpful to her and that, once the parents said it was a bilingual/bicultural situation, she was immediately able to reframe the situation. Things improved at school for Brian.

Brian's parents offered a family sign language class for parents, teachers, and children at the school. As a result, the school environment became more welcoming, and Brian's friends and their parents used their basic sign skills to communicate with Brian and his parents as they were able.

During the summer months, Brian and Chelsea attended a summer camp for deaf and hearing children at the deaf school near their home. This allowed Brian to continue his friendships with other CODA children. He felt at home in this environment, but as a teenager, he began to feel like he had a second home among his hearing peers from school. Brian always appreciated and enjoyed the deaf aspect of his identity. He was proud of it, and as he developed through life, he was comfortable telling his new hearing friends in middle school, high school, and college that his parents were deaf and that he was fluent in ASL. He taught his friends how to communicate with his parents when they visited their home.

Even with Brian's comfort in his identity as a child of deaf parents, he recognized the discrimination that his parents faced in various life situations. He had many stories to share about how sales clerks in stores would try to get him to interpret for his parents or how people calling the house would not believe him if he answered the phone and told them his parents were deaf. His parents were always strict about not allowing others to put him in an interpreting role. He and his parents had talks about this, and he understood their reasoning, even though there were times when he actually wanted to experience being an interpreter. In middle school, there was a period of time when he felt uncomfortable with the stares that he and his parents received in public places when they signed. As he grew older, it stopped bothering him as he gained a different perspective on why that happened, just as deaf adults do.

Brian went on to become a dentist with a respected practice. Many members of the deaf community and their families are his patients. He is engaged to be married, and his fiancé is now taking her second ASL class in order to be able to communicate more easily with Brian's parents.

Activities for Further Learning and Questions for Discussion

1. Do an Internet search to find at least three resources on CODA issues. How might these resources be helpful to this family or other deaf-parented families with hearing children?
2. What other "CODA behaviors" might a hearing child of deaf parents exhibit?
3. How might the teacher's responses to Brian's "disruptive" behaviors have affected him?
4. How are the bilingual/bicultural issues of hearing children of deaf adults similar to and different from the bilingual/bicultural issues of other groups for children beginning school?
5. What may have contributed to Brian and Chelsea's advanced language skills? What does research say about how common this is in deaf-parented families?
6. Discuss issues of identity development for hearing children of Deaf adults. What identity development theories help to explain Brian's sense of self in relation to both deaf and hearing worlds?
7. Discuss the reasons behind Brian's parents not wanting him to interpret for them. Do you agree or disagree with this decision? Why or why not?
8. How might Brian's experiences have been different if his parents did not have the educational, financial, or language resources they had available to them?
9. How does social construction theory play into the teacher's perceptions of Brian's behaviors, his parents' decisions and responses to various situations in his life and upbringing, and to Brian's perceptions of himself and others?
10. Where does Brian's pride and comfort in his identity come from? How might this have been affected differently in a different family?
11. What other stories can you find in the literature and on the Internet about CODA experiences?

Issues for Deaf Immigrants

Dr Martha Sheridan

Sofia Vasquez is a 56-year-old deaf Guatemalan woman who was brought to the United States by her husband Rodolfo (also deaf) in 1976. At the time of her arrival, Sofia was 20 years old and Rodolfo was 47. Rodolfo had come to the U.S. 4 years earlier on his own and was able to secure seasonal and construction work on an inconsistent basis. He saved enough money to return to Guatemala to bring Sofia back with him. The couple left Guatemala for economic, health, and safety reasons in the midst of Guatemala's civil war, devastation from an earthquake, abuse, and human rights violations against people with disabilities.

Sofia's and Rodolfo's parents had no guidance or support for their deaf children, and there were no educational opportunities available to them. They thought that there was no hope for their children. Young men in the neighborhood molested Sofia, and adults and children alike made fun of her.

Sofia's parents arranged for her to marry Rodolfo so that he could accompany her to the United States in search of new opportunities. Upon arrival in the United States, Sofia and Rodolfo had very limited written Spanish skills and communicated in Guatemalan Sign Language. They had no written or spoken English skills and no skills in American Sign Language (ASL). Like most people with disabilities in Guatemala, Sofia and Rodolfo had never attended school and had lived in poverty.

In 1979, Rodolfo found his way to a social service agency that offered resettlement assistance to the couple. The agency was able to help Rodolfo find a full-time, permanent custodial position. Rodolfo was grateful for the work and took pride in his ability to provide for Sofia, whom he loved. Gradually, the two of them learned ASL.

Sofia was unemployed and spent her days alone in the couple's apartment in the large metropolitan area where they lived. She cooked and cleaned their apartment but had no transportation, no social opportunities, and no other family for interaction. Rodolfo did not allow her to work or spend money. She grew increasingly bored and recognized that Rodolfo kept her isolated and controlled everything about their lives. Sofia had never been attracted to Rodolfo but was dependent on him for finances, food, health care, transportation, etc. Eventually, the couple met a young deaf man, Stephen, who lived in their apartment complex. Stephen introduced them to other deaf people and social events. Sofia and Stephen had an affair, and Sofia became pregnant. Sofia decided to leave Rodolfo for Stephen, the father of their baby girl, Alondra.

Alondra, who is also deaf, attended a residential school for deaf students and is now 35 years old. She works for a nonprofit organization helping deaf immigrants from South and Central America seeking economic, health, educational, and human rights opportunities in the U.S. just as her mother did. She notes that many of them experienced abuse and discrimination in their home countries and did not have access to the same opportunities as people without disabilities. Many of the immigrants she works with are applying for asylum. They fear deportation back to their home countries and the human rights violations and abuses they experienced there. Alondra works closely with an attorney who assists them through the application process. Today, education and social service programs for children with disabilities and their families are developing in some Central and

South American countries through the works of charitable organizations and volunteers. However, opportunities remain scarce, and human rights violations persist.

Activities for Further Learning and Questions for Discussion

1. Do an Internet search and

    a. Identify at least two special education, social service, and employment programs for deaf people in South and Central America. What is the history behind these programs, what are their missions, and whom do they serve? Who established the programs? What is their funding base? Do they receive any government support? Discuss their successes and the challenges they face.

    b. Identify two organizations in the United States that assist deaf immigrants and their families. Describe their history, mission, service population, services, and funding base. Describe their successes and challenges.

2. Using this book, the Internet, and additional literature, discuss educational and social policies and laws supporting the well-being of deaf people in the U.S. and whether or not similar policies exist in any of the Central and South American countries. What are the human rights violations that deaf people in Central and South American countries may experience?

3. What professional knowledge, skills, and values are needed to work successfully with these families?

4. Discuss the psychological, social, and language factors that make Sofia and other immigrant Deaf women vulnerable to physical, sexual, and psychological abuse?

5. Identify, compare, and contrast the applicability of psychological, sociological, or educational theories that help you to assess and understand the experiences of the family and individuals depicted in this case.

6. If you were a professional working with Sofia, what educational, social, or psychological services do you think should be provided for her?

7. What kinds of social networks in the Deaf community could you recommend for Deaf immigrant men and women (e.g., schools for the deaf, sports events, and/or church services that have Deaf people in the ministry, etc.)?

Impact of Being Black and Deaf

Irene W. Leigh

Malia, born to a single mother, Keisha, who had three other children as well, did not pass the hearing screening that was done at the hospital right after she was born. Keisha was anxious to get home as she needed to check on her oldest girl, who was watching the other two younger children while Keisha was in the hospital. With so much on her mind, and the need to go back to work as a staff member at a day care center, she forgot that she needed to bring Keisha to the audiology center at the hospital for follow-up testing.

When Malia was 2 and not talking or responding to sound, Keisha realized something was wrong. She took Malia to the hospital audiology center for follow-up testing. The audiologist confirmed that Malia was profoundly deaf and that Keisha needed to bring her to the early intervention program provided by the school for the deaf, which was some distance away. Keisha felt overwhelmed by all this information. She brought Malia for an intake evaluation but felt that the staff member talked over her head and did not understand her needs and difficult situation with going to work and caring for her other children. She was not motivated or able to bring Malia for regular weekly sessions as public transportation took a long time and necessitated Keisha missing too much work. Instead, attendance was intermittent, when Keisha could get off work.

When Malia was old enough for school, she was found to have significant language delay. She was placed in a public school that had a day class for deaf students. Because of the needs of other students, Malia did not get the attention she needed, and her language development lagged. Additionally, since the focus was on spoken language, and since Malia's hearing aids were broken, she missed out on a lot. Also, the home language was Black English, and the family used a lot of basic gestures plus single words to communicate with Malia. There were no books in the home, so Malia did not have any materials for reading and writing. Malia felt lost at home and did not understand the conversation around her, especially during holiday dinners when her aunts and uncles and grandparents would come to visit and tell family stories.

When Malia was in the 5th grade, she came to school one day very sad after being out for two weeks. When the teacher asked what the matter was, Malia started crying. She explained that her oldest sister had been killed as she walked to the food store to pick up milk. A bunch of boys had started shooting at each other, and the sister got caught in the crossfire. Because of her limited language, Malia used words and gestures to explain the situation.

After this incident, Malia became more subdued. The teacher strongly felt that Malia was depressed and also had more potential than what her language reflected. She requested a comprehensive psychological evaluation for Malia. The evaluation, done by a school psychologist who had never tested a deaf child and did not request sign language interpreting services for the assessment session, resulted in a IQ score of 72. The school administration felt that Malia was getting maximum benefit from her self-contained classroom. Malia's teacher disagreed and advised Keisha to look into the residential school for the deaf. She took Keisha and Malia to the school for a visit. Keisha was concerned because the students and teachers were communicating using ASL and Malia would be left out as she did not know the language. Also, most of the students were White, and Malia had never been in a White-only environment. But Keisha was starting to have significant health problems and felt that sending Keisha to this school would lessen stress on the family and possibly help Malia. She decided to give this placement a try and told Malia she would be sleeping away at the school.

Malia was placed in a class for slow learners. She was able to learn ASL more quickly than expected. However, she continued to be withdrawn and was not willing to do the schoolwork. During free time, she would go on the swings by herself rather than play with the other children. They did not try to include her in their activities. The classroom teacher had very little experience with Black students but tried her best to get Malia involved in classroom activities with only occasional success. When there was a celebration of Martin Luther King's life, the teacher gave Malia the responsibility of explaining who he was. For the first time, she noted Malia's enthusiasm.

Activities for Further Learning and Questions for Discussion

1. What systems are in place to encourage Keisha to follow up after Malia's initial hearing screening? Check the Internet to see what different states are doing to implement better follow-up practices.
2. The family is using a Black English dialect in the home. What is the best advice that early interventionists could give the mother regarding ways to include Malia in the language environment of the home?
3. What services should the public school provide for the self-contained classroom so that Malia could advance in her language learning?
4. There obviously were problems with the psychological evaluation. List these and describe approaches that should be used to ensure that evaluation results truly reflect Malia's potential and limitations.
5. Do you believe that Malia's cultural needs were respected? If so, how? If not, what should have been done?
6. How could the teacher use Malia's family photo album to share with the class and help Malia feel a part of the school community?
7. What Black role models would you introduce Malia to if you were her teacher? For example, what about a unit posting pictures and stories about President Obama, Michelle Obama, and their family?
8. What kinds of stories about famous Black Deaf Americans would you recommend that Malia's teacher use in the classroom?
9. What is the school's role, if any, in dealing with Malia's mental health needs?
10. Research the educational attainment results for Black Deaf students. What would you recommend in order to improve the educational situation for these students?
11. Are there organizations for Black Deaf students that could help Malia with her issues as a Black Deaf female growing up in the United States? How can these organizations help her?

Life as a DeafBlind Person[1]

Dr Martha Sheridan

Growing up in rural Wisconsin, Arthur Roehrig spent much of his time helping his father on the family farm. Art was born deaf and was the only deaf person in his family. As he and his family had never met another deaf person, they developed a system of homemade signs, including what he refers to as alphabet "sky-writing" to communicate. Many of the signs they created were specific to farming tools and processes such as hay baling and raking. Outside of the family, Art used a pen and paper to write for communication purposes. He credits this process of written communication with teaching him to read. Art's memories of his family reflect close, loving, and supportive bonds, and he credits this bond with influencing his strong sense of self-esteem.

In 1947, when Art was 3 years old, his mother confided in a Catholic priest that she was worried about finding a school for him. The priest told her about St. John's School for the Deaf, in Milwaukee, Wisconsin. St. John's used an oral approach to education that supported speech- and lipreading rather than American Sign Language. When Art and his parents went to visit, they were impressed with the school and the children there. He eventually learned American Sign Language at the age of 8 when a group of signing Deaf children transferred from a school in Chicago that had closed. Art excelled academically at St. John's in all subject areas. Since St. John's did not have a high school, like many of his friends, Art transferred to St. Rita School for the Deaf in Cincinnati, Ohio, for his high school years. Art read the daily newspaper. His GPA at St. John's had been in the 4.8–5.0 range. Although Art remained at the top of his class at St. Rita's, noting Art's intelligence and his strong academic potential, the staff there challenged him to further his academic achievements. Art rose to the challenge, graduating from high school with standardized testing scores at the college level.

Growing up, as Art's vision deteriorated, his performance and needs in various situations changed. As a child, Art enjoyed solitary play centered on popular television shows of the day including the many "western" shows that aired at the time. He watched these shows on television and bought and read cowboy-themed books over and over again. Night vision was becoming more of a problem for Art. Because of this, he hated camping with his peers. It was hard to see at night, and lanterns weren't bright enough to be of any help. He preferred staying in cabins with electricity on camping trips. His interest in sports developed when he was 10 years old, and he wanted to be a successful athlete, but he found participation frustrating. When he joined his peers playing football, tag, baseball, and basketball, he wasn't able to see well enough to excel. This was disappointing for him because he wanted to do well. He was able to play softball because it was slower, which made it easier for him to see the ball. However, he remembers not being picked for teams because his peers knew he couldn't see well and called him "blind.": "They knew I had a problem. . . . [T]hose were tough years." Despite his difficulty participating in sports, he developed a fascination with baseball at age 12 from watching the World Series, and to this day, he enjoys supporting his home teams in both baseball and football.

When he was 5 years old, Art was beginning to realize that he had vision problems, but he didn't think much of it until he developed tunnel vision and night blindness.

A gradual collection of experiences in his developmental years, such as learning that not everyone bumped into people and things as frequently as he did, helped him to realize that his vision was different from others. Art didn't have a proper diagnosis and wasn't aware that his vision would continue to deteriorate. Although Art saw a teacher helping a DeafBlind woman once when he was in elementary school, he did not have a reference group of DeafBlind people when he was growing up. Thus, when he learned of his own vision difficulties, he was frightened because he didn't know how others succeeded. It wasn't until adulthood that Art became consciously aware of the seriousness of his situation.

Art entered Gallaudet University in 1963. There, he majored in mathematics and participated on the wrestling team. Upon graduation in 1968, he taught math at the Maryland School for the Deaf. While there, he learned he had retinitis pigmentosa, a genetic progressive deterioration of vision that includes tunnel vision and night blindness. At that point, he realized he needed to consider a career change. Upon leaving his position with Maryland School for the Deaf in 1971, Art's vocational rehabilitation counselor guided Art to the National Center for Deaf-Blind, now called the Helen Keller National Center for Deaf-Blind Youth and Adults (HKNC). While there, in 1972 and 1973, Art had the opportunity to meet and interact with many other DeafBlind individuals. He recalled that many of them were concerned about their lack of employment and communication with their parents. He was shocked at the lack of services available for DeafBlind people and their families. He was then invited to serve on HKNC's advisory board. Through this, he developed a network of peers and professionals. He credits HKNC and American Association of the Deaf-Blind (AADB) with helping many DeafBlind individuals improve their self-esteem and develop opportunities for advancement.

In 1972, Art returned to Gallaudet for his master's degree. It was in one of his graduate classes that he learned he had Usher syndrome. Dr. McCay Vernon, a noted psychologist and researcher on DeafBlindness, had come to present in one of Art's classes. His presentation touched on Usher syndrome, and this was a turning point for Art in his understanding of his own DeafBlindness and what this meant for him. Until that time, he was not aware that his deafness and vision loss were connected. He followed up on this presentation by reading Dr. Vernon's National Institute of Health-sponsored research. He identified with the symptoms of Usher syndrome, being congenitally deaf, having retinitis pigmentosa and cerebral ataxia, which affects his balance. Art shared Dr. Vernon's work with his parents who, until that time, did not understand why their son was deaf.

Looking back on his life, Art is able to reflect on the process of his developing awareness of his vision loss. In a 1973 symposium on Usher syndrome, Art presented three levels of awareness of this process. The unconscious is when the person realizes only a difficulty with night vision. Semiconscious awareness happens when noticing continued visual deterioration. Finally, conscious awareness occurs upon receiving a confirmed diagnosis of Usher syndrome.

When he finished graduate school, Art served in various administrative positions at Gallaudet University that focused on the development and provision of services to DeafBlind individuals, families, and professionals. These positions included serving as Coordinator of Deaf-Blind Programs. In that position, Art traveled extensively, providing training, consultation, materials development, family education, adult education, and advocacy related to DeafBlindness. During the last 15 years of his employment, Art worked as a counselor and coordinator of students with disabilities in the university's Office for Students with Disabilities. In this position, he was expected to work with DeafBlind students; however, he was also very successful in his work with students with other disabilities such as learning disabilities and mobility impairments. He worked with approximately 130 students each semester. Art's professional achievements include developing guidelines on interpreting for DeafBlind people as well as a screening program for Usher syndrome and authoring publications on Usher syndrome (e.g., Roehrig, 1973; 1977).

Aside from his professional positions, Art served as president and then two terms as vice president of the AADB. In his position with AADB, he became the first DeafBlind person to coordinate the AADB conference twice and succeeded in reaching out to many DeafBlind individuals to increase AADB's membership.

Art considers one of his greatest strengths to be his self-esteem. He believes self-esteem is a key factor in adapting to Usher syndrome. He reports he developed his sense of self-esteem from the experiences he had at home and school and his communication experiences. He communicates in ASL and in writing.

> I meet many people with Usher syndrome who have a hard time accepting it. I've noticed that those with a strong sense of self-esteem and greater communication with their families have an easier time. People with low self-esteem often had poor communication at home, and they seem to have a harder time adapting.

When asked how things have changed over the years, Art reports that employment has improved because of the Rehabilitation Act of 1973, the Americans with Disabilities Act of 1990 (ADA), the Twenty-First Century Communications and Video Accessibility Act, the actions of the Federal Communications Commission, research, and the availability of funds for adaptive equipment. Many parents of DeafBlind children have joined The National Consortium on Deaf-Blindness, which has been helpful in providing resources and information. This consortium, as well as the World Deaf-Blind Federation and AADB, have helped to improve the quality of life for DeafBlind people. However, Art notices that many DeafBlind individuals are currently taking early retirement because of ongoing work-related barriers and stressors. Some of these individuals have deteriorating vision and are not able to obtain support from their supervisors to go to HKNC for adaptive training. In addition, in the current economy, some programs and services that were thriving in the 1990s and early 2000s are no longer operational.

Since Art's retirement from Gallaudet in 2011, he remains involved with AADB and represents AADB at the Deaf Hard of Hearing Consumer Advocacy Network (DHHCAN) meetings. DHHCAN is a national coalition of deaf and hard-of-hearing consumer organizations that advocates for accessibility in various sectors of society. He also volunteers on a universal design team for Gallaudet University, advising the group of access issues for DeafBlind people such as street crossings and other mobility and communication issues. He continues to travel and give workshops on DeafBlindness and accessibility. In addition, he is working on his autobiography, home improvements, and keeps up with his favorite sports teams.

Note

1 Author Note: Used with permission.

References

Roehrig, A. (1973). *Coping with Usher syndrome. Gallaudet University public service programs symposium on Usher syndrome.* Washington, DC: Gallaudet University.

Roehrig, A. (1977). Living with Usher syndrome. In N. L. Tully (Ed.), *Helen Keller National Center workshop on Usher syndrome* (pp. 23–27). Washington, DC: Gallaudet University.

Activities for Further Learning and Questions for Discussion

1. Do a literature search on Usher syndrome and answer the following questions:

    a. What is Usher syndrome? Describe the symptoms, types, progression, and potential psychosocial impact on the individual and on the family.

    b. What types of accommodations may be needed in the educational setting for a student with Usher syndrome?

    c. What factors should be considered in determining when and how to share the diagnosis of Usher syndrome with a 10-year-old child and his or her family?

2. Research various psychosocial theories (e.g., ecological theory and systems theory, family systems theory, grief theories, developmental theories, identity theories) and discuss the potential for application of these theories to individuals with DeafBlindness.

3. Do a literature search on DeafBlindness. What are some other types of DeafBlindness besides Usher syndrome? How provalent are they?

4. Do an Internet search to determine what legislation and technologies exist to support people who are DeafBlind?

5. Do an Internet search and identify national, state, and local resources for individuals who are DeafBlind.

Sudden Hearing Loss

Dr Martha Sheridan

Steven was a 37-year-old employee at an appliance manufacturing plant where he had worked for 15 years. He was married and had three children. Steven and his family lived in a quiet middle-class community in a large city in the Southeast. Steven's wife, children, and his family of origin are all hearing. The only known history of hearing loss in his family was his maternal grandfather who began wearing a hearing aid at age 72.

Steven overslept one morning when he didn't hear his alarm clock. When he woke up he experienced tinnitus and vertigo. He was confused when he didn't hear the lamp light click when he turned it on, and other normal morning household sounds such as the toilet flushing and water running were soft and muffled. Confused, and alarmed, he went to find his wife, Cassandra, who was in the kitchen getting breakfast and preparing their children's school lunches. Telling her about this experience, they both thought he must have a cold or an ear infection and that it was just a temporary situation.

Although he was worried, Steven decided to go to work that day, thinking his hearing would come back. Driving to work he felt disoriented not hearing the car radio, the traffic, etc. He became increasingly concerned, feeling he might be in danger and turned around to go back home.

Cassandra called Steven's employer and informed them that Steven would be staying home sick and going to the doctor. After dropping the children off at school, Steven and Cassandra proceeded to the local emergency room. There, they were referred to the hospital's otolaryngologist and audiologist for an examination. The audiology test confirmed a profound hearing loss in one ear and a moderate loss in the other. A medical history, magnetic resonance imaging, a balance test, and a blood test were performed. The otolaryngologist could not determine the cause of Steven's hearing loss and prescribed antibiotics and steroids as a precaution. Steven took his medication, but his hearing did not return.

He returned to work the next day, still disoriented and scared but feeling he needed to be there since he was the only working parent in their family and they depended on his income. At work, it was difficult to communicate with his coworkers who were not patient with him. He was missing announcements, instructions, etc. As time went on, Steven continued to believe his hearing would eventually return. He tried acupuncture, herbal medications, and special diets to no avail.

Cassandra and the children were growing frustrated with communication with Steven. They were talking slowly, repeating things several times for him as he tried to adjust to speechreading. Cassandra became depressed and was feeling increased responsibilities for communication at home and dealing with many of the business aspects of their family life that Steven used to take care of. Steven was becoming angry, lashing out at his children and wife. He stopped attending church with the family since he was uncomfortable with his inability to participate. He became angry with the members of his golf group as well and withdrew. Steven's children became increasingly dependent on their mother for their parenting needs.

After 4 years of continued communication difficulties at work and home, Steven succumbed to his wife's encouragement to see an audiologist and consider a hearing aid.

After obtaining his hearing aids, he learned his employer forbade the use of hearing aids in the plant where he worked for "safety reasons." As Steven's employer was in the process of downsizing, Steven was concerned that he would be one of the first to be laid off and would have a hard time finding a new job. Unfortunately, Steven was laid off from his job. With this, Steven became even more sullen and withdrawn, had difficulty sleeping, lost his appetite, lost weight, and continued to keep a distance from his normal activities.

After a couple of months, his wife's return to work, and increasing financial difficulties, Steven began to feel a sense of urgency and started searching for resources. At this time, he learned about a local self-help organization for people with hearing loss and attended one of their meetings. Finding some support in this group and seeing how people had adapted to hearing loss, he felt he had learned some things but needed time to digest it. He still wasn't sure that he was "like them." He missed the next two monthly meetings but returned again in a few months with his wife. It was then that he began to slowly but surely adapt, purchase assistive technology, etc. Things began to change for Steven and his family, not in the direction that he had hoped they would, but he was finding hope on a different level, in his adaptations. In time, Steven and his family began to take classes in American Sign Language (ASL). He thought that learning to sign would expand his opportunities for communication, work, and self-advocacy.

Activities for Further Learning and Questions for Discussion

1. In addition to the information discussed in this text about grief reactions, do a literature and Internet search on theories related to psychosocial transitions, crisis, and loss (e.g., Kübler Ross, 1969; Neimeyer, 2001; Raporport, 1970; Schlossberg, 1981) as well as resilience theory. Discuss how these theories relate to Steven's experience and that of his family. Critique the strengths and limitations and research on the theories. What pathways did Steven and his family take when he became deaf? What factors contributed to the grief, adaptation, and resilience responses for Steven and his family. Discuss how their responses might be similar to or different from that of other individuals and families. Prepare a PowerPoint presentation for a class report on your findings.

2. What opportunities existed in this crisis for Steven?

3. Identify, create a list of, and describe resources in your community that might be helpful to Steven and the process he experienced. How might they be helpful to him and his family and coworkers?

4. Do a literature and Internet search on sudden hearing loss. Create an annotated bibliography and share your findings with your class.

5. Steven and his family decided to take an ASL class. As Steven begins to meet deaf and hard-of-hearing people who are ASL users, what might this experience be like for him? What psychosocial experiences and processes might he encounter? Support your ideas with references.

6. What do you imagine Steven might experience in terms of his identity and roles?

7. What are Steven's strengths?

8. How might the Americans with Disabilities Act or other disability laws have been helpful to Steven?

Health Care and Deaf Patients

Dr Martha Sheridan

Evonne was a 25-year-old deaf woman expecting her first child. She lived with her 29-year-old hearing husband, Tyler, the father of her baby. Four months before the baby's due date, Evonne and Tyler began to "shop" for a pediatrician. The provision of American Sign Language (ASL) interpreters was one of their criteria for selecting a doctor. They spoke with friends and relatives who had children and with Evonne's obstetrician for recommendations. They also began researching the recommendations and found that Evonne's health insurance would cover each of these providers. Evonne used a video relay service to call each of the providers to inquire about their Open Houses for prospective parents and to see if they were taking new patients. Each of them confirmed that they were accepting new patients and were covered by her insurance. Upon confirming that she would be attending the Open Houses, she requested a sign language interpreter. Each provider put her on hold and came back to tell her that their office does not provide sign language interpreters. When Evonne cited the Americans with Disabilities Act (ADA) and said she would be unable to participate without an interpreter, each of the providers indicated that their lawyers told them if a patient could read and write they were not under any obligation to provide interpreters. They also asked if Tyler, her husband, could interpret for her. Frustrated and concerned, Evonne contacted the National Association of the Deaf Law and Advocacy Center for advice. Following this advice, they were finally able to reach an agreement for the provision of sign language interpreters with a pediatrician who accepted them into their practice. Evonne and Tyler were able to maintain a positive relationship with their pediatrician in the care of their healthy baby girl.

Two years later, Tyler was rushed to the emergency room with chest pains. Once there, the hospital staff went right to work and conducted a series of tests on Tyler. Evonne requested an interpreter at the front desk when they arrived at the ER, and Tyler gave the hospital permission to share information with Evonne. The staff person said she would look into finding an interpreter. The testing took several hours, and Evonne kept checking back about an interpreter because she was in the dark about her husband's condition and was very concerned about him. When she attempted to ask the medical staff how he was doing, she told them she had requested an interpreter. Their response was that they could not get her an interpreter because she was not the patient and it would be a breach of the Health Insurance Portability and Accountability Act (HIPPA) for them to share information with her about her husband's status, even though Tyler had granted the hospital permission to share information with Evonne. This response was a violation of the ADA. This was the same hospital ER that had treated Evonne a year earlier for an injury and insisted that her hearing husband interpret rather than calling for a professional interpreter as required by law.

Meanwhile, Evonne learned that a friend's elderly father who is deaf was in need of nursing care. This was a man she recalled as being very socially active in the deaf community. Her friend was concerned that, if her father was placed in a nursing facility where he had no peers or medical staff that he could communicate with, his health might deteriorate rapidly.

Evonne was determined to fight all of this discrimination and took her concerns to a meeting of representatives from her state Association of the Deaf. She detailed her experiences and presented a proposal to establish a coalition of other local organizations and legal advocates to respond to discrimination against deaf and hard-of-hearing people in the health care system. She learned that she was not alone and that every deaf person in the room that evening had similar experiences. The coalition was established and worked with local hospitals and health care centers to help them write policies and procedures for communication with deaf and hard-of-hearing people. Another responsibility of the coalition was to provide education on the legal rights for deaf and hard-of-hearing people in health care. These efforts took several years, and Evonne stayed involved to support them. One of their successes was the eventual hiring of a health care advocate in a local social service agency to ensure the continuation of these efforts and to provide case advocacy as the need arose. The coalition also began offering sign language classes in nursing programs in colleges and universities in the area. They recognized that while they were making progress, this was a long-term effort.

Activities for Further Learning and Questions for Discussion

1. Review the National Association of the Deaf's Position Statement on Health Care Access for Deaf Patients at https://nad.org/issues/health-care/position-statement-health-care-access-deaf-patients. Discuss how this position statement relates to Evonne's case. What do you see as the strengths and limitations of the statement? Is it universal for all deaf and hard-of-hearing people, including those who do not use ASL?

2. Describe the feelings of anxiety and anger that Evonne must have felt when she did not have an interpreter during her husband's emergency hospital admittance while he was undergoing tests she did not understand.

3. Describe how writing notes is not an effective mode of communication for even highly educated deaf persons when they or their family members are under duress in a highly charged emotional situation due to a medical condition in the hospital.

4. Were Evonne's techniques of self-advocacy effective? What might she and Tyler have done differently? Can you think of additional interventions that the coalition could have adopted for enhanced patient access?

5. Research lawsuits against medical facilities and hospitals that refused to provide interpreters for deaf persons. Provide a description of court decisions on these lawsuits.

6. Research and list organizations and resources in your local area that can be used to make health care more accessible for deaf and hard-of-hearing people. If you were to create a local coalition such as the one Evonne established, who should be involved? What might your goals be?

7. What specialized training should a medical sign language interpreter have?

A Young Deaf Adult with Mental Illness

Dr Martha Sheridan

Ashley first began to hallucinate at age 22. She was born deaf from unknown causes and uses American Sign Language (ASL). Her parents are hearing. Ashley grew up in a residential school for deaf students on the West Coast. She was the second of four children and the only deaf member of her family. Her parents are high school graduates and have always struggled financially to support their family. Her father, a dockworker, was recently laid off from the shipping company he worked for, and her mother is a nursing assistant in a nearby nursing home.

Ashley's parents did not know she was deaf until she was nearly two-and-a-half years old. Her parents noticed she was not developing spoken language like her older brother did and suspected she was not hearing. Her pediatrician referred the family for a hearing test, and it was discovered that Ashley was profoundly deaf. Ashley was fitted with hearing aids and began an oral preschool program. She then began her elementary education in a mainstream, oral school. At age 6, she transferred to the state school for the deaf.

These early years without formal language at home led to language and academic delays that required concerted academic support and resources at her new school where she began to learn ASL. Ashley struggled with language and math throughout her school years. She remained a student at her school until the age of 21. Her academic achievement was not strong enough to be awarded a diploma at graduation with her classmates, but she did receive a certificate of completion. As her high school years progressed, Ashley seemed to become more socially withdrawn. In her elementary and middle school years, she enjoyed bike riding, and with encouragement from her teachers, she joined the girls' basketball team. She began to withdraw from these activities in high school and was not responsive to her coach's attempts to encourage her to stay on the basketball team. Her affect began to change, and at times, she seemed almost emotionless. Classmates at school thought she was "strange" and made fun of her, particularly the increasingly bizarre comments she would make and her lack of self-care.

Following graduation, Ashley was evaluated for vocational rehabilitation services by her state Bureau of Vocational Rehabilitation counselor. Although the counselor specialized in working with adults with disabilities, she was not specifically trained to work with deaf clients and used a certified sign language interpreter in her meetings with Ashley. The counselor noticed that, on several occasions, Ashley looked away from her and signed things that seemed to be off topic. The interpreter had a difficult time making sense of what Ashley was signing. The counselor referred Ashley for a psychiatric evaluation with a psychiatrist who also did not have the communication skills or training and expertise required for work with deaf people. The psychiatrist did secure a certified sign language interpreter and proceeded to conduct a mental status exam. During this exam, Ashley indicated that she could hear voices. However, he was not aware of any mental health services that were designed specifically for deaf clients so he discharged her and asked her to return in a week for a follow-up appointment.

Ashley's speech and behavior were becoming increasingly disorganized and impulsive. Her parents and neighbors were becoming fearful of and worried about her, yet never having learned to sign, they were unable to communicate with her. She was often seen walking down the street signing to herself and at times seemed hostile. Her self-care deteriorated further, and she forgot her appointment with her psychiatrist. Her parents wanted to take her to the hospital but were afraid to. Instead, they called the police.

Activities for Further Learning and Questions for Discussion

1. What do you think may have happened when the police arrived at Ashley's home? Check your local city jail and found out how psychiatric cases are handled with persons who do not break the law but are considered a danger to themselves, family, and society.

2. What biopsychosocial factors may have contributed to Ashley's language delays and educational challenges? Consider possible etiologies that may have impacted her neurological development.

3. What types of educational and supportive services might a school provide to a child like Ashley to help foster her language, psychological, and social development? Check the Internet for resources for Deaf students with psychiatric disorders.

4. Do a literature search on language dysfluency and mental health assessments with deaf clients. What challenges exist, and what professional skills and accommodations must be accessed to obtain an accurate assessment of deaf clients who are mentally ill? Discuss the parts of the mental status examination and implications for its use with deaf clients. What does the literature say about the types of hallucinations that deaf people who are schizophrenic may experience?

5. Discuss why Ashley may have stayed in school until age 21 and obtained a certificate of completion rather than a diploma at graduation. What does the literature tell us about the graduation and academic achievement rates of deaf high school students? What factors may contribute to this?

6. Do an Internet search for deaf-related resources in your state and create a list of services that could have been helpful to Ashley and her family at various points in her life from birth through young adulthood. Include services for infants, children, families, and young adults. Consider all of her needs from biological, psychological, social, language, educational, and vocational perspectives. Discuss the strengths and limitations of these resources for helping Ashley. What gaps exist? What laws and policies may have helped or hindered her ability to receive appropriate services? What services would you want to add, and how would you consider staffing these services (e.g., types of staff, qualifications, etc.)? Check the NAD website on their position on mental health services for Deaf to assist you (https://nad.org/issues/health-care/mental-health-services/position-statement).

7. Discuss the strengths and limitations of various psychological and language assessments for use with deaf children and young adults and their usefulness for helping Ashley.

8. Discuss the role of sign language interpreters in mental health settings.

9. How will Ashley's language levels in sign and English affect her abilities to succeed during a treatment program?

A Deaf Suspect Caught in the Criminal Justice System

Jean F. Andrews

One summer night, the police arrested Gerald P., a young Hispanic American Deaf man in his early twenties, for an alleged criminal offense. The police drove the young man, who was handcuffed and placed in the back seat of the patrol car, to the jail. As a pre-trial detainee, Gerald spent one month in solitary confinement. While incarcerated, Gerald committed suicide.

What went wrong?

It started at the arrest. When the police apprehended Gerald and realized he was deaf, they did not call in a sign language interpreter. Instead, they relied on his lipreading and their writing notes to question him.

Before the patrol car pulled into the jail parking lot, the police informed the dispatcher that the suspect in custody was deaf. Even with this information, the jail officials did not call an interpreter. After Gerald was fingerprinted and his picture taken, the jail official pulled out a written form and began to ask him about his medical and psychological history. He read the form out loud while pointing to the sentences so Gerald could read them along with him. Because no interpreter was provided, Gerald could not give any pertinent information regarding medication or suicide risk, neither could he request assistive devices that he would need in jail (e.g., visual alerting devices, visual fire alarm, captioned TV, videophone, a sign language interpreter for important meetings and grievances, and ASL translations for jail documents, etc.). Deaf inmates, like Gerald may nod "yes" to all of the jail official's questions and sign documents such as the medical/psychological question-naire form. A signature typically signals the deaf person wants to cooperate, not that the suspect understands the information.

The jail official later testified in deposition that he assumed that Gerald could read the medical/psychological document as well as read his lips as the jail official read aloud. This assumption is wrong. An expert later determined that Gerald's reading level was so low that he could not read or comprehend the documents as they are written above his reading level and are filled with complex vocabulary and grammar structures.

The jail officials reported that they placed Gerald in a solitary cell because they felt that this placement would protect him from bullying by the hearing prisoners. They did not consider that being deaf in jail was isolation in itself and to place a deaf person in solitary confinement is even more isolating.

Jail records indicate that Gerald was frequently moved from cell to cell but no one could determine why. He had to endure countless hours with nothing to do, because he had no access to programs and services that hearing inmates have. Even if books and magazines were made available to him, he could not read them. He probably felt isolated and confused by what was happening around him because he did not know the routines and rules. In fact, he was never given a copy of the jail inmate handbook to learn about jail protocol in the first place. Worst of all, Gerald did not have anyone with whom to communicate. His only outlet was exchanging a few written letters with his family. Here is an example of Gerald's writing and drawing for his brother, which reflects his sadness and desperation.

> *Hi, I Do to me it cry. My family Sweet.*
> *Do can you want come to See to me.*
> *My mother want Buy out But Bound high very money $100,000.00.*
> *Do it Wash Buy at Out!!!*
> *Sweet You Miss I Love you.*
> *Smile*
> *(He inserted a picture of himself with sad face and tears coming from his eyes.)*

In his cell, after one month, Gerald hung himself using bed sheets.

A lawsuit followed, brought by his mother, Ms. P. In order to determine if Gerald received appropriate accommodations to ensure effective communication, Ms. P's lawyer requested a review of Gerald's school records, including audiology reports, his reading test scores, nonverbal IQ scores, school attendance, and a description of his primary language. The purpose of this investigation was to see, if in fact, English reading, speaking, lipreading, and writing, as put forth by the jail officials, did indeed constitute effective communication.

The investigation determined that Gerald was prelingually and profoundly deaf, was of low-average cognitive functioning, read at the 2nd-grade reading level, and used ASL as his primary language as he attended a school for the deaf for 15 years. They learned that even though he "graduated" from high school, his achievement level was not similar to the level of a hearing high school graduate and that Gerald was placed in a program at the school for the deaf that emphasized functional living skills, rather than academics due to his low cognitive and language levels.

The lawyer also requested that readability analyses be done on all the documents that Gerald was required to read while incarcerated. In the analyses, the following reading grade levels were found: medical/psychological intake form (8.4), the jail inmate handbook (18.4), the Miranda Warning (6.0), and the prearraignment detention facility rules (13.9). Clearly, with Gerald's 2nd-grade reading level, it would be impossible for him to read and comprehend those documents. He would need an ASL interpreter to translate them. And even with the ASL translation, there may be some terminology that, with Gerald's limited world knowledge as indicated by his low academic achievement, would be incomprehensible to him. For instance, the Miranda Warning is full of abstract concepts that Gerald might have difficulty comprehending (e.g., you have the right to remain silent; whatever you say can be held against you, and so on) (see Seaborn, Andrews, & Martin, 2010).

Based on objective evidence found in the school records and the readability analyses, the expert determined that ASL constituted effective communication for Gerald and that he should have been provided with a qualified sign language interpreter at critical junctures during his interactions with the criminal justice system.

One can only imagine the acute distress, emotional, and psychological pain that Gerald endured alone in jail. He was not provided with mental health services. He was not provided with appropriate supervision to ensure his safety. He was isolated from other inmates, thus exacerbating his anxiety and fear of what was going on. And he was not provided with appropriate assistive technology and interpreters in order to contact and communicate with family, friends, or legal counsel.

This tragedy could very well have been averted if police and jail officials followed ADA and Section 504 mandates.

Questions for Reflections

1. Reflect on how Gerald P. could use cognitive abilities such as memory, Theory of Mind, and executive functioning to work with different attorneys (see Chapter 4).
2. What kind of training about Deaf culture, ASL, the ADA, and Section 504 should criminal justice officials have in order to work effectively with Deaf suspects and offenders? What kind of policies and procedures should they have in place to avert a tragedy such as in Gerald's case?
3. One large federal prison system at the Estelle Unit, Huntsville, Texas, has a large deaf prison population who are housed in one unit. Describe the advantages for the Deaf inmates in placing them together. How can this help the system cut down costs in providing accommodations? If a jail or prison system does centralize their services, what disadvantages does this impose on families?
4. What is the NAD's position on the rights of deaf and hard-of-hearing inmates? How does Section 504 and ADA protect deaf prisoners' rights? To what agency can deaf prisoners complain if they believe their rights have been violated?
5. How can schools prevent the "school-to-prison pipeline" that we see in America, today, particularly among Hispanic and African American youth? What kinds of services can be provided to deaf juveniles who get into trouble?
6. Check out the blog, www.deafinprison.com. Read about one issue related to deaf inmates and present it to your study group.

Resources

Accessibility Resources

Captionfish: www.captionfish.com
   Captionfish provides a listing of theaters that provide captioned films, show times, and captioned trailers. The website will specify what type of captions are provided.

Described and Captioned Media Program: www.dcmp.org
   DCMP is a free library of several thousand media files that are mainly for use in the K-12 educational system. Users can select clips that are either closed captioned for deaf or hard-of-hearing viewers or include image descriptions for blind viewers. The media files can be watched online or users can request a DVD copy.

National Captioning Institute, Incorporated: www.ncicap.org
   The National Captioning Institute is a nonprofit organization that provides captioning services for television, web media, home video, and government programming.

American Sign Language (ASL)

The ASL App: http://theaslapp.com/#about
   The ASL App is an easy-to-use app for iOS that teaches users conversational ASL. There are over 800 signs and phrases signed by a variety of native Deaf signers.

ASL & Foreign Country Signs: www.aslresource.net/index.html
   This website displays both ASL and indigenous signs for different countries.

ASL University: www.lifeprint.com
   ASL University is a resource site for ASL students, teachers, and anyone who is interested in learning sign language. Dr. Bill Vicars adapted his in-class curriculum for online learners and provides a syllabus, suggests books/resources, and has videos of signs/phrases as well as various worksheets and exercises.

Handspeak: www.handspeak.com
   Handspeak is an ASL resource site created by a culturally Deaf native signer and ASL instructor. Featured on the website are an ASL dictionary, phrases, fingerspelling, Deaf culture information, and extracurricular activities.

American Sign Language Writing

ASL Write: www.aslwrite.com
   ASL Write, created by Adrean Clark, is a sign language writing system originally known as the American Sign Language Writing Dictionary. ASL Write is committed to keeping written ASL freely available to the public domain and encouraging the natural development of written ASL through regular usage.

Si5s: www.si5s.com
   Si5s is a sign language writing system proposed and developed by Robert Augustus as a way to transpose American Sign Language onto paper. Si5s is taught at Gallaudet University and Mt. San Antonio College in Walnut, California.

SignWriting: www.signwriting.org

> SignWriting is a writing system that uses visual symbols to represent the handshapes, movements, and facial expressions of signed languages. It is an "alphabet"—a list of symbols used to write any signed language in the world.

Art

ASL Films: www.aslfilms.com

> ASL Films is a deaf-owned production company that creates feature films. Their feature films star deaf actors and use American Sign Language.

Deaf Art: www.deafart.org

> This website provides information about De'VIA art and the National Touring Exhibit of Deaf Culture Art that occurred between 1999 and 2001. It features information about De'VIA art, the artists involved in the tour, and their artwork.

Deaf Artists: www.rit.edu/ntid/dccs/dada/dada.htm

> This website features profiles of over 40 deaf and hard-of-hearing artists in various fields. In addition, there are links to numerous resources, articles, and materials.

Deaf Arts Festival: http://infodeafartsfestiv.wix.com/deaf-arts-festival

> Deaf Arts Festival celebrates the arts by exhibiting diverse, quality visuals and performing arts through the support of the Deaf and Hard-of-Hearing population. The essence of this organization is to enrich and educate the audience through personal interaction among Deaf and Hard-of-Hearing artists.

Deaf Movies: www.johnlubotsky.com/deafcinema/

> This website provides a comprehensive list of feature length films and short films in ASL and other sign languages. Also listed are Deaf film festivals, spoken language movies that feature some degree of ASL or deaf culture, and various ASL film resources.

HandsOn: http://handson.org/node/933

> HandsOn provides interpreting for Broadway and Off-Broadway performances in New York City, has established a theater company for young people, and maintains a comprehensive listing of cultural events for the Deaf community in New York City.

National Theatre of the Deaf: www.ntd.org

> National Theatre of the Deaf is a theatre company that produces plays that utilize both American Sign Language and spoken English. Both deaf and hearing actors are involved in their productions, and their productions have been performed in all 50 states and in several countries.

Civil Rights and Forensics

Civil Rights Education and Enforcement Center: http://creeclaw.org

> CREEC is a law firm that also focuses on education and advocacy regarding disability rights laws and have litigated class action and individual civil rights cases.

Deaf in Prison: www.deafinprison.com

> Deaf in Prison is a blog that accepts contributions from different writers on the topic of deaf individuals in prison and in the criminal justice system.

Helping Educate to Advance the Rights of the Deaf: www.behearddc.org

> HEARD is a nonprofit organization that promotes equal access to the legal system for deaf, hard-of-hearing, DeafBlind, and disabled individuals. HEARD works on reversing wrongful convictions, stopping prisoner abuse and isolation, decreasing recidivism rates, and increasing the number of deaf professionals in the justice system.

National Association of the Deaf Law and Advocacy Center: https://nad.org/issues/about-law-and-advocacy-center

> The NAD Law and Advocacy Center advocates on public policy issues of concern to the deaf and hard-of-hearing community, particularly at the national level, and often in collaboration with other

national organizations. They provide general legal information about deaf-related issues and discrimination law. NAD attorneys represent individuals who are deaf or hard of hearing in selected disability discrimination civil rights cases.

CODA

Children of Deaf Adults, Inc.: www.coda-international.org
CODA International is a nonprofit organization that celebrates the heritage and multicultural identities of adult hearing children of deaf parents. The work of CODA International includes conferences, retreats, publications, scholarships, resource development, and fundraising.

Common Core

About the Common Core State Standards: www.corestandards.org/about-the-standards/
This website explains the rationale for development and implementation of the Common Core State Standards as well as an explanation of the standards.

Common Core for Teachers of the Deaf and Hard of Hearing: www.csun.edu/education/innovated/spring13/?page=3
The authors, faculty members at Eisner College of Education, explain how they are teaching their students how to apply Common Core standards in English-Language Arts to deaf and hard-of-hearing students.

Education Week Article on Common Core: www.edweek.org/ew/articles/2013/06/05/33cain.h32.html
The author posits an argument that despite its controversy, common-core testing needs to be implemented.

Deaf Organizations

Alexander Graham Bell Association for the Deaf and Hard of Hearing: www.agbell.org
The AG Bell Association is a nonprofit organization that serves oral deaf and hard-of-hearing individuals. They believe that every child and adult with hearing loss should be able to use oral language to live in a mainstream society.

Association of Late-Deafened Adults: www.alda.org
The Association of Late-Deafened Adults is a nonprofit organization that is a place for late-deafened adults to confront and accept their deafness and socialize with other adults and families.

Deaf Latino Organizations: www.councildemanos.org
This website lists different local organizations and resources for Deaf and Hard-of-Hearing Latinos and Latinas.

Deaf Women United: http://dwu.org
Deaf Women United is a nonprofit organization that encourages the personal growth, empowerment, and leadership training for deaf women. The services they provide include tools, information, training, networking opportunities, and scholarships.

DeafNation: www.deafnation.com
DeafNation is a media company that creates short films about Deaf culture, communities, and people. DeafNation also sponsors expos in different cities.

Hands and Voices: www.handsandvoices.org
Hands and Voices is a nonprofit organization that provides families of deaf and hard-of-hearing children with information about the different communication options available. This organization is also a place for families to seek support from other families with shared experience.

Hearing Loss Association of America: www.hearingloss.org
The Hearing Loss Association of America provides assistance of people with hearing loss and their families. They also work towards eradicating stigma, raising awareness, and changing public policy.

Intertribal Deaf Council: http://deafnative.com
The Intertribal Deaf Council provides education, information, and training about and for American Indians with hearing loss. The organization works with individuals, family members, and tribal councils to improve the well-being of American Indians.

National Asian Deaf Congress: www.nadcusa.org
The National Asian Deaf Congress is a nonprofit organization that aims to educate, empower, and provide leadership for members of the Asian Deaf and Hard-of-Hearing Community. NADC provides resources, training opportunities, networking opportunities, and immigration and acculturation assistance.

National Association of the Deaf: www.nad.org
The National Association of the Deaf is a civil rights organization that works to influence public policy in a broad range of topics, including education, employment, health care, and technology. NAD also works with other deaf and hard-of-hearing organizations, as well as cross-disability organizations, to advocate for the collective interest of the American Deaf community.

Rainbow Alliance of the Deaf: www.deafrad.org
The Rainbow Alliance of the Deaf is a nonprofit organization that promotes the educational, economical, and welfare of Deaf and Hard-of-Hearing LGBTQ individuals. RAD has over 20 chapters in the United States and Canada and has an annual convention.

DeafBlind

DeafBlind International: www.deafblindinternational.org
DeafBlind International promotes awareness of DeafBlindness and the implementation of appropriate support and services. DBI members include professionals, families, organizations, and DeafBlind individuals.

Lighthouse for the Blind, Inc.: www.deafblindlh.org/seabeck/index.html
The Lighthouse for the Blind, Inc., is a Seattle-based DeafBlind advocacy organization that also works with national and international DeafBlind organizations. This organization also organizes a week-long retreat for DeafBlind individuals that has activities, relaxation, and communication/support for campers.

National Center on DeafBlindness: https://nationaldb.org
The National Center on DeafBlindness is a federally funded technical assistance center that aims to improve the quality of life for DeafBlind children and their families. Their initiatives include creating visibility, establishing partnerships, encouraging innovation, and maintaining a database of information.

National Family Association for Deaf-Blind: http://nfadb.org
NFADB is a nonprofit organization that works to empower and advocate for DeafBlind individuals and their families. They aim to ensure provision of proper support, promote awareness, and disseminate information.

Diversity/Multicultural Resources

Info-to-Go Selected Readings: www.gallaudet.edu/clerc-center/info-to-go/multicultural-considerations/multicultural-issues.html
The Clerc Center has compiled a list of articles and books related to multicultural issues for deaf and hard-of-hearing students.

Understanding Deafness and Diversity: www.understandingdad.net
D.A.D. is a resource for parents, teachers, and other professionals who work with deaf and hard-of-hearing children who are deaf and diverse. Their definition of deaf and diverse includes children with additional disabilities and children who speak a language other than English or ASL at home.

Early Infant Hearing Detection

American Academy of Pediatrics: www.aap.org/en-us/advocacy-and-policy/aap-health-initiatives/PEHDIC/pages/early-hearing-detection-and-intervention.aspx
The AAP provides a list of state, federal, and other resources for parents looking for guidance on hearing screening and early intervention organizations.

American Society for Deaf Children: www.deafchildren.org
The American Society for Deaf Children is a nonprofit organization that works with families to ensure that children with hearing loss are given opportunities to access language. Their objectives include ensuring optimal intellectual, social, and emotional development through early identification; fluency in ASL and English; and access to deaf mentors.

American Speech-Language-Hearing Association: www.asha.org/Advocacy/federal/Early-Hearing-Detection-and-Intervention
ASHA provides a list of state, federal, and other resources for parents looking for guidance on hearing screening and early intervention organizations.

Early Intervention Position Papers

American Speech and Hearing Association: www.asha.org/policy/PS2008–00291/

Conference of Educational Administrators of Schools and Programs for the Deaf (CESAD): www.ceasd.org/acrobat/CEASD_EHDI.pdf

Division of Early Childhood Code of Ethics: http://dec.membershipsoftware.org/files/Position%20Statement%20and%20Papers/Inclusion%20Position%20statement.pdf

National Association for Education of Young Children: www.naeyc.org/files/naeyc/file/positions/position_statement.pdf

National Association of the Deaf: https://nad.org/issues/early-intervention/position-statement-early-hearing-detection-and-intervention

Education

American Association for the Advancement of Science. www.aaas.org
The AAAS is an organization that seeks to advance science, innovation, and engineering by providing a voice for science in societal issues, strengthen support for science education, and increase public engagement with science and technology.

Association of College Educators - Deaf & Hard-of-Hearing: www.acedhh.org
ACE-DHH is an organization of university professors of future teachers of the deaf and hard of hearing. ACE-DHH hosts an annual conference that is attended by university faculty, doctoral degree candidates, and sign language interpreters.

Auditory/Oral Education: www.handsandvoices.org/comcon/articles/aud_oral_edu.htm
Hands and Voices explains auditory/oral education and provides links to parental resources.

Center on Literacy and Deafness: http://clad.education.gsu.edu
CLAD aims to identify factors that affect reading growth in deaf and hard-of-hearing children and develop successful interventions for struggling readers in grades K-2.

Classroom Acoustics Fact Sheet: http://web.archive.org/web/20050329084534/www.njhighperformanceschools.org/PDF/acoustic/p_AB_Disability_factsheet.pdf
This fact sheet describes the progress made by the U.S. Access Board (www.access-board.gov) to develop a new standard for classroom acoustics. The fact sheet also incorporates general information on acoustics. The U.S. Access Board is an interdepartmental federal agency that coordinates and oversees development of standards for accessible design for people with disabilities.

Common Ground Project: www.ceasd.org/child-first/common-ground-project/vision-purpose-goals
The Common Ground Project is a collaboration between CESAD and Options Schools, Inc., that aims to ensure that all deaf and hard-of-hearing children receive services and supports they need to

succeed in school and life. Through this collaboration, they will share resources, models, strategies, and promote family education and advocacy.

Conference of Educational Administrators of Schools and Programs for the Deaf: www.ceasd.org
CESAD is an association of schools and educational programs for deaf and hard-of-hearing children. CESAD strives for excellence in educational opportunities and advocates for deaf and hard-of-hearing children in educational policy.

Convention of American Instructors of the Deaf: www.caid.org
The Convention of American Instructors of the Deaf is an organization of teachers and educational professionals that promotes student learning and development.

Council for Exceptional Children: www.cec.sped.org
The Council for Exceptional Children is dedicated to improving the education for children with disabilities and other needs. CEC advocates for appropriate policies, standards, and provides professional development opportunities.

Council on Education of the Deaf (CED): http://councilondeafed.org
CED promotes quality education for deaf and hard-of-hearing children by promoting nationally recognized standards for teachers of deaf and hard-of-hearing students, accrediting university programs, and collaborating with a variety of related organizations.

Curriculum and Evaluation Standards for School Mathematics: www.mathcurriculumcenter.org/PDFS/CCM/summaries/standards_summary.pdf
These NCTM-created standards were designed to guide revision of school mathematics curriculum and to define mathematics literacy.

Educational Enhancement for the Field of Deaf Education: www.deafed.net
This website is a collaboration between DeafEd.net and Hands and Voices that serves as a compilation of resources to support the educational possibilities for deaf and hard-of-hearing children.

Info to Go: Deaf Students with Additional Disabilities: www.gallaudet.edu/clerc-center/info-to-go/deaf-students-with-disabilities.html
The Clerc Center has compiled a list of resources to support deaf and hard-of-hearing students with additional disabilities.

International Congress for Education of the Deaf: www.iced2015.com/en/content.php
ICED is an international gathering of individuals who are involved in deaf education, including researchers, teachers, administrators, parents, and other professionals. The link takes you to the website for the 2015 ICED event.

Listen-up Listserv: www.listen-up.org/htm2/list.htm
The Listen-up Listserv is a resource for parents of deaf and hard-of-hearing children to support their informative and emotional needs. Parents of all deaf and hard-of-hearing children are welcome, inclusive of all communication and education choices.

National Clearinghouse for ESL Literacy Education: www.cal.org/what-we-do/projects/ncela
NCELA collects, analyzes, synthesizes, and disseminates information about English language acquisition by English second language learners.

National Council for the Social Studies: www.socialstudies.org/
NCSS is an organization that supports educators in strengthening social studies education. NCSS membership includes elementary, secondary, and college teachers of history, civics, geography, and other social studies courses.

National Council of Teachers of Mathematics: www.nctm.org
NCTM is an organization that supports teachers by promoting high-quality mathematics learning for all students. This vision is realized by providing leadership, professional development, and research.

National Deaf Education Project: www.ndepnow.org
NDEP aims to ensure a quality communication and language-driven educational delivery system for students who are deaf or hard of hearing.

National Task Force on Equity in Testing Deaf Individuals: http://research.gallaudet.edu/NTFETDHHI/index2.html#mission

The task force is a group of deaf, hard-of-hearing, and hearing individuals who strive to increase the number of deaf and hard-of-hearing professionals providing service and leadership and to promote equity in testing deaf and hard-of-hearing individuals.

NCSS Expectations of Excellence: Curriculum Standards for Social Studies: http://files.eric.ed.gov/fulltext/ED378131.pdf
These NCSS-created standards were designed to guide social studies curriculum development, decision, and creation of classroom activities.

Option Schools, Inc.: www.optionschools.org
Option Schools, Inc., is a group of schools in the United States, Canada, England, and Argentina that use a listening and spoken language approach to deaf education.

Schools and Programs for D/HH Students in the US: www.gallaudet.edu/clerc-center/info-to-go/national-resources-and-directories/schools-and-programs.html
Victorian Deaf Education Institution: www.deafeducation.vic.edu.au/Pages/home.aspx
VDEI aims to support deaf education in Victoria (Australia) via professional learning programs, research, curriculum improvement, and networking amongst professionals.

General Information on Deafness

Culturally and Linguistically Appropriate Services: http://clas.uiuc.edu/techreport/tech6.html
CLAS published a guide for professionals serving hearing children with deaf parents and the best practices.

Gallaudet University Info to Go: www.gallaudet.edu/clerc-center/info-to-go.html
Info to Go has a wide range of information and resources for parents of and professionals working with deaf and hard-of-hearing children.

Hearing and Speech

American Speech-Language and Hearing Association: www.asha.org
ASHA is the national association of audiologists; speech-language pathologists; speech, language, and hearing scientists; audiology and speech-language pathology support personnel; and students.

Audiology Online: www.audiologyonline.com/about-us
Audiology Online provides continuing education opportunities by leading experts in the field to enhance audiological clinical knowledge and skills. It connects quality professionals to jobs and enhances students' knowledge and skills to contribute to the profession.

Better Hearing Institute: www.betterhearing.org
The BHI is a resource for children and adults with hearing loss. BHI contains information about research, medical technology, and other skills that help people make the most of their hearing.

Cochlear Implant Education Center at Gallaudet: www.gallaudet.edu/clerc-center/our-resources/cochlear-implant-education-center.html
The Cochlear Implant Education Center is a resource center created by the Clerc Center at Gallaudet University. The CIEC explores and shares considerations and best practices for language use for children with cochlear implants.

Cochlear Implant Information: www.nidcd.nih.gov/health/hearing/pages/coch.aspx
The National Institutes of Health explains how a cochlear implant works and provides links to other resources and articles on cochlear implants.

Educational Audiology Association: www.edaud.org
A professional association of educational audiologists that can help you locate an educational audiologist in your area.

Financial Assistance for Assistive Devices: www.hearingloss.org/content/financial-assistance-programs-foundations
The Hearing Loss Association of America provides a list of various resources for assistance with the cost of hearing aids.

Hearing Health Magazine: www.hearinghealthmag.com
Hearing Health Magazine is a publication of the Hearing Health Foundation, a research organization with a mission to prevent and cure hearing loss and tinnitus.

MedlinePlus site on Cochlear Implants: www.nlm.nih.gov/medlineplus/cochlearimplants.html
MedlinePlus explains basic information about how a cochlear implant works and provides links to more resources.

National Center for Hearing Assessment and Management: www.infanthearing.org
The NCHAM aims to ensure early identification of all infants and toddlers with hearing loss and the implementation of appropriate early intervention services, including audiological, educational, and medical intervention.

SLPDEAF: http://groups.yahoo.com/group/slpdeaf
SLPDEAF is a listserv for speech pathologists working with deaf and hard-of-hearing children and also provides links to other resources. For local resources, contact your state's commission for deaf and hard-of-hearing services.

International

Discovering Deaf Worlds: www.discoveringdeafworlds.org
The DDW aims to advance the autonomy and independence of signing Deaf communities worldwide by collaborating with community members to develop and sustain self-advocacy and equal access.

Global Reach Out Initiative: www.globalreachout.org
The GRO Initiative works in India to promote high-quality leadership and management skills training for Deaf individuals. Their ultimate goal is to create strong leaders who enact positive change in their community.

International Deaf and Disability Organizations: www.gallaudet.edu/rsia/world-deaf-information-resource/deaf-orgs/international-deaf-and-disability-organizations.html
Gallaudet University has compiled a list of various international Deaf and disability organizations.

World Federation of the Deaf: http://wfdeaf.org
The WFD supports and promotes in its work the many United Nations conventions on human rights, with a focus on Deaf people who use sign language and their friends and family. The WFD works with the aim of solidarity and unity to make the world a better place.

Language Assessment Resources (ASL and English)

American Sign Language: Receptive Skills Test: www.northernsignsresearch.com
The American Sign Language Receptive Skills test is an ASL receptive test that measures vocabulary and eight different ASL grammatical structures for children from 8 to 12 years old.

ASL, English, and Neurocognitive Assessments in *Assessing Literacy in Deaf Individuals: Neurocognitive Measurement and Predictors*, edited by Morere and Allen: www.springer.com/us/book/9781461452683
This book provides a battery of clinical and educational tests developed for the VL2 Toolkit providing assessments in both ASL and English in general cognitive functioning, academic achievement, linguistic function including expressive and receptive language, fingerspelling, ASL assessment, and lipreading and writing.

The Visual Sign Communication and Sign Language Checklist (VSCL): http://vl2.gallaudet.edu/resources/vcsl/
The VCSL is a standardized visual communication and sign language checklist for signing children. It is designed to track and evaluate young children's language development from birth to age 5.

Programs to Prepare Professionals Working with Deaf People

Gallaudet University Clinical (Ph.D.) and School (Psy.D.) Psychology Programs: www.gallaudet.edu/psychology/graduate-programs.html

Lamar University Deaf Studies and Deaf Education (Ed.D.) Program: http://fineartscomm.lamar.edu/
deaf-studies-deaf-education/academic-programs/ed.d.-in-deaf-studies-deaf-education.html
National Institute for the Deaf School Psychology (M.S.) Program: www.rit.edu/cla/psychology/graduate/
ms-school-psych/overview
University of California, San Diego Teaching and Learning: Emphasis in American Sign Language—
English Bilingual Education of Deaf Children (M.A.) Program: www-tep.ucsd.edu/graduate/asl/index.
html

Psychology

American Psychological Association: www.apa.org
APA is a national organization for researchers, educators, clinicians, consultants, and students in the
psychology field.

Internet Mental Health: www.mentalhealth.com
Internet Mental Health is an encyclopedia of mental health information created by a psychiatrist.

National Institute of Mental Health: www.nimh.nih.gov/
The NIMH is the federal agency for research on mental disorders, conducting clinical research on the
understanding and treatment of mental illnesses.

National Library of Medicine: www.nlm.nih.gov
The NLM is the world's largest biomedical library with a vast print and electronic library.

Religion and Organizations

Deaf Churches: http://members.aol.com/deaflist/deafch.htm
Episcopal Conference of the Deaf: www.ecdeaf.org
International Catholic Deaf Association: www.icda-us.org
Jewish Deaf Congress: http://jewishdeafcongress.org
National Catholic Office for the Deaf: www.ncod.org
United Methodist Congress of the Deaf: www.UMCD.org

Professional and Service Organizations

American Counseling Association: www.counseling.org
ACA is the world's largest professional organization for counselors. They strive for the promotion of
professional counselors and the counseling profession and advocate for respect for human dignity and
diversity.

American Deafness and Rehabilitation Association: www.adara.org
ADARA aims to enrich the professional competency of service professionals that work with deaf and
hard-of-hearing individuals.

American Psychological Association: www.apa.org
The APA is the largest professional organization for psychologists in the United States. Their mission
is to advance the role psychology plays in improving people's lives by encouraging development and
application of psychology, research, and establishing high ethical and conduct standards.

National Alliance of Black Interpreters: www.naobidc.org
The NAOBI-DC provides professional training and networking opportunities for African American
interpreters.

National Association of Social Workers: www.socialworkers.org
NASW is the largest professional organization for social workers. They encourage professional development, establish professional standards, and advance social policies.

Office of Special Education and Rehabilitative Services: www2.ed.gov/about/offices/list/osers/index.html
The OSERS aims to improve the results of persons with disabilities by promoting inclusion and equity,
as well as creating opportunities for inclusion.

Registry of Interpreters for the Deaf, Inc.: www.rid.org/
   The RID advocates for best practices in sign language interpreting, professional development opportunities, and the implementation of high performance standards in order to ensure access for deaf individuals.

TDI: https://tdiforaccess.org/
   The TDI advocates for equal access to telecommunication, media, and information technology for deaf and hard-of-hearing people.

Special Education

ADA and Disabilities Information: www.ada.gov
   The Americans with Disabilities Act is a federal law that prohibits discrimination against and mandates appropriate accommodations be made for people with disabilities in employment, government services, facilities, and transportation.

The Center for Parent Information and Resources: www.parentcenterhub.org
   CIPR supports professionals working with and parents of children with disabilities with products and materials, education, and coordination of service provision.

Council for Exceptional Children: www.cec.sped.org
   The CEC advocates for government policies, sets professional standards, and helps obtain needed resources in order to improve the quality of education for individuals with disabilities.

Postsecondary Education Consortium: www.pepnet.org
   PEPNET aims to improve the postsecondary and vocational outcomes for deaf and hard-of-hearing individuals both with and without additional disabilities.

SERI: Special Education Resources on the Internet: http://seriweb.com
   SERI is a collection of special education resources in a variety of topics, including law, technology, specific disability information, and literature.

Summer Camps and Programs

Aspen Camp: www.aspencamp.org
   Aspen Camp provides year-round programs to Deaf, hard-of-hearing, and CODA youth, adults, and their family members. The camp emphasizes the power of community and provides services to local citizens through ASL classes, advocacy, and cultural training.

Deaf Film Camp: www.deaffilmcamp.com
   Deaf Film Camp is a two-week summer program for deaf and hard-of-hearing teenagers interested in filmmaking.

List of Summer Camps and Programs for Children and Adolescents: www.agbell.org/SummerCampsListing/
Youth Leadership Camp: https://nad.org/youthleadershipcamp
   YLC is a month-long summer camp for deaf and hard-of-hearing students that aims to develop scholarship, leadership, and citizenship. Campers participate in a variety of activities that contribute to self-discovery and growth, confidence, and interpersonal skills.

Sports

European Deaf Sport Organization: www.edso.eu
   The EDSO organizes sporting competitions for deaf and hard-of-hearing Europeans.

International Committee of Sports for the Deaf: www.deaflympics.com/icsd.asp
   The ICSD coordinates the annual Summer and Winter Deaflympics for deaf and hard-of-hearing athletes.

USA Deaf Sports Federation: www.usdeafsports.org
   The USADF is the national governing body of deaf sport organizations and coordinates sporting events and fundraisers for deaf athletes to attend the Deaflympics.

Research Labs and Organizations

American Sign Language Linguistic Research Project: www.bu.edu/asllrp/
   The ASLLRP researches the syntactic structure of ASL, develops multimedia tools for sign language research, and explores computer recognition and production of sign language.

Brain Language Laboratory for Neuroimaging: http://petitto.gallaudet.edu
   BL2 conducts neuroimaging and behavioral studies to better understand the impact of bilingualism on the brain and the developmental stages of bilingual language and reading acquisition.

Center for Education Research Partnerships: www.rit.edu/ntid/cerp/
   CERP promotes collaboration of researchers and research organizations investigating development and learning among deaf and hard-of-hearing students.

Center Research in Language: http://crl.ucsd.edu
   The CRL is a multidisciplinary center that studies signed and spoken languages, language disorders, literacy between deaf mothers and children, and the neuroimaging of language.

Gallaudet Research Institute: http://research.gallaudet.edu
   The GRI oversees the Priority Research Fund and Small Grant Programs, maintains a database of research at Gallaudet University, and conducts the Annual Survey of Deaf and Hard of Hearing Children and Youth.

House Ear Institute: www.hei.org
   The HEI researches the causes of hearing and balance disorders and explores potential treatments and novel diagnostic technologies.

Laboratory for Cognitive Neuroscience: http://lcn.salk.edu/lm_index.html
   The LCN investigates the nature of sign language processing and the impact of the different modality on neural organization and language acquisition.

National Institute on Deafness and Other Communication Disorders: www.nidcd.nih.gov
   The NIDCD researches the processes of hearing, balance, taste, smell, voice, speech, and language.

National Rehabilitation Information Center: www.naric.com
   NARIC houses and disseminates all the publications from the National Institute on Disability, Independent Living, and Rehabilitation Research.

Rochester Bridges to the Doctorate: http://deafscientists.com
   The Bridges program provides master's level mentoring and guidance toward admission to a doctoral degree program in biomedical and behavioral science disciplines.

Sign Language Linguistics Laboratory: https://signlanguagelab.uchicago.edu
   The SLLL researches sign languages from all over the world to better understand their similarities and differences. Also, SLLL strives to better understand the human language capacity and the properties that all languages share, whether spoken or signed.

Sign Language Linguistics Society: http://slls.eu
   The SLLS is a resource for sign language linguistics researchers and sponsors a tri-annual international sign language research conference.

Visual Language and Visual Learning Laboratory: http://vl2.gallaudet.edu
   VL2 investigates the effect of visual processes, visual language, and visual social experience.

References

Acredolo, L., & Goodwyn, S. (1994). Sign language among hearing infants: The spontaneous development of symbolic gestures. In V. Volterra & C. Erting (Eds.), *From gesture to language in hearing children* (pp. 68–78). Washington, DC: Gallaudet University Press.

Adam Walsh Child Protection and Safety Act, 42 U.S.C. § 16901 (2006).

Aguayo, M., & Coady, N. (2005). The experience of deafened adults: Implications for rehabilitative services. In F. Turner (Ed.), *Social work diagnosis in contemporary practice* (pp. 387–394). New York, NY: Oxford.

Aikins v. St. Helena Hospital, 843 F. Supp. 1329 (N.D Cal 1994).

Ainsworth, M., Blehar, M., Waters, E., & Wall, S. (1978). *Patterns of attachment: A psychological study of the strange situation.* Hillsdale, NJ: Erlbaum.

Alberti, P. (1998). Noise-induced hearing loss: A global problem. In L. Luxon & D. Prasher (Eds.), *Advances in noise research: Protection against noise* (Vol. 1, pp. 7–15). London, UK: Whurr.

Albrecht, G., Seelman, K., & Bury, M. (Eds.). (2001). *Handbook of disability studies.* Thousand Oaks, CA: Sage.

Alexander Graham Bell Association for the Deaf and Hard of Hearing. (2008). *Position statement: American Sign Language.* Retrieved from www.listeningandspokenlanguage.org/Document.aspx?id=387

Alexander Graham Bell Association for the Deaf and Hard of Hearing. (n.d.). *Position statement: Cochlear implants in children.* Retrieved from www.listeningandspokenlanguage.org/Document.aspx?id=386

Alford, R., Arnos, K., Fox, M., Lin, J., Palmer, C., Pandya, A., . . ., Yoshinaga-Itano, C. (2014). American College of Medical Genetics and Genomics guideline for the clinical evaluation and etiologic diagnosis of hearing loss. *Genetics in Medicine*, 16(4), 347–355.

Allen, T. E. (2015). ASL skills, fingerspelling ability, home communication context and early alphabetic knowledge of preschool-aged deaf children. *Sign Language Studies*, 15(3), 233–265.

Allen, T. E., Letteri, A., Choi, S. H., & Dang, D. (2014). Early visual language exposure and emergent literacy in preschool deaf children: Findings from a national longitudinal study. *American Annals of the Deaf*, 159(4), 346–358.

Altshuler, K., & Rainer, J. (1966). *Comprehensive mental health services for the deaf.* New York, NY: New York Psychiatric Institute, Department of Medical Genetics, Columbia University.

American Academy of Audiology. (1995). *Cochlear implants in children.* Retrieved from www.audiology.org/publications-resources/document-library/cochlear-implants-children

American Civil Liberties Union (ACLU). (2016). *ACLU National Prison Project.* Retrieved from www.aclu.org/aclu-national-prison-project

American Educational Research Association (AERA), American Psychological Association (APA), & National Council on Measurement in Education (NCME). (2014). *Standards for educational and psychological testing.* Washington, DC: AERA.

American Psychiatric Association. (2000). *Diagnostic and statistical manual of mental disorders* (4th ed., text rev.). Washington, DC: Author.

American Psychiatric Association. (2013). *Diagnostic and statistical manual of mental disorders* (5th ed.). Washington, DC: Author.

American Psychological Association. (2012). Guidelines for assessment of and intervention with persons with disabilities. *American Psychologist*, 67(1), 43–62.

American Speech-Language-Hearing Association. (2004). *Scope of practice in audiology* [scope of practice]. Retrieved from www.asha.org/policy

Americans with Disabilities Act of 1990 (Public Law 101–336).

Ammons, D. K. (2009). International Committee of Sports for the Deaf and Deaflympics. In D. F. Moores & M. S. Miller (Eds.), *Deaf people around the world* (pp. 368–373). Washington, DC: Gallaudet University Press.

Anderson, D., & Reilly, J. (2002). The MacArthur communicative development inventory: Normative data for American Sign Language. *Journal of Deaf Studies and Deaf Education, 7*(2), 83–106.

Anderson, G. (2006). *Still I rise! The enduring legacy of Black Deaf Arkansans before and after integration.* [Book/DVD]. Little Rock, AR: Arkansas Association of the Deaf.

Anderson, M., Leigh, I. W., & Samar, V. (2011). Intimate partner violence against Deaf women: A review. *Aggression and Violent Behavior, 16*(3), 200–206. DOI: 10:1016/j.avb.2011.02.006.

Andrews, J. F. (1992). Equal access for deaf teachers in Texas. *Viewpoints on Deafness: A Deaf American monograph, 42,* 13–18.

Andrews, J. F. (2011). Deaf inmates: Cultural and linguistic challenges and comprehending the inmate handbook. *Corrections Compendium, 36*(1), 1–6.

Andrews, J. F. (2012). Reading to Deaf children who sign: A response to Williams (2012) and suggestions for future research. *American Annals of the Deaf, 157*(3), 307–319.

Andrews, J. F. (2013). *Deaf juvenile sex offenders.* Unpublished raw data.

Andrews, J. F., Byrne, A., & Clark, M. D. (2015). Deaf scholars on reading: A historical review of 40 years of dissertation research (1973–2013): Implications for research and practice. *American Annals of the Deaf, 159*(5), 393–418.

Andrews, J. F., & Covell, J. A. (2006/2007). Preparing future teachers and doctoral level leaders in deaf education: Meeting the challenge. *American Annals of the Deaf, 151*(5), 464–475.

Andrews, J. F., & Dionne, V. (2008). Audiology and Deaf education: Preparing the next generation of professionals. *ADVANCE for Speech-Language Pathologists & Audiologists, 18*(18), 10–13.

Andrews, J. F., Ferguson, C., Roberts, S., & Hodges, P. (1997). What's up, Billy Jo?: Deaf children and bilingual-bicultural instruction in east-central Texas. *American Annals of the Deaf, 142*(1), 16–25.

Andrews, J. F., & Franklin, T. C. (1997, March). Why hire deaf teachers? *Texas Journal of Speech and Hearing (TEJAS), XXII*(1), 12013.

Andrews, J. F., & Jaussi, K. (1993). Teacher education in deafness in Appalachian Kentucky. *Special Education Quarterly, 12*(4), 8–21. (ERIC document: ED 425 600).

Andrews, J. F., Leigh, I. W., & Weiner, M. T. (2004). *Deaf people: Evolving perspectives from psychology, education and sociology.* Boston, MA: Allyn & Bacon.

Andrews, J.F., Liu, H., Liu, C., Gentry, M., & Smith, Z. (2016). Increasing early reading skills in young signing deaf children using shared book reading: A feasibility study. *Early Child Development and Care,* Special Issue. Manuscript accepted for publication.

Andrews, J. F., Logan, R., & Phelan, J. (2008). Milestones of language development for speech, hearing & ASL. *ADVANCE for Speech-Language Pathologists and Audiologists, 18*(2), 16–19.

Andrews, J. F., & Lokensgard, L. (2010). The visual language of art, ASL, and English. *Multicultural Review, 19*(3), 37–44.

Andrews, J. F., & Mason, J. M. (1986). How do deaf children learn about prereading? *American Annals of the Deaf, 131*(3), 210–217.

Andrews, J. F., & Rusher, M. (2010). Codeswitching techniques: Evidence-based instructional practices for the ASL/English bilingual classroom. *American Annals of the Deaf, 155*(4), 407–424.

Andrews, J. F., Shaw, P., & Lomas. (2011). Deaf and hard of hearing students. In J. M. Kauffman & D. Hallahan (Eds.), *Handbook of special education* (pp. 233–246). New York, NY: Routledge.

Andrews, J. F., Vernon, M., & LaVigne, M. (2006, May). The deaf suspect/defendant and the Bill of Rights. *Views,* 7–10.

Andrews, J. F., Vernon, M., & LaVigne, M. (2007, Summer). The Bill of Rights, due process and the deaf suspect/defendant. *Journal of Interpretation,* 9–38.

Annual Disability Statistics Compendium. (2014). *Table 2.3.* Retrieved from www.disabilitycompendium. org/compendium-statistics/employment/2–3-civilians-with-hearing-disabilities-ages-18–64-living-in-the-community-for-the-u-s-

Anthony, D. (1971). *Seeing Essential English* (Vol. 1 & 2). Anaheim, CA: Education Services Division, Anaheim School District.

Antia, S., & Kreimeyer, K. (2015). *Social competence of deaf and hard of hearing children.* New York, NY: Oxford.

Antia, S., Kreimeyer, K., Metz, K., & Spolsky, S. (2010). Peer interactions of deaf and hard-of-hearing children. In M. Marschark & P. Spencer (Eds.), *Oxford handbook of deaf studies, language, and education* (2nd ed., Vol. 1, pp. 173–187). New York, NY: Oxford.

Antia, S., & Metz, K. K. (2014). Co-enrollment in the United States: A critical analysis of benefits and challenges. In M. Marschark, G. Tang, & H. Knoors (Eds.), *Bilingualism and bilingual deaf education* (pp. 424–441). New York, NY: Oxford.

Appleman, K., Callahan, J., Mayer, M., Luetke, B., & Stryker, D. (2012). Education, employment, and independent living of young adults who are deaf and hard of hearing. *American Annals of the Deaf, 157*(3), 264–275.

Archbold, S., Harris, M., O'Donoghue, G., Nikolopoulos, T., White, A., & Richmond, H. L. (2008). Reading abilities after cochlear implantation: The effect of age at implantation on outcomes at 5 and 7 years after implantation. *International Journal of Pediatric Otorhinolaryngology, 72*(10), 1471–1478.

Archbold, S., & Mayer, C. (2012). Deaf education: The impact of cochlear implantation. *Deafness and Education International, 14*(1), 2–15.

Archbold, S., Sach, T., Lutman, M., & Gregory, S. (2006). Deciding to have a cochlear implant and subsequent after-care: Parental perspectives. *Deafness and Education International, 8*(4), 190–206.

Armstrong, D. (2014). Deaf president now and the struggle for deaf control of Gallaudet University. *Sign Language Studies, 15*(1), 42–56.

Arnett, J. J. (2006). Emerging adulthood: Understanding the new way of coming of age. In J. J. Arnett & J. L. Tanner (Eds.). *Emerging adults in America* (pp. 3–19). Washington, DC: American Psychological Association.

Arnos, K. (2002). Genetics and deafness: Impacts on the deaf community. *Sign Language Studies, 2*, 150–168.

Arnos, K., & Pandya, A. (2004). Genes for deafness and the genetic program at Gallaudet University, In J. Van Cleve (Ed.), *Genetics, disability, and deafness* (pp. 111–126). Washington, DC: Gallaudet University Press.

Arnos, K., & Pandya, A. (2011). Advances in the genetics of deafness. In M. Marschark & P. Spencer (Eds.), *The Oxford handbook of Deaf studies, language, and education* (pp. 412–424. New York, NY: Oxford.

Atkins, S. (2013). A study into the lived experiences of deaf entrepreneurs: Considerations for the professional. *JADARA, 47*(2), 222–236.

Ausbrooks, M., Baker, S., & Daugaard, J. (2012). Recruiting deaf and diverse teachers: Priorities of pre-service teachers in deaf education, *ADARA, 46*(1), 369–398.

Ausbrooks, M. M., Gentry, M. A., & Martin, G. (2014). Exploring linguistic interdependence between American Sign Language and English through correlational and multiple regression analyses of the abilities of biliterate deaf adults. *International Journal of English Linguistics, 4*(1), 1–18.

Bahan, B. (2008). Upon the formation of a visual variety of the human race. In H-D. Bauman (Ed.), *Open your eyes: Deaf studies talking* (pp. 83–99). Minneapolis, MN: University of Minnesota Press.

Bailes, C. N. (1998). Primary-grade teachers' strategic use of ASL in teaching English literacy in a bilingual setting. (Unpublished doctoral dissertation, University of Maryland, College Park, MD).

Bailey, K., & Miner, I. (2010). Psychotherapy for people with Usher syndrome. In I. W. Leigh (Ed.), *Psychotherapy with deaf clients from diverse groups* (2nd ed., pp. 136–158). Washington, DC: Gallaudet University Press.

Baker, L. (2002). Metacognition in comprehension instruction. In C. Block & M. Pressley (Eds.), *Comprehension instruction: Research-based best practices* (pp. 77–95). New York, NY: Guilford Press.

Baker, S. (2010, July). The importance of fingerspelling for reading. Visual Language and Visual Learning Science of Learning Center. Washington, DC. Retrieved from http://vl2.gallaudet.edu/files/7813/9216/6278/research-brief-1-the-importance-of-fingerspelling-for-reading.pdf

Baldwin, S. (1993). *Pictures in the air: The story of the National Theater of the Deaf.* Washington, DC: Gallaudet University Press.

Bandurski, M., & Galkowski, T. (2004). The development of analogical reasoning in deaf children and their parents' communication mode. *Journal of Deaf Studies and Deaf Education, 9*(2), 153–175.

Barber, S., Wills, D., & Smith, M. (2010). Deaf survivors of sexual assault. In I. W. Leigh (Ed.), *Psychotherapy with Deaf clients from diverse groups* (pp. 320–340). Washington, DC: Gallaudet University Press.

Barbour County Bd. of Educ. v. Parent. (1999). 29 IDELR 848. *Individuals with Disabilities Act Law Report, 29*(7), 848–852.

Barker, D., Qittner, A., Fink, N., Eisenberg, L., Tobey, E., & Niparko, J. (2009). Predicting behavior problems in deaf and hearing children: The influences of language, attention, and parent-child communication. *Development and Psychopathology, 21*(2), 373–392.

Barnartt, S. (2006). Deaf women and inequality in educational attainment and occupational status. In B. J. Brueggemann & S. Burch (Eds.), *Women and deafness* (pp. 57–77). Washington, DC: Gallaudet University Press.

Barnett, S., & Franks, P. (1999). Deafness and mortality: Analyses of linked data from the National Health Interview Survey and National Death Index. *Public Health Reports, 114*(4), 330–336.

Barnett, S., Klein, J., Pollard, R., Samar, V., Schlehofer, D., Starr, M., . . ., Pearson, T. (2011). Community participatory research with Deaf sign language users to identify health inequities. *American Journal of Public Health, 101*(12), 2235–2238.

Barnett, S., McKee, M., Smith, S., & Pearson, T. (2011). Deaf sign language users, health inequities, and public health: Opportunity for social justice. *Preventing Chronic Disease, 8*(2), A45.

Basilier, T. (1964). The psychic consequences of congenital or early acquired deafness. *Acta Psychiatrica Scandinavia, 40*(Suppl. 180), 362–374.

Bat-Chava, Y. (1993). Antecedents of self-esteem in deaf people: A meta-analytic review. *Rehabilitation Psychology, 38,* 221–234.

Bat-Chava, Y. (2000). Diversity of deaf identities. *American Annals of the Deaf, 145,* 420–428.

Bathard, H. (2014). *Intricate identities: Cochlear implant users negotiating lives between d/Deaf and hearing worlds* (Master's thesis). Victoria University of Wellington, Wellington, NZ. Retrieved from http://researcharchive.vuw.ac.nz/xmlui/bitstream/handle/10063/3475/thesis.pdf?sequence=2

Batten, G., Oakes, P., & Alexander, T. (2014). Factors associated with social interactions between deaf children and their hearing peers: A systematic literature review. *Journal of Deaf Studies and Deaf Education, 19*(3), 285–302.

Bauman, H-D. (2008a). On the disconstruction of (sign) language in the Western tradition: A Deaf reading of Plato's Cratylus. In H-D. Bauman (Ed.), *Open your eyes: Deaf Studies talking* (pp. 1–32). Minneapolis, MN: University of Minnesota Press.

Bauman, H-D. (2008b). Preface. In H-D. Bauman (Ed.), *Open your eyes: Deaf Studies talking* (pp. vii–ix). Minneapolis, MN: University of Minnesota Press.

Bauman, H. (2014). Deaf space: An architecture toward a more livable and sustainable world. In H. Bauman & J. Murray (Eds.), *Deaf gain* (pp. 375–401). Minneapolis, MN: University of Minnesota Press.

Bauman, H-D., & Murray, J. (2010). Deaf studies in the 21st century: "Deaf-gain" and the future of human diversity. In M. Marschark & P. Spencer (Eds.), *The Oxford handbook of Deaf studies, language, and education* (Vol. 2, pp. 210–225). New York, NY: Oxford.

Bauman, H-D., & Murray, J. (Eds.). (2014). *Deaf gain: Raising the stakes for human diversity.* Minneapolis, MN: University of Minnesota Press.

Bauman, S., & Pero, H. (2011). Bullying and cyberbullying among deaf students and their hearing peers: An exploratory study. *Journal of Deaf Studies and Deaf Education, 16*(2), 236–253.

Bavelier, D., Brozinsky, C., Tomann, A., Mitchell, T., Neville, H., & Guoying, L. (2001). Impact of early deafness and early exposure to sign language on the cerebral organization for motion processing. *Journal of Neuroscience, 21*(22), 8931–8942.

Baynton, D. (1993). Savages and deaf mutes: Evolutionary theory and the campaign against sign language in the nineteenth century. In J. Van Cleve (Ed.). *Deaf history unveiled: Intepretations from the new scholarship* (pp. 92–112). Washington, DC: Gallaudet University Press.

Baynton, D., Gannon, J., & Bergey, J. (2007). *Through deaf eyes: A photographic history of an American history.* Washington, DC: Gallaudet University Press.

Bechter, F. (2008). The Deaf convert culture and its lessons for Deaf theory. In H-D. Bauman (Ed.), *Open your eyes: Deaf studies talking* (pp. 60–79) Minneapolis, MN: University of Minnesota Press.

Bell, C. (2014). *El deafo.* New York, NY: Amulet Books.

Bellugi, U., Marks, S., Bihrle, A., & Sabo, H. (1994). Dissociation between language and cognitive functions in Williams Syndrome. In D. Bishop & K. Mogford (Eds.), *Language development in exceptional children* (pp. 177–189). Mahwah, NJ: Erlbaum Associates.

Benedict, B., & Sass-Lehrer, M. (2007). Deaf and hearing partnerships: Ethical and communication considerations. *American Annals of the Deaf, 152*(3), 275–282.

Bennett, B., Spencer, D., Bergmann, J., Cockrum, T., Musallam, R., Sams, A., . . ., Overmyer, J. (2013). *The flipped classroom manifest*. Retrieved from www.thedailyriff.com/articles/the-flipped-class-manifest-823.php

Berens, M. S., Kovelman, I., & Petitto, L. A. (2013). Should bilingual children learn reading in two languages at the same time or in sequence?. *Bilingual Research Journal, 36*(1), 35–60.

Berke, M. (2013). Reading books with young deaf children: Strategies for mediating between American Sign Language and English. *Journal of Deaf Studies and Deaf Education, 18*(3), 299–311.

Berkowitz, M., & Jonas, J. (2014). *Deaf and hearing siblings in conversation*. Jefferson, NC: McFarland & Co.

Berlin, F., & Krout, E. (1986). Pedophilia: Diagnostic concepts, treatment and ethical considerations. *American Journal of Forensic Psychiatry, 7*(1), 13–30.

Best, H. (1943). *Deafness and the deaf in the United States*. New York, NY: Macmillan.

Bickley, C., Moseley, M., & Stansky, A. (2012). Analysis of responses to lipreading prompts as a window to deaf students' writing strategies. In D. Morere & T. Allen (Eds.), *Assessing literacy in deaf individuals: Neurocognitive measurement and predictors* (pp. 209–227). New York, NY: Springer.

Biesold, H. (1999). *Crying hands: Eugenics and deaf people in Nazi Germany*. Washington, DC: Gallaudet University Press.

Binnie, C., Montgomery, A., & Jackson, P. (1974). Auditory and visual contributions to the perception of consonants. *Journal of Hearing and Speech Research, 1*(17), 619–630.

Bishop, K. (2013). Culturally affirmative adaptations to trauma treatment with deaf children in a residential setting. In N. Glickman (Ed.), *Deaf mental health care* (pp. 268–297). New York, NY: Routledge.

Bishop, M., & Hicks, S. (2008). *Hearing, mother father deaf: Hearing people in Deaf families*. Washington, DC: Gallaudet University Press.

Bitner-Glindzicz, M., & Rahman, S. (2007). Ototoxicity caused by aminoglycosides. *BMJ, 335*(7624), 784–785.

Black, P. A., & Glickman, N. S. (2006). Demographics, psychiatric diagnoses, and other characteristics of North American deaf and hard-of-hearing inpatients. *Journal of Deaf Studies and Deaf Education, 11*(3), 303–321.

Blackwell, D. L., Lucas, J. W., & Clarke, T. C. (2014). Summary health statistics for US adults: National health interview survey, 2012. *Vital and health statistics. Series 10, Data from the National Health Survey, 260*, 1–161.

Blamey, P., & Sarant, J. (2011). Development of spoken language by deaf children. In M. Marschark & P. Spencer (Eds.), *The Oxford handbook of Deaf studies, language, and education* (2nd ed., Vol. 1, pp. 241–257). New York, NY: Oxford.

Blanchfield, B., Feldman, J., Dunbar, J., & Gardner, E. (2001). The severely to profoundly hearing impaired population in the United States: Prevalence estimates and demographics. *Journal of the American Academy of Audiology, 12*, 183–189.

Blankmeyer Burke, T. (2014). Armchairs and stares: On the privation of deafness. In H-D. Bauman & J. Murray (Eds.), *Deaf gain* (pp. 3–22). Minneapolis, MN: University of Minnesota Press.

Board of Education v. Rowley, 458 U. S. 176: Vol. 458 (1982). *US Supreme Court Cases from Justia & Oyez*. N.p., n.d. Retrieved from the web. 21 June 2016.

Boboltz, S. (2015). In defense of closed captioning, which is entirely under rated. *The Huffington Post*. Retrieved from www.huffingtonpost.com/entry/closed-captioning-is-underrated_559d67c7e4b05b1d028f8af5

Bohlin, G., Hagekull, B., & Rydell, A. (2000). Attachment and social functioning: A longitudinal study from infancy to middle childhood. *Social Development, 9*(1), 24–39. DOI: 10.1111/1467-9507.00109

Bornstein, H. (1982). Toward a theory of use of signed English: From birth through adulthood. *American Annals of the Deaf, 127*, 69–72.

Borum, V. (2008). African American parents with deaf children: Reflections on spirituality. *JADARA, 41*(3), 207–226.

Bourzac, K. (2014). Cochlear implant also uses gene therapy to improve hearing. *Biomedicine News*. Retrieved from www.technologyreview.com/news/526906/cochlear-implant-also-uses-gene-therapy-to-improve-hearing/

Bouton, K. (2013). Quandary of hidden disabilities: Conceal or reveal. *The New York Times*. Retrieved from www.nytimes.com/2013/09/22/business/quandary-of-hidden-disabilities-conceal-or-reveal.html?_r=0

Bovet, D. (1990). *The path to language: Bilingual education for deaf children*. Cleveton, UK: Multilingual Matters.

Bowe, F. (1991). *Approach equality: Education of the deaf*. Silver Spring, MD: T. J. Publishers.

Bowlby, J. (1958). The nature of the child's tie to his mother. *International Journal of Psycho-Analysis, 39*, 350–373.

Braden, J. (1994). *Deafness, deprivation, and IQ*. New York, NY: Plenum.

Braden, J. (2001). The clinical assessment of deaf people's cognitive abilities. In M. Clark, M. Marschark, & M. Karchmer (Eds.), *Context, cognition, and deafness* (pp. 14–37). Washington, DC: Gallaudet University Press.

Bradham, T., Caraway, T., Moog, J., Houston, T., & Rosenthal, J. (2015). *Facts about pediatric hearing loss*. Retrieved from www.asha.org/aud/Facts-about-Pediatric-Hearing-Loss/

Bramley, S. (2007). Working with deaf people who have committed sexual offenses against children: The need for an increased awareness. *Journal of Sexual Aggression, 13*(1), 59–69.

Brannon, G. (2015). *History and mental status examination*. Retrieved from http://emedicine.medscape.com/article/293402-overview

Branson, J., & Miller, D. (2002). *Damned for their difference: The cultural construction of deaf people as disabled*. Washington, DC: Gallaudet University Press.

Brentari, D. (1990). *Theoretical foundations in American Sign Language phonology*. (Unpublished doctoral dissertation. University of Chicago, Chicago. IL).

Brentari, D. (1998). *A prosodic model of sign language phonology*. Cambridge MA: MIT Press.

Brentari, D. (2001). Handshape in sign language phonology. In M. van Oostendorp, C. J. Ewen, E. Hume, & K. Rice (Eds.), *The Blackwell companion to phonology* (pp. 195–222). Oxford, England: Blackwell.

Brentari, D. (Ed.). (2010). *Sign languages*. New York, NY: Cambridge University Press.

Brice, P., & Adams, E (2011). Developing a concept of self and other: Risk and protective factors. In D. Zand & K. Pierce (Eds.), *Resilience in deaf children* (pp. 115–137). New York, NY: Springer.

Brice, P., Leigh, I. W., Sheridan, M., & Smith, K. (2013). Training of mental health professionals: Yesterday, today, and tomorrow. In N. Glickman (Ed.), *Deaf mental health care* (pp. 298–322). New York, NY: Routledge.

Brougham v. Town of Yarmouth. (1993). 20 IDELR 12. *Individuals with Disabilities Law Report, 20*(1), 12–18.

Brouwer, M., McIntyre, P., Prasad, K., & van de Beek, D. (2013). Corticosteroids for bacterial meningitis. *The Cochrane Library*, 9. DOI: 10.1002/14651858.CD004405.pub4

Brown, E., Chau, J., Atashband, S., Westerberg, B., & Kozak, F. (2009). A systematic review of neonatal toxoplasmosis exposure and sensorineural hearing loss. *International Journal of Pediatric Otorhinolaryngology, 73*(5), 707–711.

Brown, M., & Mkhize, Z. (2014). Perceptions of HIV/AIDS: A conversation with deaf adults in Kwa Zulu-Natal Province, South Africa. *JADARA, 49*(1), 27–40.

Brown, P. M., & Cornes, A. (2015). Mental health of deaf and hard-of-hearing adolescents: What the students say. *Journal of Deaf Studies and Deaf Education, 20*(1), 75–81.

Brueggemann, B. (1999). *Lend me your ear*. Washington, DC: Gallaudet University Press.

Buchanan, R. (1999). *Illusions of equality*. Washington, DC: Gallaudet University Press.

Buchman, C., Copeland, B., Yu, K., Brown, C., Carrasco, V., & Pillsbury, H. (2004). Cochlear implantation in children with congenital inner ear malformations. *The Laryngoscope, 114*, 309–316.

Buck, D. (2000). *Deaf peddler: Confessions of an inside man*. Washington, DC: Gallaudet University Press.

Burch, S. (2002). *Signs of resistance: American Deaf cultural history, 1900 to 1942*. New York, NY: New York University Press.

Burch, S., & Joyner, H. (2007). *Unspeakable*. Chapel Hill, NC: University of North Carolina Press.

Burch, S., & Kafer, A. (2010). *Deaf and disability studies: Interdisciplinary perspectives*. Washington, DC: Gallaudet University Press.

Bureau of Justice Statistics. (2014). Correctional Populations in the United States. Retrieved from www.bjs.gov/index.cfm?ty=pbdetail&iid=5519

Burton, S., Withrow, K., Arnos, K., Kalfoglou, A., & Pandya, A. (2006). A focus group study of consumer attitudes toward genetic testing and newborn screening for deafness. *Genetics in Medicine, 8*(12), 779–783.

Byrd, Todd. (2007). *Deaf space*. Retrieved from www.gallaudet.edu/university_communications/gallaudet_today_magazine/deaf_space_spring_2007.html

Byrne, A. (2013). *American Sign Language (ASL) literacy and ASL literature: A critical appraisal* (Unpublished doctoral dissertation). York University, Toronto, ON.

Calderon, R., & Greenberg, M. (2011). Social and emotional development of deaf children: Family, school, and program effects. In M. Marschark & P. Spencer (Eds.), *The Oxford handbook of Deaf studies, language, and education* (2nd ed., Vol. 1, pp. 188–199). New York, NY: Oxford.

Callaway, A. (2000). *Deaf children in China*. Washington, DC: Gallaudet University Press.

Callis, L. (2015). *Let's see more #Deaftalent in Hollywood*. Retrieved from www.huffingtonpost.com/lydia-l-callis/lets-see-more-deaftalent-_b_6690324.html

Calvet, L. J. (1998). *Language wars and linguistic politics*. New York, NY: Oxford University Press on Demand.

Camenisch v. Univ. of Tex., 616 F.2d 127 (5th Cir.1980).

Campbell, R., MacSweeney, M., & Waters, D. (2008). Sign language and the brain: A review. *Journal of Deaf Studies and Deaf Education, 13*(1), 3–20.

Cannon, J. E., & Guardino, C. (2016). A new kind of heterogeneity: What we can learn from d/Deaf and hard of hearing multilingual learners. *American Annals of the Deaf, 161*(1), 8–16.

Cantor, D., & Spragins, A. (1977). Delivery of service to the hearing impaired child in the elementary school. *American Annals of the Deaf, 122*(5), 330–336.

Carr, A. (2011). *Positive psychology and human strengths* (2nd ed.). New York, NY: Routledge.

Carver, L. (2011, May 25). Jury finds against Texas Tech in employee case. *Lubbock Avalanche Journal*. Retrieved from http://lubbockonline.com/local-news/2011–05–25/jury-finds-against-texas-tech-employee-case#.VjbmoaSBL0t

Caserta, M. (2013a). Congenital rubella. *The Merck Manual Professional Edition*. Retrieved from www.merckmanuals.com/professional/pediatrics/infections_in_neonates/congenital_rubella.html

Caserta, M. (2013b). Congenital toxoplasmosis. *The Merck Manual Professional Edition*. Retrieved from www.merckmanuals.com/professional/pediatrics/infections_in_neonates/congenital_toxoplasmosis.html

Castillo, M. (2011). Claiming persecution, deaf immigrants seek U.S. asylum. *CNN*. Retrieved from www.cnn.com/2011/10/04/us/california-deaf-asylum-seekers/

Cawthon, S. (2011). *Accountability-based reforms*. Washington, DC: Gallaudet University Press.

Cawthon, S., & Leppo, R. (2013). Assessment accommodations on tests of academic achievement for students who are deaf or hard of hearing: A qualitative meta-analysis of the research literature. *American Annals of the Deaf, 158*(3), 363–376.

Cawthon, S. W., Schoffstall, S. J., & Garberoglio, C. L. (2014). How ready are postsecondary institutions for students who are D/deaf or hard-of-hearing?. *Education Policy Analysis Archives, 22*(13). DOI: dx.doi.org/10.14507/epaa.v22n13.2014

Census. (2010). *2010 Census shows American's diversity*. Retrieved December 9, 2014 from www.census.gov/newsroom/releases/archives/2010_census/cb11-cn125.html

Center on the Developing Child. (2012). *Executive function* (InBrief). Retrieved from www.developingchild.harvard.edu

Centers for Disease Control and Prevention (CDC). (2014). *Summary of 2012 national CDC EHDI data*. Retrieved from www.cdc.gov/ncbddd/hearingloss/2012-data/2012_ehdi_hsfs_summary_b.pdf

Chamberlain, C., & Mayberry, R. I. (2000). Theorizing about the relation between American Sign Language and reading. In J. P. Morford & R. I. Mayberry (Eds.), *Language acquisition by eye* (pp. 221–259). Mahwah, NJ: Lawrence Erlbaum.

Chapman, R. S. (2000). Children's language learning: An interactionist perspective. *Journal of Child Psychology and Psychiatry, 41*(1), 33–54.

Chase, P., Hall, J., & Werkhaven, J. (1996). Sensorineural hearing loss in children: Etiology and pathology. In F. Martin & J. Clark (Eds.), *Hearing care for children* (pp. 73–91). Boston, MA: Allyn and Bacon.

Chia, E., Mitchell, P., Rochtchina, E., Foran, S., Golding, M., & Wang, J. (2006). Association between vision and hearing impairments and their combined effects on quality of life. *Archives of Ophthalmology, 124*(10), 1465–1470.

Chomsky, N. (1959). A review of B.F. Skinner's verbal behavior. *Language, 35*(1), 26–58.

Chomsky, N. (1965). *Aspects of the theory of syntax*. Cambridge, MA: MIT Press.

Christiansen, J. (2010). *Reflections: My life in the deaf and hearing worlds*. Washington, DC: Gallaudet University Press.

Christiansen, J. B., & Barnartt, S. (1995). *Deaf president now! The 1988 revolution at Gallaudet University*. Washington, DC: Gallaudet University Press.

Christiansen, J. B., & Leigh, I. W. (2002/2005). *Cochlear implants in children: Ethics and choices*. Washington, DC: Gallaudet University Press.

Christiansen, J. B., & Leigh, I. W. (2011). Cochlear implants and deaf community perspectives. In R. Paludneviciene & I. W. Leigh (Eds.), *Cochlear implants: Evolving perspectives* (pp. 39–55). Washington, DC: Gallaudet University Press.

Clark, J. G. (1981). Uses and abuses of hearing loss classification. *ASHA, 23,* 493–500.

Clark, J. L. (2009). *Deaf American poetry: An anthology*. Washington, DC: Gallaudet University Press.

Clark, M. D., Galloza-Carrero, A., Keith, C. L., Tibbitt, J. S., Wolsey, J.L.A., & Zimmerman, H. G. (2015). Eye-gaze development in infants: Learning to look-and looking to learn. *Advance for Speech and Hearing*. Retrieved from http://speech-language-pathology-audiology.advanceweb.com/Features/ Articles/Eye-Gaze-Development-in-Infants.aspx

Clark, M. D., Hauser, P., Miller, P., Kargin, T., Rathmann, C., Guidenoglu, B., & . . ., Israel, E. (2016). The importance of early sign language acquisition for deaf readers. *Reading & Writing Quarterly: Overcoming Learning Difficulties, 32*(2), 127–151.

Cobb, A., Green, B., Gill, D., Ayliffe, P., Lloyd, T., Bulstrode, N., & Dunaway, D. (2014). The surgical management of Treacher Collins Syndrome. *British Journal of Oral and Maxillofacial Surgery, 52*(7), 581–589.

Cohen, H., & Jones, E. (1990). Interpreting for cross-cultural research: Changing written English to American Sign Language. *JADARA, 24,* 41–48.

Cohrrsen, C., Church, A., & Tayler, C. (2009). *Victorian early years learning and development framework: Evidence paper*. Melbourne, Australia: University of Melbourne Department of Education and Early Childhood Development. Retrieved from www.eduweb.vic.gov.au/edulibrary/public/earlylearning/ respectful-relns.pdf

Cokely, D. (2005). Shifting positionality: A critical examination of the turning point in the relationship of interpreters and the Deaf community. In M. Marschark, R. Peterson, & E. Winston (Eds.), *Sign language interpreting and interpreter education* (pp. 3–28). New York, NY: Oxford University Press.

Cole, K. (2003). Using the MMPI-2 with deaf individuals: A test of the test. *Dissertation Abstracts International: Section B, 64*(2), 957.

Coll, K., Cutler, M., Thobro, P., Haas, R., & Powell, S. (2009). An exploratory study of psychosocial risk behavior of adolescents who are deaf or hard of hearing: Comparisons and recommendations. *American Annals of the Deaf, 154*(1), 30–35.

Common Core State Standards Initiative. (2012). *Adoption by states*. Retrieved from www.corestandards. org/in-the-states

Cone, B. (2011). Screening and assessment of hearing loss in infants. In M. Marschark & P. Spencer (Eds.), *Oxford handbook of Deaf studies, language, and education* (2nd ed., Vol. 1, pp. 439–451). New York, NY: Oxford.

Cone-Wesson, B. (2005). Prenatal alcohol and cocaine exposure: Influences on cognition, speech, language, and hearing. *Journal of Communication Disorders, 38,* 279–302.

Connor, C., Hieber, S., Arts, H., & Zwolan, T. (2000). Speech, vocabulary, and the education of deaf children using cochlear implants: Oral or total communication? *Journal of Speech, Language, and Hearing Research, 43*(5), 1185–1204.

Connor, C. M., & Zwolan, T. A. (2004). Examining multiple sources of influence on the reading comprehension skills of children who use cochlear implants. *Journal of Speech, Language, and Hearing Research, 47*(3), 509–526.

Conrad, R. (1979). *The deaf school child*. London, UK: Harper & Row Ltd.

Convertino, C., Borgna, G., Marschark, M., & Durkin, A. (2014). Word and world knowledge among deaf learners with and without cochlear implants. *Journal of Deaf Studies and Deaf Education, 19*(4), 471–483.

Conway, C. M., Pisoni, D. B., Anaya, E. M., Karpicke, J., & Henning, S. C. (2011). Implicit sequence learning in deaf children with cochlear implants. *Developmental Science, 14*(1), 69–82.

Cooper, A., & Rashid, K. (2015). *Citizenship, politics, difference: Perspectives from sub-Saharan signed language communities*. Washington, DC: Gallaudet University Press.

Corballis, M. (2002). *From hand to mouth: The origins of language*. Princeton, NJ: Princeton University Press.

Corbett, C. (2010). Mental health issues for African American Deaf people. In I. W. Leigh (Ed.), *Psychotherapy with Deaf clients from diverse groups* (2nd ed., pp. 161–182). Washington, DC: Gallaudet University Press.

Corker, M. (1996). *Deaf transitions*. London, UK: Jessica Kingsley.

Corker, M. (1998). *Deaf and disabled, or deafness disabled?* Buckingham, UK: Open University Press.

Cornett, O. (1967). Cued speech. *American Annals of the Deaf, 112*(1), 3–13.

Crenshaw, K. (1989). Demarginalizing the intersection of race and sex: A black feminist critique of antidiscrimination doctrine, feminist theory, and antiracist politics. *University of Chicago Legal Forum*, 139–167.

Cripps, J., & Supalla, S. (2012). The power of spoken language in schools and deaf students who sign. *International Journal of Humanities and Social Sciences, 2*(16), 86–102.

Crume, P. (2013). Teachers perceptions of promoting sign language phonological awareness in an ASL/English bilingual program. *Journal of Deaf Studies and Deaf Education*. DOI: 10.1093/deafed/ent023

Cuijpers, P., Sijbrandij, M., Koole, S., Andersson, G., Beekman, A., & Reynolds, C. (2013). The efficacy of psychotherapy and pharmacotherapy in treating depressive and anxiety disorders: A meta-analysis of direct comparisons. *World Psychiatry, 12*(2), 137–148.

Cummins, J. (1979). Linguistic interdependence and the educational development of bilingual children. *Review of Educational Research, 49*(2), 222–251.

Cummins, J. (1981). *Bilingualism and minority-language children. Language and literacy series*. Toronto, ON: The Ontario Institute for Studies in Education.

Cupples, L., Ching, T.Y.C., Crowe, K., Day, J., & Seeto, M. (2014). Predictors of early reading skill in 5-year-old children with hearing loss who use spoken language. *Reading Research Quarterly, 49*(1), 85–104.

CVAA. (2010, 2012, 2013, 2014). *Twenty-first Century Communications and Video Accessibility Act*. Public Law 111-260. Retrieved from www.fcc.gov/consumers/guides/21st-century-communications-and-video-accessibility-act-cvaa

Daigle, B. (1994). *An analysis of a deaf psychotic inpatient population* (Unpublished master's thesis). Western Maryland College (now McDaniel College), Westminster, MD.

Dammeyer, J. (2010). Psychosocial development in a Danish population of children with cochlear implants and deaf and hard-of-hearing children. *Journal of Deaf Studies and Deaf Education, 15*(1), 50–58.

Davidson, K., Lillo-Martin, D., & Chen-Pichler, D. C. (2014). Spoken English language development in native signing children with cochlear implants. *Journal of Deaf Studies and Deaf Education, 19*(2), 238–250.

Davis, L. (1995). *Enforcing normality: Disability, deafness, and the body*. London: Versace.

Davis, L. (2008). Postdeafness. In H-D. Bauman (Ed.), *Open your eyes: Deaf studies talking* (pp. 314–325). Minneapolis, MN: University of Minnesota Press.

Dawes, S. E., Palmer, B. W., & Jeste, D. V. (2008). Adjudicative competence. *Current Opinion in Psychiatry, 21*(5), 490–494.

Deaf American. (1969). Deaf post office clerks being trained in Ohio. *The Deaf American, 22*, 29.

Deaf American. (1970). New Orleans post office employs deaf workers. *The Deaf American, 22*, 34.

DeLana, M., Gentry, M. A., & Andrews, J. (2007). The efficacy of ASL/English bilingual education: Considering public schools. *American Annals of the Deaf, 152*(1), 73–87.

Delich, N. (2014). Spiritual direction and Deaf spirituality: Implications for social work practice. *Journal of Religion & Spirituality in Social Work: Social Thought, 33*(3–4), 317–338.

DeLuca, D., Leigh, I. W., Lindgren, K., & Napoli, D. (2008). *Access: Multiple avenues for deaf people*. Washington, DC: Gallaudet University Press.

Denoyelle, F., Weil, D., Maw, M. A., Wilcox, S. A., Lench, N. J., Allen-Powell, D. R., . . ., Dodé, C. (1997). Prelingual deafness: high prevalence of a 30delG mutation in the connexin 26 gene. *Human Molecular Genetics, 6*(12), 2173–2177.

Denworth, L. (2014). *I can hear you whisper*. New York, NY: Dutton.

Department of Counseling, Gallaudet University and Gallaudet Research Institute. (2015). *Mental health services for Deaf people: A resource directory* (5th ed). Retrieved from http://research.gallaudet.edu/resources/mhd/

DesJardin, J. L., Ambrose, S. E., & Eisenberg, L. S. (2009). Literacy skills in children with cochlear implants: The importance of early oral language and joint storybook reading. *Journal of Deaf Studies and Deaf Education, 14*(1), 22–43.

Dillon, C., F., Gu, Q., Hoffman, H., & Ko, C. W. (2010). *Vision, hearing, balance, and sensory impairment in Americans aged 70 years and over: United States, 1999–2006* (NCHS Data Brief No. 31). Hyattsville, MD: National Center for Health Statistics.

Dodd, B. (1977). The role of vision in the perception of speech. *Perception, 6*(1), 31–40.

Dollard, S., Grosse, S., & Ross, D. (2007). New estimates of the prevalence of neurological and sensory sequelae and mortality associated with congenital cytomegalovirus infection. *Medical Virology, 17*(5), 355–363.

Dolman, D. (2013). The Common Core Standards: Why they matter to teachers and parents of children with hearing loss. *Volta Voices, 20*(4), 24–27. Retrieved from www.agbell.org/uploadedFiles/Connect/Publications/Volta_Voices/AGBellVVJulyAug_4.pdf

Donaldson, J. D. (2014). *Acute otitis media.* Retrieved from http://emedicine.medscape.com/article/859316-overview#a0156

Dostal, H. M., & Wolbers, K. A. (2014). Developing language and writing skills of deaf and hard of hearing students: A simultaneous approach. *Literacy Research and Instruction, 53*(3), 245–268.

Drasgow, E., & Paul, P. V. (1995). A critical analysis of the use of MCE systems with deaf students: A review of the Literature. *ACEHI Journal/Revue ACEDA, 21*, 80–93.

Drolsbaugh, M. (2000, November). You deaf people. *Silent News, 32*, 12.

Druchen, B. (2014). The legacy of Deaf President Now in South Africa. *Sign Language Studies, 15*(1), 74–86.

Du, Y., Wu, H., & Li, L. (2006). Mechanisms of bacterial meningitis-related deafness. *Drug Discovery Today: Disease Mechanisms, 3*(1), 115–118.

Dube, W. (2011). Study: Abuse rates higher among deaf and hard-of-hearing children compared with hearing youth. *RIT University News.* Retrieved from www.rit.edu/news/story.php?id=48054

du Feu, M., & Chovaz, C. (2014). *Mental health and deafness.* New York, NY: Oxford.

Dusky v. United States, 362 U.S. 402, 402(1960).

Dye, M.W.G., & Bavelier, D. (2010). Attentional enhancements and deficits in deaf populations: An integrative review. *Restorative Neurology and Neuroscience, 28*, 181–192.

Easterbrooks, S. R., & Beal-Alvarez, J. (2012). States' reading outcomes of students who are d/Deaf and hard of hearing. *American Annals of the Deaf, 157*(1), 27–40.

Easterbrooks, S. R., & Beal-Alvarez, J. (2013). *Literacy instruction for students who are deaf and hard of hearing.* New York, NY: Oxford University Press.

Easterbrooks, S. R., Lederberg, A. R., Antia, S., Schick, B., Kushalnagar, P., Webb, M. Y., . . ., Connor, C. M. (2015). Reading among diverse DHH learners: What, how, and for whom?. *American Annals of the Deaf, 159*(5), 419–432.

Easterbrooks, S., Lytle, L., Sheets, P., & Crook, B. (2004). Ignoring free, appropriate, public education, a costly mistake: The case of F.M. & L.G. *Journal of Deaf Studies and Deaf Education, 9*(2), 219–227.

Eckert, R. (2010). Toward a theory of Deaf ethnos: Deafnicity ≈ D/deaf (Hómaemon. Homóglosson. Homóthreskon). *Journal of Deaf Studies and Deaf Education, 15*(4), 317–333.

Eckert, R., & Rowley, A. (2013). Audism: A theory and practice of audiocentric privilege. *Humanity and Society, 37*(2), 101–130.

Eckhardt, E., Goldstein, M., Creamer, P., & Berry, R. (2013). *A culturally and linguistically specific deaf depression screener: Results of prototype development.* Paper presented at the 141st American Public Health Association Annual Meeting, Boston, MA.

Ehrlichmann, M. (2013, March 4). *I Don't Know.* Retrieved from https://deafinprison.wordpress.com/2013/03/04/the-theft-of-dignity-by-pastor-mark-ehrlichmann/

Eldredge, N. (2010). Culturally responsive psychotherapy with Deaf American Indians. In I. W. Leigh (Ed.), *Psychotherapy with Deaf clients from diverse groups* (pp. 183–209). Washington, DC: Gallaudet University Press.

Emery, S., Middleton, A., & Turner, G. (2010). Whose deaf genes are they anyway? The Deaf community's challenge to legislation on embryo selection. *Sign Language Studies, 10*(2), 155–169.

Emmorey, K. (2002). *Language, cognition and the brain: Insights from sign language research.* Mahwah, NJ: Lawrence Erlbaum.

Emmorey, K. (2015). *The neural underpinnings of reading skill in profoundly deaf adults*. Keynote presented at the 22nd International Congress on the Education of the Deaf, Athens, Greece.

Emmorey, K., & McCullough, S. (2009). The bimodal bilingual brain: Effects of sign language experience. *Brain and Language, 109*(2), 124–132.

Emmorey, K., & Petrich, J. A. (2012). Processing orthographic structure: Associations between print and fingerspelling. *Journal of Deaf Studies and Deaf Education, 17*(2), 194–204.

Enns, E., Boudreault, P., & Palmer, C. (2010). Examining the relationship between genetic counselors' attitudes toward Deaf people and the genetic counseling session. *Journal of Genetic Counseling, 19*(2), 161–173.

Enns, C. J., Zimmer, K., Boudreault, P., Rabu, S., & Broszeit, C. (2013). *American sign language: Receptive skills test*. Winnipeg, MB: Northern Signs Research.

Erikson, E. (1980). *Identity and the life cycle*. New York, NY: W. W. Norton.

Erting, C., Prezioso, C., & Hynes, M. (1990). The interactional context of deaf mother-infant communication. In V. Volterra & C. Erting (Eds.), *From gesture to language in hearing and deaf children*. Washington, DC: Gallaudet University Press.

Ertner, D., & Iyer, S. N. (2010). Prelinguistic vocalizations in infants and toddlers with hearing loss: Identifying and stimulating auditory-guided speech development. In M. Marschark & P. Spencer (Eds.), *The Oxford handbook of Deaf studies, language, and education* (Vol. 2, pp. 360–375). New York, NY: Oxford.

Ervin, S. (2015). *Assessment tools: Introduction to the anatomy and physiology of the auditory system*. Retrieved from www.workplaceintegra.com/hearing-articles/Ear-anatomy.html

Esmail, J. (2013). *Reading Victorian deafness*. Athens, OH: University of Ohio Press.

Estrada, A. B. (2015). Mental health services in Mexico: Challenges and proposals. In A. B. Estrada & I. Sleeboom-Van Raaij (Eds.), *Mental health services for deaf people* (pp. 41–47). Washington, DC: Gallaudet University Press.

Estrada, A. B., & Sleeboom-Van Raaij, I. (Eds.). (2015). *Mental health services for deaf people*. Washington, DC: Gallaudet University Press.

Evans, C., & Seifert, K. (2000). Fostering the development of ESL/ASL bililnguals. *TESL Canada Journal, 18*(1), 1–16.

Every Student Succeeds Act (ESSA). (2015). Pub.L. 114-95 (http://legislink.org/us/pl-114–95).

Farley, L. (2008). The Adam Walsh Act: The scarlet letter of the twenty-first century. *Washburn Law Review, 47*(2), 471–503.

Feldman, D. (2010). Psychotherapy and Deaf elderly clients. In I. W. Leigh (Ed.), *Psychotherapy with Deaf clients from diverse groups* (pp. 281–299). Washington, DC: Gallaudet University Press.

Feldman, D., & Kearns, W. (2007). Mental health needs and perspectives of culturally deaf older adults living in two counties in Florida. *JADARA, 40*(2), 5–18.

Fellinger, J. (2015). Public health of deaf people. In A. B. Estrada & I. Sleeboom-Van Raaij (Eds.), *Mental health services for deaf people* (pp. 111–130). Washington, DC: Gallaudet University Press.

Fellinger, J., Holzinger, D., Dobner, U., Gerich, J., Lehner, R., Lenz, G., & Goldberg, D. (2005). Mental distress and quality of life in a deaf population. *Social Psychiatry and Psychiatric Epidemiology, 40*(9), 737–742.

Fellinger, J., Holzinger, D., & Pollard, R. (2012). Mental health of deaf people. *The Lancet, 379*(9820), 1037–1044.

Feuerstein, R. (1980). *Instrumental enrichment*. Baltimore, MD: University Park Press.

Fischer, L. (2000). *Cultural identity development and self-concept of adults who are deaf: A comparative analysis* (Doctoral dissertation, Arizona State University, Tempe). Retrieved from Dissertation Abstracts International (61-10B, 5609).

Fischer, L., & McWhirter, J. (2001). The Deaf Identity Development Scale: A revision and validation. *Journal of Counseling Psychology, 48*, 355–358.

Fish, S. & Morford, J. (2012, June). Visual Language and Visual Learning Science of Learning Center. *The Benefits of Bilingualism* (Research Brief No. 7). Washington, D.C.

Framingham, J. (2013). What is psychological assessment? *Psych Central*. Retrieved from http://psychcentral.com/lib/what-is-psychological-assessment/

Frank, S. M. (2015). Deafness is having a cultural moment. So why are deaf roles still handed to hearing actors? *The Washington Post*. Retrieved from www.washingtonpost.com/posteverything/wp/2015/12/08/deafness-is-having-a-cultural-moment-so-why-are-deaf-roles-still-handed-to-hearing-actors/

Freel, B. L., Clark, M. D., Anderson, M. L., Gilbert, G., Musyoka, M. M., & Hauser, P. C. (2011). Deaf individuals' bilingual abilities: American Sign Language proficiency, reading skills, and family characteristics. *Psychology*, 2(1), 18–23.

Friedlander, H. (2002). Holocaust studies and the deaf community, In D. Ryan & J. Schuchman (Eds.), *Deaf people in Hitler's Europe* (pp. 15–31). Washington, DC: Gallaudet University Press.

Friedner, M., & Kusters, A. (Eds.). (2015). *It's a small world: International Deaf spaces and encounters.* Washington, DC: Gallaudet University Press.

Fromkin, V., Krashen, S., Curtiss, S., Rigler, D., & Rigler, M. (1974). The development of language in Genie: a case of language acquisition beyond the "critical period." *Brain and Language*, 1(1), 81–107.

Fuller, S. (1889). *An illustrated primer.* Boston, MA: D.C. Heath & Co.

Furth, H. (1964). Research with deaf persons: Implications for language and cognition. *Psychological Bulletin*, 63(3), 145–164.

Furth, Hans. (1966). *Thinking without language: Psychological implications of deafness.* New York, NY: The Free Press.

Gable, S., & Haidt, J. (2005). What (and why) is positive psychology? *Review of General Psychology*, 9(2), 103–110.

Gallaudet Research Institute. (2013). *Regional and national summary report of data from the 2011–12 annual survey of deaf and hard of hearing children and youth.* Washington, DC: GRI, Gallaudet University.

Gárate, M. (2011). Educating children with cochlear implants in an ASL/English bilingual classroom. In R. Paludneviciene & I. W. Leigh (Eds.), *Cochlear implants: Evolving perspectives* (pp. 206–228). Washington, DC: Gallaudet University Press.

Garate, M. (2012, June). *ASL/English Bilingual Education* (Research Brief No. 8). Washington, D.C. Visual Language and Visual Learning Science of Learning Center. Available at http://vl2.gallaudet.edu/files/3813/9216/6289/research-brief-8-asl-english-bilingual-education.pdf

Gárate, M., & Lenihan, S. (2016). Collaboration for communication, language, and cognitive development. In M. Sass-Lehrer (Ed.), *Deaf and hard-of-hearing infants, toddlers, and their families: Interdisciplinary perspectives* (pp. 233–273). New York, NY: Oxford.

Garberoglio, C., Cawthon, S., & Bond, M. (2014). Assessing English literacy as a predictor of postschool outcomes in the lives of deaf individuals. *Journal of Deaf Studies and Deaf Education*, 19(1), 50–67.

García, A.M.G., & Bravo, J. M. (2015). Mental health care for deaf people: An approach based on human rights. In A. B. Estrada & I. Sleeboom-Van Raaij (Eds.), *Mental health services for deaf people* (pp. 3–14). Washington, DC: Gallaudet University Press.

García, G. E., Pearson, P. D., & Jimenez, R. T. (1994). *The at-risk situation: A synthesis of the reading literature (Special Report).* Urbana-Champaign: University of Illinois. Center for the Study of Reading.

García, O., & Baker, C. (Eds.). (2007). *Bilingual education: An introductory reader.* Clevedon, UK: Multilingual Matters Limited.

García, O., & Kleifgen, J. A. (2010). *Educating emergent bilinguals: Policies, programs, and practices for English language learners.* New York, NY: Teachers College Press.

Geers, A. E. (2003). Predictors of reading skill development in children with early cochlear implantation. *Ear and Hearing*, 24(1), 59S–68S.

Geers, A. E., Brenner, C., & Tobey, E. A. (2011). Article 1: Long-term outcomes of cochlear implantation in early childhood: Sample characteristics and data collection methods. *Ear and Hearing*, 32(1), 2–12.

Geers, A. E., & Hayes, H. (2011). Reading, writing, and phonological processing skills of adolescents with 10 or more years of cochlear implant experience. *Ear and Hearing*, 32(1), 49S–59S.

Geers, A. E., & Sedey, A. L. (2011). Language and verbal reasoning skills in adolescents with 10 or more years of cochlear implant experience. *Ear and Hearing*, 32(1 Suppl), 39S–48S.

Geers, A., Tobey, E., Moog, J., & Brenner, C. (2008). Long-term outcomes of cochlear implantation in the preschool years: From elementary grades to high school. *International Journal of Audiology*, 47(Sup 2), S21–S30.

Genetics Home Reference. (2016). *What is gene therapy?* Retrieved from http://ghr.nlm.nih.gov/handbook/therapy/genetherapy

Gentry, M. A., Andrews, J., & DeLana, M. (2007). The efficacy of ASL/English bilingual education: Considering public schools. *American Annals of the Deaf*, 152(1), 73–87.

Gertz, G. (2008). Dysconscious audism: A theoretical proposition. In H-D. Bauman (Ed.), *Open your eyes: Deaf studies talking* (pp. 219–234). Minneapolis, MN: University of Minneapolis Press.

Geslin, J. (2007). *Deaf bilingual education: A comparison of the academic achievement of deaf children of deaf parents and deaf children of hearing parents* (Doctoral dissertation). Indiana University, Bloomington, IN.

Gilman, R., Easterbrooks, S., & Frey, M. (2004). A preliminary study of multidimensional life satisfaction among Deaf/Hard-of-Hearing youth across environmental settings. *Social Indicators Research, 66*, 143–164.

Gleason, M. (2014). A different way of life. *The Endeavor, Fall 2014*, 37–38.

Glickman, N. (1996). The development of culturally deaf identities. In N. Glickman & M. Harvey (Eds.), *Culturally affirmative psychotherapy with Deaf persons* (pp. 115–153). Mahwah, NJ: Erlbaum.

Glickman, N. (2009). *Cognitive-behavioral therapy for Deaf and hearing persons with language and learning challenges*. New York, NY: Routledge.

Glickman, N. (Ed.). (2013a). *Deaf mental health care*. New York, NY: Routledge.

Glickman, N. (2013b). Lessons learned from 23 years of a Deaf psychiatric inpatient unit. In N. Glickman (Ed.), *Deaf mental health care* (pp. 37–68). New York, NY: Routledge.

Glickman, N., & Heines, W. (2013). Creating Deaf residential treatment programs. In N. Glickman (Ed.), *Deaf mental health care* (pp. 181–233). New York, NY: Routledge.

Glickman, N. S., Lemere, S., & Smith, C. M. (2013). Engaging deaf persons with language and learning challenges and sexual offending behaviors in sex offender-oriented mental health treatment. *JADARA, 47*(2), 168–203.

Glickman, N., & Pollard, R. (2013). Deaf mental health research. In N. Glickman (Ed.), *Deaf mental health care* (pp. 358–387). New York, NY: Routledge.

Goldberg, D., & Flexer, C. (1993). Outcome survey of auditory-verbal graduates: Study of clinical efficacy. *Journal of the American Academy of Audiology, 4*, 189–200.

Goldin-Meadow, S. (2003). *The resilience of language: What gesture creation in deaf children can tell us about how all children learn language*. New York, NY: Psychology Press.

Goldring, R., Gray, L., & Bitterman, A. (2013). Characteristics of Public and Private Elementary and Secondary School Teachers in the United States: Results from the 2011–12 Schools and Staffing Survey. First Look. NCES 2013-314. *National Center for Education Statistics*.

Gonsoulin, T. (2001). Cochlear implant/Deaf world dispute: Different bottom elephants. *Otolaryngology-Head and Neck Surgery, 125*, 552–556.

Goodstein, H. (2006). *The Deaf way II reader*. Washington, DC: Gallaudet University Press.

Gournaris, M. J. (2009). Preparation for the delivery of telemental health services with individuals who are deaf. *JADARA, 43*(1), 34–51.

Gournaris, M. J. (2016). Certified peer support specialists: Advancing peer support services in deaf mental health care. *JADARA, 50*(1). Retrieved from http://repository.wcsu.edu/jadara/vol50/iss1/1

Gournaris, M. J., & Aubrecht, A. (2013). Deaf-hearing cross-cultural conflicts. In N. Glickman (Ed.), *Deaf mental health care* (pp. 69–106). New York, NY: Routledge.

Gournaris, M. J., Hamerdinger, S., & Williams, R. (2013). Creating a culturally affirmative continuum of mental health services. In N. Glickman (Ed.), *Deaf mental health care* (pp. 138–180). New York, NY: Routledge.

Grantham v. Moffett, 101 F.3d 698 (5th Cir. 1998).

Greenberg, M. & Kusche, M. (1998). Preventive intervention for school-age deaf children: The PATHS curriculum. *Journal of Deaf Studies and Deaf Education, 3*(1), 49–63.

Greenwald, B. (2014). Introduction. *Sign Language Studies, 15*(1), 5–9.

Griest, S. E., Folmer, R. L., & Martin, W. H. (2007). Effectiveness of "Dangerous Decibels,": A school-based hearing loss prevention program. *American Journal of Audiology, 16*(2), S165–S181.

Grosjean, F. (1998). Living with two languages and two cultures. In I. Parasnis (Ed.), *Cultural and language diversity and the deaf experience* (pp. 20–37). New York, NY: Cambridge University Press.

Grosjean, F. (2010). *Bilingual: Life and reality*. Cambridge, MA: Harvard University Press.

Groth-Marnat, G. (2009). *Handbook of psychological assessment*. New York, NY: Wiley.

Grushkin, D. (2003). A dual identity for hard of hearing students: Good for the world, good for the community, critical for students. *Odyssey, 4*(2), 30–35.

Guardino, C., & Cannon, J. (2015). Theory, research, and practice for students who are deaf and hard of hearing with disabilities: Addressing the challenges from birth to secondary school. *American Annals of the Deaf, 160*(4), 347–355.

Gustason, G., Pfetzing, D., & Zawolkow, E. (1978). *Signing exact English.* Silver Spring, MD: Modern Signs Press.

Guthman, D., Sandberg, K., & Dickinson, J. (2010). Chemical dependency: An application of a treatment model for deaf people. In I. W. Leigh (Ed.), *Psychotherapy with deaf clients from diverse groups* (pp. 341–371). Washington, DC: Gallaudet University Press.

Guthman, D., & Sternfeld, C. (2013). Substance abuse treatment and recovery. In N. Glickman (Ed.), *Deaf mental health care* (pp. 234–267). New York, NY: Routledge.

Gutman, V., & Zangas, T. (2010). Therapy issues with lesbians, gay men, bisexuals, and transgender individuals who are deaf. In I. W. Leigh (Ed.), *Psychotherapy with deaf clients from diverse groups* (2nd ed., pp. 85–108). Washington, DC: Gallaudet University Press.

Hadadian, A. (1995). Attitudes toward deafness and security of attachment relationships among young deaf children and their parents. *Early Education and Development, 6*(2), 181–191.

Hadjikakou, K., & Papas, P. (2012). Bullying and cyberbullying and deaf and hard of hearing children: A review of the literature. *International Journal on Mental Health and Deafness, 2,* 18–32.

Hakuta, K., Bialystok, E., & Wiley, E. (2003). Critical evidence: A test of the critical-period hypothesis for second language acquisition. *Psychological Science, 14*(1), 31–38.

Hall, M. L., & Bavelier, D. (2010). Working memory, deafness, and sign language. In M. Marschark & P. Spencer (Eds.), *The Oxford handbook of Deaf studies, language, and education* (Vol. 2, pp. 458–472). New York, NY: Oxford University.

Hamdan, N., McKnight, P., McKnight, K., & Arfstrom, K. M. (2013). A review of flipped learning. *Flipped Learning Network.* Retrieved from www.flippedlearning.org/review

Hamilton, H. (2011). Memory skills of deaf learners: Implications and applications. *American Annals of the Deaf, 156*(4), 402–423.

Hansen, V. J. (1929). *Beretning om sindslidelse blaudt Danmarks d ovstumme.* Copenhagen, Denmark: Johansens Bogtrykkej.

Haptonstall-Nykaza, T. S., & Schick, B. (2007). The transition from fingerspelling to English print: Facilitating English decoding. *Journal of Deaf Studies and Deaf Education, 12*(2), 172–183.

Hardonk, S., Daniels, S., Desnerck, G., Loots, G., Van Hove, G, Van Kerschaver, E., . . ., Louckx, F. (2011). Deaf parents and pediatric cochlear implantation: An exploration of the decision-making process. *American Annals of the Deaf, 156*(3), 290–304.

Harmon, K., & Nelson, J. (2012). *Deaf American prose.* Washington, DC: Gallaudet University Press.

Harris, M. (2010). Early communication in sign and speech. In M. Marschark & P. Spencer (Eds.), *The Oxford handbook of Deaf studies, language, and education* (Vol. 2, pp. 316–330). New York, NY: Oxford.

Harris, M. (2016). The impact of cochlear implants on deaf children's literacy. In M. Marschark & P. Spencer (Eds.), *Oxford handbook of Deaf studies in language* [Kindle version]. New York: Oxford.

Harris, M., & Terlektsi, E. (2010). Reading and spelling abilities of deaf adolescents with cochlear implants and hearing aids. *Journal of Deaf Studies and Deaf Education, 16*(1), 24–34.

Harris, R. L. (2011). *A case study of extended discourse in an ASL/English bilingual preschool classroom* (Unpublished doctoral dissertation), Gallaudet University, Washington, DC.

Harris, R. L. (2013, March 22). Fingerspelling strategies. *National American Sign Language and English Bilingual Early Childhood Education Summit,* Austin, TX.

Harter, S. (1997). The personal self in social context. In R. D. Ashmore & L. Jussim (Eds.), *Self and identity* (pp. 81–105). New York, NY: Oxford.

Harvey, M. (2003). *Psychotherapy with deaf and hard of hearing persons: A systematic model* (2nd ed.). Mahwah, NJ: Erlbaum.

Hassanzadeh, S. (2012). Outcomes of cochlear implantation in deaf children of deaf parents: comparative study. *Journal of Laryngology and Otology, 126*(10), 989.

Haualand, H. (2008). Sound and belonging: What is a community? In H-D. Bauman (Ed.), *Open your eyes: Deaf studies talking* (pp. 111–123). Minneapolis, MN: University of Minnesota Press.

Hauser, P., Finch, K., & Hauser, A. (Eds.). (2008). *Deaf professionals and designated interpreters.* Washington, DC: Gallaudet University Press.

Hauser, P., Lukomski, J., & Hillman, T. (2008). Development of deaf and hard of hearing students' executive function. In M. Marschark & P. Hauser (Eds.), *Deaf cognition: Foundations and outcomes* (pp. 286–308). New York, NY: Oxford.

Hauser, P., Paludneviciene, R., Riddle, W., Kurz, K., Emmorey, K., & Contreras, J. (2016). American Sign Language comprehension test: A tool for sign language researchers. *Journal of Deaf Studies and Deaf Education, 21*(1), 64–69.

Hauser, P.C., O'Hearn, A., McKee, M., & Thew, D. (2010). Deaf epistemology: Deafhood and deafness. *American Annals of the Deaf,* 154(5), 486–496.

Hayes, H., Geers, A. E., Treiman, R., & Moog, J. S. (2009): Receptive vocabulary development in deaf children with cochlear implants: Achievement in an intensive auditory-oral setting. *Ear & Hearing,* 30(1), 128–135.

Hearing Loss Association of America. (2007). *Policy statement: Cochlear implants.* Retrieved from www.hearingloss.org/sites/default/files/docs/HLAA_POLICYSTATEMENT_Cochlear_Implants.pdf

Helping Educate to Advance the Rights of the Deaf (HEARD). (2016). Retrieved from www.beheard.org

Herbold, J. (2008). *Emergent literacy development: Case studies of four deaf ASL-English bilinguals* (Unpublished doctoral dissertation). University of Arizona, Tucson, AZ.

Hermans, D., Knoors, H., Ormel, E., & Verhoeven, L. (2008). The relationship between the reading and signing skills of deaf children in bilingual education programs. *Journal of Deaf Studies and Deaf Education,13*(4), 518–530. DOI:10.1093/deafed/enn009

Herzig, M., & Malzkuhn, M. (2015). Bilingual storybook apps: An interactive reading experience for children. *Odyssey: New Directions in Deaf Education, 16,* 40–44.

Hidalgo, L., & Williams, S. (2010). Counseling issues for Latino Deaf individuals and their families. In I. W. Leigh (Ed.), *Psychotherapy with Deaf clients from diverse groups* (2nd ed., pp. 237–257). Washington, DC: Gallaudet University Press.

Hidden curriculum. (2014, August 26). In S. Abbott (Ed.), *The glossary of education reform.* Retrieved from http://edglossary.org/hidden-curriculum

Hille, E., van Straaten, H., & Verkerk, P. (2007). Prevalence and independent risk factors for hearing loss in NICU infants, *Acta Pædiatrica,* 96, 1155–1158.

Hintermair, M. (2008). Self-esteem and satisfaction with life of deaf and hard-of-hearing people: A resource-oriented approach to identity work. *Journal of Deaf Studies and Deaf Education, 13*(2), 278–300.

Hintermair, M. (2011). Health-related quality of life and classroom participation of deaf and hard-of-hearing students in general schools. *Journal of Deaf Studies and Deaf Education, 16*(2), 254–271. DOI: 10.1093/deafed/enq045

Hintermair, M. (2013). Executive functioning and behavioral problems in deaf and hard of hearing students at general and special schools. *Journal of Deaf Studies and Deaf Education, 18*(3), 344–359.

Hintermair, M. (2014). Psychosocial development in deaf and hard-of-hearing children in the twenty-first century. In M. Marschark, G. Tang, & H. Knoors (Eds.), *Bilingualism and bilingual deaf education* (pp. 152–186). New York, NY: Oxford.

Hirshorn, E. (2011). *Visual selective attention and deafness.* NSF Science of Learning Center on Visual Language and Visual Learning, Research Brief No. 3. Retrieved from http://vl2.gallaudet.edu/files/4613/9216/6284/research-brief-3-visual-attention-and-deafness.pdf

HM Inspectorate of Prisons. (2009). *Disabled prisoners: A short thematic review on the care and support of prisoners with a disability,* London, UK: HM Inspectorate of Prisons.

Hoffman, M., Quittner, A., & Cejas, I. (2014). Comparisons of social competence in young children with and without hearing loss: A dynamic systems framework. *Journal of Deaf Studies and Deaf Education,* 20(2), 115–124.

Hoffmeister, R. (2008). Border crossings by hearing children of deaf parents: The lost history of Codas. In H-D. Bauman (Ed.), *Open your eyes: Deaf studies talking* (pp. 189–215). Minneapolis, MN: University of Minnesota Press.

Hoffmeister, R. J., & Caldwell-Harris, C. L. (2014). Acquiring English as a second language via print: The task for deaf children. *Cognition, 132*(2), 229–242.

Hoffmeister, R. J., & Harvey, M. (1996). Is there a psychology of the hearing? In N. Glickman & M. Harvey (Eds.), *Culturally affirmative psychotherapy with deaf persons* (pp. 73–97. Mahwah, NJ: Erlbaum.

Holcomb, T. K. (1997). Development of deaf bicultural identity. *American Annals of the Deaf, 142*(2), 89–93.

Holcomb, T. K. (2012). Paving the way for reform in deaf education. In P. Paul & D. Moores (Eds.), *Deaf epistemologies: Multiple perspectives on the acquisition of knowledge* (pp. 125–145). Washington, DC: Gallaudet University Press.

Holcomb, T. K. (2013). *Introduction to American Deaf culture.* New York, NY: Oxford University Press.

Horejes, T. (2012). *Social constructions of deafness: Examining deaf languacultures in education.* Washington, D.C.: Gallaudet University Press.

Hoskins, B., Cramer, C., Silvius, D., Zou, D., Raymond, R., Orten, D., . . ., Friedhelm, H. (2007). Transcription factor *SIX5* is mutated in patients with Branchio-Oto-Renal syndrome. *American Journal of Human Genetics, 80*(4), 800–804.

Hrastinski, I., & Wilbur, R. (2016). Academic achievement of deaf and hard of hearing students in an ASL/English bilingual program. *Journal of Deaf Studies and Deaf Education.* DOI: 10.1093/deafed/env072

Hsu, A. S., Chater, N., & Vitányi, P. M. (2011). The probabilistic analysis of language acquisition: Theoretical, computational, and experimental analysis. *Cognition, 120*(3), 380–390.

Hu, M. (2015). *The study of deaf people since Braden (1994).* Retrieved from http://humanvarieties. org/2014/09/21/the-study-of-deaf-people-since-braden-1994/

Humphries, T. (2008). Scientific explanation and other performance acts in the reorganization of DEAF. In K. Lindgren, D. DeLuca, & D. J. Napoli (Eds.), *Signs and voices: Deaf culture, identity, language, and arts* (pp. 3–20). Washington, DC: Gallaudet University Press.

Humphries, T. (2014). Our time: The legacy of the twentieth century. *Sign Language Studies, 15*(1), 57–73.

Humphries, T. (2016, February 13). *Beyond bilingual education: Transformational deaf education.* Presentation at the 42nd Annual ACE-DHH Conference, New York City, New York.

Humphries, T., & Allen, B. M. (2008). Reorganizing teacher preparation in deaf education. *Sign Language Studies, 8*(2), 160–180.

Humphries, T., Kushalnagar, P., Mathur, G., Napoli, D. J., Padden, C., Pollard, R., . . ., Smith, S. (2014b). What medical education can do to ensure robust language development in deaf children. *Medical Science Educator, 24*(4), 409–419.

Humphries, T., Kushalnagar, P., Mathur, G., Napoli, D. J., Padden, C., & Rathmann, C. (2014a). Ensuring language acquisition for deaf children: What linguists can do. *Language, 90*(2), e31–e52.

Humphries, T., Kushalnagar, P., Mathur, G., Napoli, D. J., Padden, C., Rathman, C., & Smith, S. (2014c). Bilingualism: A pearl to overcome certain perils of cochlear implants. *Journal of Medical Speech-Language Pathology, 21*(2), 107–125.

Humphries, T., & MacDougall, F. (1999). "Chaining" and other links: Making connections between American Sign Language and English in Two Types of School Settings. *Visual Anthropology Review, 15*(2), 84–94.

Hyde, M., Punch, R., & Komesaroff, L. (2010). Coming to a decision about cochlear implantation: Parents making choices for their deaf children. *Journal of Deaf Studies and Deaf Education, 15*(2), 162–178.

Individuals with Disabilities Education Act of 1990 (IDEA), Pub. L. 101-476, U.S.C.20 §§ 1400–1485.

Ingraham, C. (2015). *An exploration of how persons with visual and auditory loss use adaptive and assistive technology for daily living and aging in place* (Unpublished doctoral dissertation). Lamar University, Beaumont, TX.

Interpreting in Health Care Settings. (2015). *Challenges and issues in medical interpreting.* Retrieved from http://healthcareinterpreting.org/faqs/lit-challenges-and-issues-in-medical-interpreting/

Invisible Disabilities Association. (2011). *People with disabilities are the largest minority group in the U.S.* Retrieved from http://invisibledisabilities.org/coping-with-invisible-disabilities/disability-benefits/disabilities-largest-minority-group-us/

Israelite, N., Ower, J., & Goldstein, G. (2002). Hard-of-hearing adolescents and identity construction: Influence of school experiences, peers, and teachers. *Journal of Deaf Studies and Deaf Education, 7*(2), 134–148.

Jackson, C. (2011). Family supports and resources for parents of children who are deaf or hard of hearing. *American Annals of the Deaf, 156*(4), 343–362.

Jacobson, R. (1995). Allocating two languages as a key feature of a bilingual methodology. *Policy and Practice in Bilingual Education: A Reader Extending the Foundations, 2,* 166.

James, W. (1893). Thought before language: A deaf mute's recollections. *American Annals of the Deaf, 38*(3), 135–145.

Jankowski, K. (1997). *Deaf empowerment.* Washington, DC: Gallaudet University Press.

Jensema, C. (1990). Hearing loss in a jail population. *JADARA, 24*(2), 49–58.

Jernigan, J. (2010). *Risk factors of deaf males at the Alabama School for the Deaf* (Unpublished doctoral dissertation). Lamar University, Beaumont, TX.

Jiménez, R. T., García, G. E., & Pearson, P. D. (1996). The reading strategies of bilingual Latina/o students who are successful English readers: Opportunities and obstacles. *Reading Research Quarterly, 31*(1), 90–112.

Johnson, C., & Goswami, U. (2010). Phonological awareness, vocabulary, and reading in deaf children with cochlear implants. *Journal of Speech, Language, and Hearing Research, 53*(2), 237–261.

Johnson, H. A. (2013). Initial and ongoing teacher preparation and support: Current problems and possible solutions. *American Annals of the Deaf, 157*(5), 439–449.

Johnson, R. E. (1994). Sign language and the concept of deafness in a traditional Yucatec Mayan village. In C. Erting, R. C. Johnson, D. Smith, & B. Snider (Eds.), *The Deaf way* (pp. 102–109). Washington, DC: Gallaudet University Press.

Johnston, T. (2006). W(h)ither the Deaf community? Population, genetics, and the future of Australian Sign Language. *Sign Language Studies, 6*(2), 137–173.

Joint Committee on Infant Hearing. (2013). Supplement to the JCIH 2007 position statement: Principles and guidelines for early intervention after confirmation that a child is deaf or hard of hearing. *Pediatrics, 131*(4), 1324–1349.

Jones, S., & McEwen, M. (2000). A conceptual model of multiple dimensions of identity. *Journal of College Student Development, 41*(4), 405–414.

Jones Thomas, A., & Schwarzbaum, S. (2006). *Culture & identity*. Thousand Oaks, CA: Sage.

Kagan, J. (1998). Is there a self in infancy? In M. Ferrari & R. Sternberg (Eds.), *Self-awareness: Its nature and development* (pp. 137–147). New York, NY: Guilford.

Kam, C.-M., Greenberg, M., & Kusche, C. (2004). *Journal of Emotional and Behavioral Disorders, 12*(2), 66–78.

Katz, D., Vernon, M., Penn, A., & Gillece, J. (1992). The consent decree: A means of obtaining mental health services for people who are deaf. *Journal of the American Deafness and Rehabilitation Association, 26*(2), 22–28.

Katz, J. (2009). Clinical audiology. In J. Katz, L. Medwetsky, R. Burkard, & L. Hood (Eds.), *Handbook of clinical audiology* (6th ed., pp. 3–6). Philadelphia, PA: Wolters Kluwer/Lippincott Williams & Wilkins.

Kelly, R. R., Quagliata, A. B., DeMartino, R., & Perotti, V. (2016). 21st Century deaf workers: Going beyond just employed to career growth and entrepreneurship In M. Marschark, V. Lampropoulou, & E. Skordilis (Eds.), *Diversity in deaf education*. New York, NY: Oxford University Press.

Kemmery, M., & Compton, M. (2014). Are you deaf or hard of hearing? Which do you go by: Perceptions of identity in families of students with hearing loss. *The Volta Review, 114*(2), 157–192.

Khairi, M., Rafidah, K., Affizal, A., Normastura, A., Suzana, M., & Normani, Z. (2011). Anxiety of the mothers with referred baby during universal newborn hearing screening. *International Journal of Pediatric Otorhinolaryngology, 75*(4), 513–517.

Kilpatrick, B. (2007). *The history of the formation of deaf children's theater in the United States* (Unpublished doctoral dissertation). Lamar University, Beaumont, TX.

Kisch, S. (2004). Negotiating (genetic) deafness in a Bedouin community. In J. V. Van Cleve (Ed.), *Genetics, disability, and deafness* (pp. 148–173). Washington, DC: Gallaudet University Press.

Klima, E. S., & Bellugi, U. (1979). *The signs of language*. Cambridge, MA: Harvard University Press.

Knight, T. (2013). *Social identity in hearing youth who have deaf parents: A qualitative study* (Unpublished doctoral dissertation). Lamar University, Beaumont, TX.

Knoors, H., & Marschark, M. (2012). Language planning for the 21st century: Revisiting bilingual language policy for deaf children. *Deaf Studies and Deaf Education, 17*(3), 291–305. DOI: 10.1093/deafed/ens018

Knoors, H., & Marschark, M. (2015). *Educating deaf learners: Creating a global evidence base*. New York, NY: Oxford.

Knoors, H., Tang, G., & Marschark, M. (2014). Bilingualism and bilingual deaf education: Time to take stock. In M. Marschark, G. Tang, & H. Knoors (Eds.), *Bilingualism and bilingual deaf education* (pp. 1–20). New York, NY: Oxford.

Koester, L., & McCray, N. (2011). Deaf parents as sources of positive development and resilience for deaf infants. In D. Zand & K. Pierce (Eds.), *Resilience in deaf children* (pp. 65–86). New York, NY: Springer.

Koester, L., Papousek, H., & Smith-Gray, S. (2000). Intuitive parenting, communication, and interaction with deaf infants. In P. Spencer, C. Erting, & M. Marschark (Eds.), *The deaf child in the family and at school* (pp. 55–71). Mahwah, NJ: Erlbaum.

Koester, L., Traci, M., Brooks, L., Karkowski, A., & Smith-Gray, S. (2004). Mother-infant behaviors at 6 and 9 months: A microanalytic view. In K. Meadow-Orlans, P. Spencer, & L. Koester (Eds.), *The world of deaf infants: A longitudinal study* (pp. 40–56). New York, NY: Oxford.

Krents, E., & Atkins, D. (1985). No-go-tell! A child protection curriculum for very young disabled children. New York, NY: Lexington Center.

Krentz, C. (2014). The hearing line: How literature gains from deaf people. In H-D. Bauman & J. Murray (Eds.), *Deaf gain* (pp. 421–435). Minneapolis, MN: University of Minnesota Press.

Kröner, S., Plass, J., & Leutner, D. (2005). Intelligence assessment with computer simulations. *Intelligence, 33*(4), 347–368.

Krywko, K. (2015). Reaching out. *Volta Voices, 22*(2), 11–15.

Kübler-Ross, E. (1969). *On death and dying*. New York, NY: Macmillan.

Kübler-Ross, E. (2000). *Life lessons*. New York, NY: Scribner.

Kuenburg, A., Fellinger, P., & Fellinger, J. (2016). Health care access among deaf people. *Journal of Deaf Studies and Deaf Education, 21*(1), 1–10.

Kuhl, P. (2007). Is speech learning 'gated' by the social brain? *Developmental Science, 10*(1), 110–120.

Kuhl, P. (2010). Brain mechanisms in early language acquisition. *Neuron, 67*(5), 713–727.

Kuhl, P. (2015). Baby talk. *Scientific American, 313*(5), 64–69.

Kuhl, P., & Rivera-Gaxiola, M. (2008). Neural substrates of language acquisition. *Annual Review of Neuroscience, 31*, 511–534.

Kuntze, M. (2000). *Literacy acquisition and deaf children: A study of the interaction between ASL and written English* (Unpublished doctoral dissertation). Stanford University, Stanford, CA.

Kuntze, M., Golos, D., & Enns, C. (2014). Rethinking literacy: Broadening opportunities for visual learners. *Sign Language Studies, 14*(2), 203–224.

Kurz, C., & Cuculick, J. (2015). International Deaf space in social media: The Deaf experience in the United States. In M. Friedner & A. Kusters (Eds.), *It's a small world: International Deaf spaces and encounters* (pp. 225–235). Washington, DC: Gallaudet University Press.

Kusche, C., & Greenberg, M. (1993). *The PATHS curriculum*. Seattle, WA: Developmental Research and Programs.

Kushalnagar, P., Draganac-Hawk, M., & Patrick, D. (2015). Quality of life of Latino deaf and hard of hearing individuals in the United States. In A. B. Estrada & I. Sleeboom-Van Raaij (Eds.), *Mental health services for Deaf people* (pp. 131–139). Washington, DC: Gallaudet University Press.

Kushalnagar, P., McKee, M., Smith, S., Hopper, M., Kavin, D., & Atcherson, S. (2014). Conceptual model for quality of life among adults with congenital or early deafness. *Disability and Health Journal, 7*(3), 350–355. DOI: 10.1016/j.dhjo.2014.04.001

Kushalnagar, P., & Rashid, K. (2008). Attitudes and behaviors of deaf professionals and interpreters. In P. Hauser, K. Finch, & A. Hauser (Eds.), *Deaf professionals and designated interpreters* (pp. 43–57). Washington, DC: Gallaudet University Press.

Kushalnagar, P., Topolski, T., Schick, B., Edwards, T., Skalicky, A., & Patrick, D. (2011). Mode of communication, perceived level of understanding, and perceived quality of life in youth who are deaf or hard of hearing. *Journal of Deaf Studies and Deaf Education, 16*(4), 512–523.

Kusters, A. (2015). *Deaf space in Adamorobe*. Washington, DC: Gallaudet University Press.

Kusters, A., & De Meulder, M. (2013). Understanding Deafhood: In search of its meanings. *American Annals of the Deaf, 158*(5), 428–438.

Kvam, M. (2004). Sexual abuse of deaf children: A retrospective analysis of abuse among deaf adults in Norway. *Child Abuse and Neglect, 28*(3), 241–251.

Kvam, M., Loeb, M., & Tambs, K. (2007). Mental health in adults: Symptoms of anxiety and depression among hearing and deaf individuals. *Journal of Deaf Studies and Deaf Education, 12*(1), 1–7.

Ladd, P. (2003). *Understanding Deaf culture: In search of Deafhood*. Clevedon, UK: Multilingual Matters.

Ladd, P. (2015). Global Deafhood: Exploring myths and realities. In M. Friedner & A. Kusters (Eds.), *It's a small world: International Deaf spaces and encounters* (pp. 274–285). Washington, DC: Gallaudet University Press.

LaFromboise, T., Coleman, H, & Gerton, J. (1993). Psychological impact of biculturalism: Evidence and theory. *Psychological Bulletin, 114*, 395–412.

Laird, G. (2015). *First in history: The first DeafBlind VRS calls were made with CAAGVRS*. Retrieved from http://deafnetwork.com/wordpress/blog/2015/01/19/first-in-history-the-first-deafblind-vrs-calls-were-made-with-caagvrs/no

Lake, N. (2002, January 21). Language wars. *Harvard Magazine*. Retrieved from http://harvardmagazine.com/2002/03/language-wars.html

Landsberger, S., & Diaz, D. (2010). Inpatient psychiatric treatment of Deaf adults: Demographic and diagnostic comparisons with hearing inpatients. *Psychiatric Services, 61*(2), 196–199.

Lane, H. (1976). *The wild boy of Aveyron.* Cambridge, MA: Harvard University Press.

Lane, H. (1992). *The mask of benevolence.* New York, NY: Alfred A. Knopf.

Lane, H. (1999). *The mask of benevolence: Disabling the Deaf community.* San Diego, CA: DawnSign Press.

Lane, H., Hoffmeister, R., & Bahan, B. (1996). *A journey into the Deaf-world.* San Diego, CA: DawnSign Press.

Lane, H., Pillard, R., & French, H. (2000). Origins of the American deaf-world: Assimilating and differentiating societies and their relation to genetic patterning. *Sign Language Studies, 1,* 17–44.

Lane, H., Pillard, R., & Hedberg, U. (2011). *The people of the eye.* New York, NY: Oxford University Press.

Lang, H., Cohen, O., & Fischgrund, J. (2008). *Moment of truth.* Rochester, NY: RIT Press.

Lang, H., & Meath-Lang, B. (1995). *Deaf persons in the arts and sciences.* Washington, DC: Gallaudet University Press.

Lange, C., Lane-Outlaw, S., Lange, W., & Sherwood, D. (2013). American sign language/English bilingual model: A longitudinal study of academic growth. *Journal of Deaf Studies and Deaf Education, 18,* 532–544.

LaSasso, C., & Crain, K. (2015). Reading for deaf and hearing readers: Qualitatively and/or qualitatively similar or different? A nature versus nurture issue. *American Annals of the deaf, 159*(5), 447–467.

LaSasso, C. J, Crain, K. L., & Leybaert, J. (2010). *Cued speech and cued language for deaf and hard of hearing children.* San Diego, CA: Plural Publishing.

LaVigne, M., and Van Rybroek, G. (2013, August 22). "He got in my face so i shot him": How defendants' language impairments impair attorney-client relationships. *CUNY Law Review* 69. Univ. of Wisconsin Legal Studies Research Paper No. 1228. Available at SSRN: http://ssrn.com/abstract=2314546

LaVigne, M., & Vernon, M. (2003). Interpreter isn't enough: Deafness, language, and due process. *Wisconsin Law Review,* 843–936.

Leigh, I. W. (1999). Inclusive education and personal development. *Journal of Deaf Studies and Deaf Education, 4,* 236–245

Leigh, I. W. (2009). *A lens on deaf identities.* New York, NY: Oxford.

Leigh, I. W. (Ed.). (2010). *Psychotherapy with deaf clients from diverse groups* (2nd ed.). Washington, DC: Gallaudet University Press.

Leigh, I. W. (2012). Not just deaf: Multiple intersections. In R. Nettles & R. Balter (Eds.), *Multiple minority identities* (pp. 59–80). New York, NY: Springer.

Leigh, I. W., & Anthony-Tolbert, S. (2001). Reliability of the BDI-II with deaf persons. *Rehabilitation Psychology, 46,* 195–202.

Leigh, I. W., Corbett, C., Gutman, V., & Morere, D. (1996). Providing psychological services to deaf individuals: A response to new perceptions of diversity. *Professional Psychology: Research and Practice, 27,* 364–371.

Leigh, I. W., & Gutman, V. (2010). Psychotherapy with deaf people: The ethical dimension. In I. W. Leigh (Ed.), *Psychotherapy with deaf clients from diverse groups* (2nd ed., pp. 3–17). Washington, DC: Gallaudet University Press.

Leigh, I. W., & Lewis, J. (2010). Deaf therapists and the deaf community. In I. W. Leigh (Ed.), *Psychotherapy with deaf clients from diverse groups* (2nd ed., pp. 39–61). Washington, DC: Gallaudet University Press.

Leigh, I. W., Marcus, A., Dobosh, P., & Allen, T. (1998). Deaf/hearing identity paradigms: Modification of the Deaf Identity Development Scale. *Journal of Deaf Studies and Deaf Education, 3,* 329–338.

Leigh, I. W., Maxwell-McCaw, D., Bat-Chava, Y., & Christiansen, J. B. (2009). Correlates of psychosocial adjustment in deaf adolescents with and without cochlear implants: A preliminary investigation. *Journal of Deaf Studies and Deaf Education, 14*(2), 244–259.

Leigh, I. W., Morere, D., & Kobek Pezzarossi, C. (2014). Deaf gain: Beyond Deaf culture. In H-D. Bauman & J. Murray (Eds.), *Deaf gain: Raising the stakes for human diversity* (pp. 356–371). Minneapolis, MN: University of Minnesota Press.

Leigh, G., Newall, J., & Newall, A. (2010). Newborn screening and earlier intervention with deaf children: Issues for the developing world. In M. Marschark & P. Spencer (Eds.), *Oxford handbook of Deaf studies, language, and education* (Vol. 2, pp. 345–359). New York, NY: Oxford.

Leigh, I. W., & Pollard, R. (2011). Mental health and deaf adults. In M. Marschark & P. Spencer (Eds.), *The Oxford handbook of Deaf studies, language, and education* (2nd ed., Vol. 1, pp. 214–226). New York, NY: Oxford.

Levine, E. S. (1974). *Lisa and her soundless world*. New York, NY: Human Sciences Press.

Levine, E. S. (1977). *The preparation of psychological service providers to the deaf*. A report of the Spartanburg Conference on the Functions, Competencies and Training of Psychological Service Providers to the Deaf. Monograph No. 4.

Levine, E. S. (1981). *The ecology of early deafness: Guides to fashioning environments and psychological assessments*. New York, NY: Columbia University Press.

Lewis-Fernández, R., Raggio, G., Magdaliz, G., Duan, N., Marcus, S, Cabassa, L., . . . Hinton, D. (2013). A checklist to assess comprehensive reporting of race, ethnicity, and culture in psychiatric publications. *Journal of Nervous and Mental Disorders, 201*(10), 860–871.

Lieberman, A. M., Hatrak, M., & Mayberry, R. I. (2011). The development of eye gaze control for linguistic input in deaf children. In *Proceedings of the 35th Boston University Conference on Language Development* (pp. 391–403). Boston, MA.

Lieberman, A.M., Hatrak, M. & Mayberry, R.I. (2014). Learning to look for language: Development of joint attention in young deaf children. *Language Learning and Development, 10*(1), 19–35.

Lin, F., Niparko, J., & Ferrucci, L. (2011, November 20). Hearing loss prevalence in the United States. *Archives of Internal Medicine, 171*(20), 1851–1852. DOI:10.1001/archinternmed.2011.506

Litchenstein, E. (1988). The relationships between reading processes and English skills of deaf college students. *Journal of Deaf Studies and Deaf Education, 3*(2), 80–134.

Lomas, G., & Johnson, H. (2012). Overlooked and unheard: Abuse of children who are deaf or hard of hearing and their experiences with CPS and foster care. *The Family Journal, 20*(4), 376–383.

Lopez, I., Ishiyama, A., & Ishiyama, G. (2012). Sudden sensorineural hearing loss due to drug abuse. *Seminars in Hearing, 33*(3), 251–260.

Lucas, B. (2012). *The Deaf and Hard of Hearing Consumers Advocacy Network*. Retrieved from www.nbda.org/blog/the-deaf-hard-of-hearing-consumers-advocacy-network-by-brian-k.-lucas

Lucas, C., & Valli, C. (1992). *Language contact in the American deaf community*. Washington, DC: Gallaudet University Press.

Lucker, J. L. (2002/2005). Cochlear implants: A technological overview. In J. B. Christiansen & I. W. Leigh (Eds.), *Cochlear implants in children: Ethics and choices* (pp 45–64). Washington, DC: Gallaudet University Press.

Luckner, J. L., & Ayantoye, C. (2013). Itinerant teachers of students who are deaf or hard of hearing: Practices and preparation. *Journal of Deaf Studies and Deaf Education, 18*(3), 409–423.

Luckner, J. L., & McNeill, J. H. (1994). Performance of a group of deaf and hard-of-hearing students and a comparison group of hearing students on a series of problem-solving tasks. *American Annals of the Deaf, 139*(3), 371–377.

Luckner, J., Sebald, A., Cooney, Young, J., & Muir, S. (2006). An examination of the evidence-based literacy research in deaf education. *American Annals of the Deaf, 150*(5), 443–456.

Luczak, R. (Ed.). (2007). *Eyes of desire 2: A deaf GLBT reader*. Minneapolis, MN: Handtype Press.

Luft, P. (2014). A national survey of transition services for deaf and hard of hearing students. *Career Development and Transition for Exceptional Individuals, 37*(3), 177–192.

McAdams, D. (2006). The redemptive self: Generativity and the stories Americans live by. *Research in Human Development, 3*(2&3), 81–100.

McCaskill, C., Lucas, C., Bailey, R., & Hill, J. (2011). *The hidden treasure of Black ASL*. Washington, DC: Gallaudet University Press.

Macaulay, C. E., & Ford, R. M. (2006). Language and theory-of-mind development in prelingually deafened children with cochlear implants: A preliminary investigation. *Cochlear Implants International, 7*(1), 1–14.

McCreery, R. (2014). Promoting connectivity for children with hearing loss. *The Hearing Journal, 67*(11), 40, 42.

McCulloch, D. (2011). *Not hearing us: An exploration of the experience of deaf prisoners in English and Welsh prisons*. London, UK: Howard League for Penal Reform.

McDonald, D. (2014). *The art of being deaf*. Washington, DC: Gallaudet University Press.

McIlroy, G., & Storbeck, C. (2011). Development of deaf identity: An ethnographic study. *Journal of Deaf Studies and Deaf Education, 16*(4), 494–511.

McIntosh, A. (2006). *Marital satisfaction and conflict styles in deaf-hearing couples*. Paper presented at the 5th Annual Hawaii International Conference on Social Sciences, Honolulu, HI.

McKay, S., Gravel, J., & Tharpe, A. (2008). Amplification considerations for children with minimal or mild bilateral hearing loss and unilateral hearing loss. *Trends in Amplification, 12*(1), 43–54.

McKee, M., Paasche-Orlow, M., Winters, P., Fiscella, K., Zazove, P., Sen, A., & Pearson, T. (2015). Assessing health literacy in Deaf American sign language users. *Journal of Health Communication: International Perspectives, 20*(Supplement 2), 92–100.

McQuarrie, L., & Parrila, R. (2014). Literacy and linguistic development in bilingual deaf children: Implications of the "and" for phonological processing. *American Annals of the Deaf, 159*(4), 372–384.

McQuiller Williams, L., & Porter, J. (2010, February). *An examination of the incidence of sexual, physical, and psychological abuse and sexual harassment on a college campus among underrepresented populations*. Paper presented at the Western Society of Criminology Conference, Honolulu, HI.

MacSwan, J. (2000). The threshold hypothesis, semilingualism, and other contributions to a deficit view of linguistic minorities. *Hispanic Journal of Behavioral Sciences, 22*, 3–45.

MacSweeney, M., Capek, C., Campbell, R., & Woll, B. (2008). The signing brain: The neurobiology of sign language. *Trends in Cognitive Sciences, 12*(11), 432–440.

Maher, J. (1996). *Seeing language in sign: the work of William C. Stokoe*. Washington, DC: Gallaudet University Press.

Mahshie, S. N. (1995). *Educating deaf children bilingually: With insights and applications from Sweden and Denmark*. Washington, DC: Pre-College Programs, Gallaudet University.

Maller, S., & Braden, J. (2011). Intellectual assessment of deaf people: A critical review of core concepts and issues. In M. Marschark & P. Spencer (Eds.), *The Oxford handbook of Deaf studies, language, and education* (pp. 473–485). New York, NY: Oxford.

Maller, S., & Immekus, J. (2005). The psychometric properties of intelligence tests when used with deaf and hard of hearing individuals: Practices and recommendations. In J. Mounty & D. Martin (Eds.), *Assessing deaf adults* (pp. 75–89). Washington, DC: Gallaudet University Press.

Mance, J., & Edwards, L. (2012). Deafness-related self-perceptions and psychological well-being in deaf adolescents with cochlear implants. *Cochlear Implants International, 13*(2), 93–104.

Marazita, M., Ploughman, I., Rawlings, B., Remington, E., Arnos, K., & Nance, W. (1993). Genetic epidemiological studies of early-onset deafness in the U.S. school-age population. *American Journal of Medical Genetics, 46*, 486–491.

Marsaja, I. G. (2008). *Desa Kolok: A deaf village and its sign language in Bali, Indonesia*. Nijmegen, Netherlands: Ishara Press.

Marschark, M. (1993). *Psychological development of deaf children*. New York, NY: Oxford.

Marschark, M. (2007). *Raising and educating a deaf child* (2nd ed.). New York, NY: Oxford.

Marschark, M., & Clark, M. D. (1987). Linguistic and nonlinguistic creativity of deaf child. *Developmental Review, 7*(1), 22–38.

Marschark, M., & Everhart, V. S. (1999). Problem-solving by deaf and hearing students: Twenty questions. *Deafness and Education International, 1*(2), 65–82.

Marschark, M., & Harris, M. (1996). Success and failure in learning to read: The special case (?) of deaf children. In C. Cornoldi & J. Oakhill (Eds.), *Reading comprehension difficulties: Processes and intervention* (pp. 279–300). Mahwah, NJ: Erlbaum.

Marschark, M., & Hauser, P. (2008). *Deaf cognition: Foundations and outcomes*. New York, NY: Oxford.

Marschark, M., & Hauser, P. (2012). *How deaf children learn: What parents and teachers need to know*. New York, NY: Oxford University Press.

Marschark, M., Knoors, H., & Tang, G. (2014). Perspectives on bilingualism and bilingual education for deaf learners In M. Marschark, G. Tang, & H. Knoors (Eds.), *Bilingualism and bilingual deaf education* (pp. 445–476). New York, NY: Oxford.

Marschark, M., Lang, H. G., & Albertini, J. A. (2002). *Educating deaf students: From research to practice*. New York, NY: Oxford.

Marschark, M., Morrison, C., Lukomski, J., Borgna, G., & Convertino, C. (2013). Are deaf students visual learners?. *Learning and Individual Differences, 25*, 156–162.

Marschark, M., Rhoten, C., & Fabich, M. (2007). Effects of cochlear implants on children's reading and academic achievement. *Journal of Deaf Studies and Deaf Education, 12*(3), 269–282.

Marschark, M., Sapere, P., Convertino, C., & Seewagen, R. (2005). Access to postsecondary education through sign language interpreting. *Journal of Deaf Studies and Deaf Education, 10*(1), 38–50.

Marschark, M., Sarchet, T., Rhoten, C., & Zupan, M. (2010). Will cochlear implants close the reading achievement gap for deaf students? In M. Marschark & P Spencer (Eds.), *The Oxford handbook of Deaf studies, language, and education* (Vol. 2, pp. 127–143). New York, NY: Oxford.

Marschark, M., Shaver, D. M., Nagle, K. M., & Newman, L. A. (2015). Predicting the academic achievement of deaf and hard-of-hearing students from individual, household, communication, and educational factors. *Exceptional Children, 81*(3), 350–369.

Marschark, M., Spencer, L. J., Durkin, A., Borgna, G., Convertino, C., Machmer, E., . . ., Trani, A. (2015). Understanding language, hearing status, and visual-spatial skills. *Journal of Deaf Studies and Deaf Education, 20*(4), 310–330.

Marschark, M., Tang, G., & Knoors, H. (Eds.). (2014). *Bilingualism and bilingual deaf education*. New York, NY: Oxford.

Marschark, M., & Wauters, L. (2008). Language comprehension and learning by deaf students. In M. Marschark & P. Hauser (Eds.), *Deaf cognition: Foundations and outcomes* (pp. 309–350). New York, NY: Oxford.

Marschark, M., & West, S. A. (1985). Creative language abilities of deaf children. *Journal of Speech, Language, and Hearing Research, 28*(1), 73–78.

Martin, D. S. (2014). Instrumental enrichment: Impacts upon learners who are deaf. *Transylvanian Journal of Psychology, XVI*, 177–194.

Martin, D., Bat-Chava, Y., Lalwani, A., & Waltzman, S. (2011). Peer relationships of deaf children with cochlear implants: Predictors of peer entry and peer interaction success. *Journal of Deaf Studies and Deaf Education, 16*(1), 108–120.

Martin, M. P., Balanzategui, M. V., & Morgan, G. (2014). Sign bilingual and co-enrollment education for children with cochlear implants in Madrid, Spain. In M. Marschark, G. Tang, & H. Knoors (Eds.), *Bilingualism and bilingual deaf education* (pp. 368–395). New York, NY: Oxford.

Mason, T., & Mounty, J. (2005). Maximizing access to licensure for deaf and hard of hearing social workers. In J. Mounty & D. Martin (Eds.), *Assessing deaf adults* (pp. 149–155). Washington, DC: Gallaudet University Press.

Mather, C. (2007). *Sign language interpreters in court: Understanding best practices*. Bloomington, IN: AuthorHouse.

Mather, M. (2009). Children in immigrant families charter new path. *Population Reference Bureau*. Retrieved from www.prb.org/pdf09/immigrantchildren.pdf

Mather, S., & Andrews, J. (2008). Eyes over ears: The development of visual strategies by hearing children of deaf parents. In M. Bishop & S. Hicks (Eds.), *Hearing, mother father deaf* (pp. 132–161). Washington, DC: Gallaudet University Press.

Mather, S., Rodriguez-Fraticelli, Y., Andrews, J. F., & Rodriguez, J. (2006). Establishing and maintaining sight triangles: Conversations between deaf parents and hearing toddlers in Puerto Rico. In C. Lucas (Ed.), *Multilingualism and sign languages: From the Great Plains to Australia* (pp. 159–187). Washington, DC: Gallaudet University Press.

Mauk, G., & Mauk, P. (1992). Somewhere, out there: Preschool children with hearing impairment and learning disabilities. *Topics in Early Childhood Special Education: Hearing Impaired Preschoolers, 12*, 174–195.

Maxwell-McCaw, D. (2001). *Acculturation and psychological well-being in deaf and hard-of-hearing people* (Doctoral dissertation, The George Washington University, Washington, DC). Retrieved from Dissertation Abstracts International (61(11-B), 6141).

Maxwell-McCaw, D., & Zea, M. C. (2011). The Deaf Acculturation Scale (DAS): Development and validation of a 58-item measure. *Journal of Deaf Studies and Deaf Education, 16*, 325–342.

Mayberry v. VonValtier, 843 F. Supp. 1160 (E. D. Mich. 1994).

Mayberry, R. I. (2002). Cognitive development of deaf children: The interface of language and perception in neuropsychology. In S. J. Segaolwitz & I. Rapin (Eds.), *Handbook of Neuropsychology*, (2nd ed., Vol. 8, Part II, 71–107). Amsterdam, NL: Elsevier.

Mayberry, R. I., del Giudice, A. A., & Lieberman, A. M. (2011). Reading achievement in relation to phonological coding and awareness in deaf readers: A meta-analysis. *Journal of Deaf Studies and Deaf Education*, 16(2), 164–188.

Mayer, C. (2010). The demands of writing and the deaf writer. In M. Marschark & P. Spencer (Eds.) *Oxford handbook of Deaf studies, language, and education* (Vol. 2, pp. 144–155). New York, NY: Oxford.

Mayer, C., & Leigh, G. (2010). The changing context for sign bilingual education programs: Issues in language and the development of literacy. *International Journal of Bilingual Education and Bilingualism*, 13(2), 175–186.

Mayer, C., & Trezek, B. J. (2015). *Early literacy development in deaf children*. New York, NY: Oxford University Press.

Mayer, C., & Wells, G. (1996). Can the linguistic interdependence theory support a bilingual-bicultural model of literacy education for deaf students?. *Journal of Deaf Studies and Deaf Education*, 1(2), 93–107.

Meadow, K. (1980). *Deafness and child development*. Berkeley, CA: University of California Press.

Meadow-Orlans, K. (1985). Social and psychological effects of hearing loss in adulthood: A literature review. In H. Orlans (Ed.), *Adjustment to adult hearing loss* (pp. 35–57). San Diego, CA: College-Hill Press.

Meadow-Orlans, K., Mertens, D., & Sass-Lehrer, M. (2003). *Parents and their deaf children: The early years*. Washington, DC: Gallaudet University Press.

Meadow-Orlans, K., Spencer, P., & Koester, L. (2004). *The world of deaf infants: A longitudinal study*. New York, NY: Oxford.

Mejstadt, L., Heiling, K., & Swedin, C. (2008/2009). Mental health and self-image among deaf and hard of hearing children. *American Annals of the Deaf*, 153(5), 504–515.

Mertens, D. M. (2014). *Research and evaluation in education and psychology: Integrating diversity with quantitative, qualitative, and mixed methods* (4th ed.). Thousand Oaks, CA: Sage.

Micro Power & Light. (1995). *Readability calculations* [Computer program]. Dallas, TX: Micro Power & Light, Co.

Middleton, A. (2004). Deaf and hearing adults' attitudes toward genetic testing for deafness. In J. Van Cleve (Ed.), *Genetics, disability, and deafness* (pp. 127–147). Washington, DC: Gallaudet University Press.

Middleton, A., Emery, S., & Turner, G. (2010). Views, knowledge, and beliefs about genetics and genetic counseling among deaf people. *Sign Language Studies*, 10(2), 170–196.

Miles, B. (2008). *Overview on deaf-blindness*. Retrieved from https://nationaldb.org/library/page/1934

Miller, E. M., Lederberg, A. R., & Easterbrooks, S. R. (2013). Phonological awareness: Explicit instruction for young deaf and hard-of-hearing children. *Journal of Deaf Studies and Deaf Education*, 18(2), 206–227.

Miller, K. R. (2001). *Forensic issues of deaf offenders* (Unpublished doctoral dissertation). Lamar University, Beaumont, TX.

Miller, K. R. (2004). Linguistic diversity in a deaf prison population: implications for due process. *Journal of Deaf Studies and Deaf Education*, 9(1), 112–119.

Miller, K. R., & Vernon, M. (2001). Linguistic diversity in deaf defendants and due process rights. *Journal of Deaf Studies and Deaf Education*, 6(3), 226–234.

Miller, K. R., & Vernon, M. (2002). Accessibility of interpreting services for deaf prison inmates at arrest and in court: A matter of basic constitutional rights. *JADARA*, 36(1), 1–11.

Miller, K., & Vernon, M. (2003). Deaf sex offenders in a prison population. *Journal of Deaf Studies and Deaf Education*, 8(3), 357–362.

Miller, K. R., Vernon, M., & Capella, M. E. (2005). Violent offenders in a deaf prison population. *Journal of Deaf Studies and Deaf Education*, 10(4), 417–425.

Mindel, E., & Vernon, M. (1971). *They grow in silence: The deaf child and his family*. Silver Spring, MD: National Association of the Deaf.

Miranda v. Arizona, 384 U.S. 436 (1966).

Mitchell, R. (2005). How many deaf people are there in the United States? Estimates from the survey of income and program participation. *Journal of Deaf Studies and Deaf Education*, 11(1), 112–119.

Mitchell, R., & Karchmer, M. (2004). Chasing the mythical ten percent: Parental hearing status of deaf and hard of hearing students. *Sign Language Studies*, 5, 83–96.

Mitchell, R., Young, T., Bachleda, B., & Karchmer, M. (2006). How many people use ASL in the United States? Why estimates need updating. *Sign Language Studies*, 6(3), 306–335.

Mitchiner, J. (2015). Deaf parents of cochlear-implanted children: Beliefs on bimodal bilingualism. *Journal of Deaf Studies and Deaf Education*, 20(1), 51–66.

Mitchiner, J., Nussbaum, D. B., & Scott, S. (2012, June). The implications of bimodal bilingual approaches for children with cochlear implants (Research Brief No. 6). Washington, DC: Visual Language and Visual Learning Science of Learning Center. Available at: http://vl2.gallaudet.edu/research/research-briefs/english/children-cochlear-implants/

Mitchiner, J., & Sass-Lehrer, M. (2011). My child can have more choices: Reflections of deaf mothers on cochlear implants for their children. In R. Paludneviciene & I. W. Leigh (Eds.), *Cochlear implants: Evolving perspectives* (pp. 71–94). Washington, DC: Gallaudet University Press.

Moeller, M. P., & Schick, B. (2006). Relations between maternal input and theory of mind understanding in deaf children. *Child Development*, 77(3), 751–766.

Monaghan, L. (2008). HIV/AIDS in the United States deaf community. In D. DeLuca, I. W. Leigh, K. Lindgren, & D. J. Napoli (Eds.), *Access: Multiple avenues for deaf people* (pp. 168–192. Washington, DC: Gallaudet University Press.

Monaghan, L., Schmaling, C., Nakamura, K., & Turner, G. (Eds.). (2003). *Many ways to be Deaf*. Washington, DC: Gallaudet University Press.

Montag, J. L., AuBuchon, A. M., Pisoni, D. B., & Kronenberger, W. G. (2014). Speech intelligibility in deaf children after long-term cochlear implant use. *Journal of Speech, Language & Hearing Research*, 57(6), 2332–2343.

Montanini Manfredi, M. (1993). The emotional development of deaf children. In M. Marschark & M. D. Clark (Eds.), *Psychological perspectives on deafness* (pp. 49–63). Hillsdale, NJ: Erlbaum.

Moog, J., Geers, A., Gustus, C., & Brenner, C. (2011). Psychosocial adjustment in adolescents who have used cochlear implants since preschool. *Ear and Hearing*, 32(1 Suppl), 75S.

Moores, D. F. (1993). Book reviews: The mask of benevolence: Disabling the deaf community. *American Annals of the Deaf*, 138(1), 4–9.

Moores, D. F. (2010). The history of language and communication issues in deaf education. In M. Marschark & P Spencer (Eds.), *Oxford handbook of Deaf studies, Language, and education* (pp. 17–30). New York, NY: Oxford.

Moores, D. F., & Miller, M. (2009). *Deaf people around the world*. Washington, DC: Gallaudet University Press.

Morere, D. (2011). Bimodal processing of language for cochlear implant users. In R. Paludneviciene & I. W. Leigh (Eds.), *Cochlear implants: Evolving perspectives* (pp. 113–141). Washington, DC: Gallaudet University Press.

Morere, D., & Allen, T. (Eds.). (2012). *Assessing literacy in deaf individuals: Neurocognitive measurement and predictors*. New York: Springer.

Morrison, H., Sherman, L., Legg, J., Banine, F. Isacke, C., Haipek, C., . . ., Herrlich, P. (2001). The NF2 tumor suppressor gene product, merlin, mediates contact inhibition of growth through interactions with CD44. *Genes and Development*, 15, 968–980.

Morton, C., & Nance, W. (2006). Newborn hearing screening: A silent revolution. *New England Journal of Medicine*, 354, 2151–2164.

Mounty, J. L., Pucci, C. T., & Harmon, K. C. (2014). How deaf American Sign Language/English bilingual children become proficient readers: An emic perspective. *Journal of Deaf Studies and Deaf Education*, 19(3), 333–346.

Mundy, L. (2002, March 31). A world of their own. *The Washington Post Magazine*, 22–29, 38, 40, 42–43.

Munro, L., Knox, M., & Lowe, R. (2008). Exploring the potential of constructionist therapy: Deaf clients, hearing therapists and a reflecting team. *Journal of Deaf Studies and Deaf Education*, 13(3), 307–323.

Munro, L., & Rodwell, J. (2009). Validation of an Australian sign language instrument of outcome measurement for adults in mental health settings. *Australian and New Zealand Journal of Psychiatry*, 43(4), 332–339.

Murphy, K. (2013, June 5). American Sign Language more popular at colleges. *Chicago Tribune*. Retrieved from http://articles.chicagotribune.com/2013–06–05/health/sc-health-0605-asl-20130605_1_american-sign-language-asl-rosemary-feal

Murray, J. (2008). Coequality and transnational studies. In H-D. Bauman (Ed.), *Open your eyes: Deaf Studies talking* (pp. 100–110). Minneapolis, MN: University of Minnesota Press.

Muse, C., Harrison, J., Yoshinaga-Itano, C., Grimes, A., Brookhouser, P. E., Epstein, S., . . ., Martin, P. (2013). Supplement to the JCIH 2007 position statement: Principles and guidelines for early intervention after confirmation that a child is deaf or hard of hearing. *Pediatrics, 131*(4), e1324–e1349.

Musyoka, M. (2015). Understanding indoor play in deaf children: An analysis of play behaviors. *Psychology,* 6(1), 10–19.

Myers, M. (2011). The relationship between English reading comprehension scores and years enrolled at a residential school for the deaf. Unpublished doctoral dissertation, Lamar University, Beaumont, Texas.

Myklebust, H. R. (1964). *The psychology of deafness.* New York, NY: Grune & Stratton.

Nance, W. (2004). *A high rate of marriage among deaf individuals can explain the increased frequency of connexin deafness in the United States.* Retrieved from www.news-medical.net/news/2004/04/27/911.aspx

Nance, W., Liu, X., & Pandya, A. (2000). Relation between choice of partner and high frequency of connexin-26 deafness. *Lancet, 356,* 500–501.

National Association of School Psychologists. (2012). *Position statement: Serving students who are deaf or hard of hearing.* Retrieved from www.nasponline.org/about_nasp/positionpapers/ServingStudents WhoAreDeaf.pdf

National Association of the Deaf. (2000). *NAD position statement on cochlear implants.* Retrieved from http://nad.org/issues/technology/assistive-listening/cochlear-implants.

National Association of the Deaf. (2003). *NAD position statement on mental health services.* Retrieved from http://nad.org/issues/health-care/mental-health-services/position-statement

National Association of the Deaf. (2008a). *Position statement on mental health for deaf children.* Retrieved from http://nad.org/issues/health-care/mental-health-services/for-deaf-children.

National Association of the Deaf. (2008b). *Position statement: VRI services in hospitals.* Retrieved from https://nad.org/issues/technology/vri/position-statement-hospitals

National Association of the Deaf. (2014a). *Highlights of NAD law and advocacy center in court.* Retrieved from http://nad.org/issues/about-law-and-advocacy-center/highlights

National Association of the Deaf. (2014b). *The battle for accessible housing.* Retrieved from https://nad.org/news/2014/1/battle-accessible-housing

National Association of the Deaf. (2015). *Legal rights: The guide for deaf and hard of hearing people* (6th ed.). Washington, DC: Gallaudet University Press.

National Association of the Deaf. (n.d.). *NAD position statement on health care access for deaf patients.* Retrieved from https://nad.org/issues/health-care/position-statement-health-care-access-deaf-patients

National Association of the Deaf (n.d.). *NAD position statement on quality foster care services continuum for deaf children.* Retrieved from http://nad.org/issues/health-care/position-statement-quality-foster-care-services-continuum-deaf-children

National Association of the Deaf Mental Health Subcommittee of the Public Policy Committee. (2008). *Position statement supplement: Culturally affirmative and linguistically accessible mental health services.* Retrieved from https://nad.org/issues/health-care/mental-health-services/position-statement-supplement

National Council on Disability. (2012). *Rocking the cradle: Ensuring the rights of parents with disabilities and their children.* Washington, DC: U.S. Government Printing Office.

National Deaf Children's Society. (1999). *PATHS: the way towards personal and social empowerment for deaf children: A report on the NDCS deaf children in mind project-personal and social initiative.* London, UK: National Deaf Children's Society.

National Early Literacy Panel. (2008). *Developing early literacy: Report of the national early literacy panel.* Washington, DC: National Institute for Literacy. Retrieved from www.nifl.gov/earlychildhood/NELP/NELReport.html.

National Institute on Deafness and Other Communication Disorders. (2014a). *Cochlear implants.* Retrieved from www.nidcd.nih.gov/health/hearing/pages/coch.aspx#e

National Institute on Deafness and Other Communication Disorders. (2014b). *Noise-induced hearing loss.* Retrieved from www.nidcd.nih.gov/health/hearing/pages/noise.aspx

National Reading Panel (NRP). (2000). *Report of the national reading panel: Teaching children to read. An evidence-based assessment of the scientific research literature on reading and its implications for reading instruction.* Jessup, MD: National Institute for Literacy at EDPubs.

National Research Council. (1929). *Research recommendations of the second conference on problems of the deaf and hard of hearing*. Series of the National Research Council (No. 88). Washington, DC: Reprint and Circular.

NCI. (2015). *National captioning institute: History of closed captioning*. Retrieved from www.ncicap.org/about-us/history-of-closed-captioning/

Neimeyer, R. A. (Ed.). (2001). *Meaning reconstruction and the experience of loss*. Washington, DC: American Psychological Association.

Nelson Schmitt, S. S., & Leigh, I.W (2015). Examining a sample of Black Deaf individuals on the Deaf Acculturation Scale. *Journal of Deaf Studies and Deaf Education, 20*(3), 283–295.

Newman, L., Wagner, M., Knokey, A.-M., Marder, C., Nagle, K., Shaver, D., . . ., Schwarting, M. (2011). *The post-high school outcomes of young adults with disabilities up to 8 years after high school. A report from the national longitudinal transition study-2 (NLTS2)*. (NCSER 2011–3005). Menlo Park, CA: SRI International

Newport, E., & Meier, R. (1985). The acquisition of American Sign Language. In D. Slobin (Ed.), *The crosslinguistic study of language acquisition* (pp. 881–938). Mahwah, NJ: Lawrence Erlbaum.

Nicholas, J. G., & Geers, A. E. (2007). Will they catch up? The role of age at cochlear implantation in the spoken language development of children with severe to profound hearing loss. *Journal of Speech, Language, and Hearing Research, 50*(4) 1048–1062.

Nikolopoulos, T. P., Dyar, D., Archbold, S., & O'Donoghue, G. M. (2004). Development of spoken language grammar following cochlear implantation in prelingually deaf children. *Archives of Otolaryngology–Head & Neck Surgery, 130*(5), 629–633.

Niparko, J. K., Tobey, E. A., Thal, D. J., Eisenberg, L. S., Wang, N. Y., Quittner, A. L., . . ., CDaCI Investigative Team. (2010). Spoken language development in children following cochlear implantation. *Jama, 303*(15), 1498–1506.

NL Association of the Deaf (n.d.). *What is the Deaf community?* Retrieved from www.nlad.org/what_is_the_deaf_com.html

No Child Left Behind Act of 2001, 20 U.S.C. 6301 *et seq.*

Noble, T. (2003). Embryos screened for deafness: A quiet first for Australia. *Sydney Morning Herald*. Retrieved from www.smh.com.au/articles/2003/07/10/1057783286800.html

Nordal, K. (2015, December). Embracing telepsychology. *Monitor on Psychology, 46*(11), 64.

Norman, N., & Jamieson, J. R. (2015). Social and emotional learning and the work of itinerant teachers of the deaf and hard of hearing. *American Annals of the Deaf, 160*(3), 273–288.

Northern, J., & Downs, M. (2014). *Hearing in children* (6th ed.). San Diego, CA: Plural Publishing.

Nover, S. (2000). *History of language planning in deaf education: The 19th century* (Unpublished doctoral dissertation). University of Arizona, Tucson, AZ.

Nover, S., & Andrews, J. (1998). *Critical pedagogy in deaf education: Bilingual methodology and staff development: Year 1 (1997–1998)*. Santa Fe, NM: Star School Project. New Mexico School for the Deaf.

Nover, S., Andrews, J., Baker, S., Everhart, V., & Bradford, M. (2002). *Staff development in ASL/English bilingual instruction for deaf students: Evaluation and impact study. Final Report 1997–2002*. Retrieved May 17, 2016, from www.gallaudet.edu/Documents/year5.pdf.

Nover, S., Christensen, K., & Cheng, L. (1998). Development of ASL and English competence for learners who are deaf. *Topics in Language Disorders, 18*(4), 61–72.

Nussbaum, D., & Scott, S. (2011). The Cochlear Implant Education Center. In R. Paludneviciene & I. W. Leigh (Eds.), *Cochlear implants: Evolving perspectives* (pp. 175–205). Washington, DC: Gallaudet University Press.

Nussbaum, D. B., Scott, S., & Simms, L. E. (2012). The "Why" and "How" of an ASL/English bimodal bilingual program. *Odyssey: New Directions in Deaf Education, 13*, 14–19.

Nwosu, C., Batalova, J., & Auclair, G. (2014). *Frequently requested statistics on immigrants and immigration in the United States. Migration information source*. Retrieved January 1, 2015 from www.migrationpolicy.org/article/frequently-requested-statistics-immigrants-and-immigration-united-states

Obinna, J., Krueger, S., Osterbaan, C., Sadusky, J., & DeVore, W. (2005). *Understanding the needs of the victims of sexual assault in the deaf community*. Retrieved June 10, 2015 from www.ncjrs.gov/pdffiles1/nij/grants/212867.pdf

O'Brien, C. (2011). *The influence of deaf culture in school culture and leadership: A case study of a school for the deaf* (Unpublished doctoral dissertation). University of Missouri, Columbia, MO.

O'Brien, C., Kuntze, M., & Appanah, T. (2015). Culturally relevant leadership: A deaf education cultural approach [Review of the book cultural proficiency: A manual for school leaders]. *American Annals of the Deaf, 159*(3), 296–301.

O'Brien, C., & Placier, P. (2015). Deaf culture and competing discourses in a residential school for the deaf: "Can do" versus "can't do." *Equity & Excellence in Education, 48*(2), 320–338.

O'Brien, L., Kenna, M., Neault, M., Clark, T., Kammerer, B., Johnston, J., . . ., Licameli, G. (2010). *International Journal of Pediatric Otorhinolaryngology, 74*(10), 1144–1148.

Oettingen, G. (2014). *Rethinking positive thinking: Inside the new science of motivation.* New York, NY: Penguin Group.

Ogunyipe, B. (n.d.). *Black Deaf culture through the lens of Black Deaf history.* Retrieved from www.dcmp.org/ai/366/

Oliva, G. (2004). *Alone in the mainstream.* Washington, DC: Gallaudet University Press.

Oliva, G., & Lytle, L. (2014). *Turning the tide: Making life better for deaf and hard of hearing schoolchildren.* Washington, DC: Gallaudet University Press.

Olkin, R. (1999). *What psychotherapists should know about disability.* New York, NY: Guilford

Olmstead, M., & Kuhlmeier, V. (2015). *Comparative cognition.* London, UK: Cambridge University Press.

Omalu, B., DeKosky, S., Minster, R., Kamboh, M., Hamilton, R., & Wecht, C. (2005). Chronic traumatic encephalopathy in a national league football player. *Congress of Neurological Surgeons, 57*(1), 128–134.

O'Rourke, S., Glickman, N., & Austen, S. (2013). Deaf people in the criminal justice system. In N. Glickman (Ed.), *Deaf mental health care* (pp. 323–357). New York, NY: Routledge.

Ostrove, J., & Oliva, G. (2010). Identifying allies: Explorations of deaf-hearing relationships. In S. Burch & A. Kaufer (Eds.), *Deaf and disability studies* (pp. 105–119). Washington, DC: Gallaudet University Press.

Ouellette, A. (2011). Hearing the deaf: Cochlear implants, the deaf community, and bioethical analysis. *Valparaiso University Law Review, 45*(3), 1247–1270.

Ouellette, S. (1988). The use of projective drawing techniques in the personality assessment of prelingually deafened young adults: A pilot study. *American Annals of the Deaf, 133,* 212–218.

Padden, C. (1980). The deaf community and the culture of deaf people. In C. Baker & R. Battison (Eds.), *Sign language and the deaf community* (pp. 89–102). Silver Spring, MD: National Association of the Deaf.

Padden, C. (2006). Learning to fingerspell twice: Young signing children's acquisition of fingerspelling. In B. Schick, M. Marschark & P. Spencer (Eds.), *Advances in the sign language development of deaf children* (pp. 189–201). New York, NY: Oxford Press.

Padden, C. (2008). The decline of Deaf clubs in the United States: A treatise on the problem of place. In H-D Bauman (Ed.), *Open your eyes: Deaf Studies talking* (pp. 169–176). Minneapolis, MN: University of Minnesota Press.

Padden, C., & Humphries, T. (1988). *Deaf in America: Voices from a culture.* Cambridge, MA: Harvard University Press.

Padden, C., & Humphries, T. (2005). *Inside Deaf culture.* Cambridge, MA: Harvard University Press.

Padden, C., & Ramsey, C. (2000). American Sign Language and reading ability in deaf children. *Language Acquisition by Eye, 1,* 65–89.

Paddock, C. (2014). Cochlear implants without external hardware: New chip looks promising. *Medical News Today.* Retrieved from www.medicalnewstoday.com/articles/272439.php

Pagliaro, C. (2015). Developing numeracy in DHH individuals. In H. Knoors & M. Marschark (Eds.), *Educating deaf learners: Creating a global evidence base* (pp. 173–195). New York, NY: Oxford.

Paijmans, R., Cromwell, J., & Austen, S. (2006). Do profoundly prelingually Deaf patients with psychosis really hear voices? *American Annals of the Deaf, 151*(1), 42–48.

Paludneviciene, R., & Leigh, I. W. (Eds.). (2010). *Cochlear implants: Evolving perspectives.* Washington, DC: Gallaudet University Press.

Parents and Families of Natural Communication, Inc. (1998). *We CAN hear and speak!* Washington, DC: Alexander Graham Bell Association for the Deaf.

Paris, D. (2012). *Factors that influence the leadership development of American Indian Deaf women* (Doctoral dissertation, Lamar University, Beaumont, TX). Retrieved from UMI (No. 3527616).

Parks, E. (2009). *Deaf and hard of hearing homeschoolers: Sociocultural motivation and approach* (Vol. 49). Work papers of the Summer Institute of Linguistics, University of North Dakota session. Retrieved from http://arts-sciences.und.edu/summer-institute-of-linguistics/work-papers/_files/docs/2009-parks.pdf

Parton, B. (2014). Facilitating exposure to sign languages of the world: The case for mobile assisted language learning. *The Journal of Information Technology Education: Innovations in Practice, 13*(1), 13–24. Retrieved from www.jite.org/documents/Vol13/JITEv13IIPp013–024Parton0396.pdf

Parton, B. (2015). Leveraging augmented reality apps to create enhanced learning environments for deaf students. *International Journal of Instructional Technology & Distance Learning, 12*(6), 21–28. Retrieved from www.itdl.org/Journal/Jun_15/Jun15.pdf

Paterson, M. M., & Cole, E. (2010). The university of Hartford and CREC Soundbridge: A new master's of education in aural habilitation and education of hearing impaired children. *The Volta Review, 110*(2), 279–291.

Paul, P. V., Wang, Y., Trezek, B. J., & Luckner, J. L. (2009). Phonology is necessary, but not sufficient: A rejoinder. *American Annals of the Deaf, 154*(4), 346–356.

Paul, P., Wang, Y., & Williams, C. (2013). *Deaf students and the qualitative similarity hypothesis: Understanding language and literacy.* Washington, DC: Gallaudet University Press.

Pediatrics Clerkship. (2013). TORCH infections. *The University of Chicago.* Retrieved from https://pedclerk.bsd.uchicago.edu/page/torch-infections

Peltz Strauss, K. (2006). *A new civil right.* Washington, DC: Gallaudet University Press.

People v. Lang, 76 Ill.2d 311, 327, 29 Ill. Dec. 87, 391 N.E.2d 350 (1979).

Pepnet 2. (n.d.) Common Core State Standards: Considerations for teachers of students who are deaf or hard of hearing (Research Brief). Retrieved from www.pepnet.org/research/researchbriefs

Percy-Smith, L., Cayé-Thomasen, P., Gugman, M., Jensen, J., & Thomsen, J. (2008). Self-esteem and social well-being of children with cochlear implant compared to normal-hearing children. *International Journal of Pediatric Otorhinolaryngology, 72,* 1113–1120.

Perfetti, C. A., & Sandak, R. (2000). Reading optimally builds on spoken language: Implications for deaf readers. *Journal of Deaf Studies and Deaf Education, 5*(1), 32–50.

Peters, C. (2000). *Deaf American literature: From carnival to cannon.* Washington, DC: Gallaudet University Press.

Peterson, N. R., Pisoni, D. B., & Miyamoto, R. T. (2010). Cochlear implants and spoken language processing abilities: Review and assessment of the literature. *Restorative Neurology and Neuroscience, 28*(2), 237–250.

Petitto, L. A. (2000). The acquisition of natural signed languages: Lessons in the nature of human language and its biological foundations. In C. Chamberlain, J. Morford, & R. Mayberry (Eds.), *Language acquisition by eye* (pp. 41–59). Manwah, NJ: Erlbaum.

Petitto, L. A. (2009). New discoveries from the bilingual brain and mind across the life span: Implications for education. *Mind, Brain, and Education, 3*(4), 185–197.

Petitto, L. A. (2012). Revolutions in the science of learning: A new view from a new center-visual language and visual learning. *Odyssey: New Directions in Deaf Education, 13,* 70–75.

Petitto, L. A., Berens, M. S., Kovelman, I., Dubins, M. H., Jasinska, K., & Shalinsky, M. (2012). The "Perceptual Wedge Hypothesis" as the basis for bilingual babies' phonetic processing advantage: New insights from fNIRS brain imaging. *Brain and Language, 121*(2), 130–143.

Petitto, L. A., & Dunbar, K. (2004). *Proceedings from the Conference on Building Usable Knowledge in Mind, Brain, & Education '04: New findings from educational neuroscience on bilingual brains, scientific brains, and the educated mind.* Cambridge, MA: Harvard Graduate School of Education.

Petitto, L. A., Holowka, S., Sergio, L. E., & Ostry, D. (2001). Language rhythms in baby hand movements. *Nature, 413*(6851), 35–36.

Petitto, L. A., & Marentette, P. F. (1991). Babbling in the manual mode: Evidence for the ontogeny of language. *Science, 251,* 1493–1496.

Piaget, J. (1929). *The child's conception of the world.* New York, NY: Harcourt, Brace.

Piaget, J. (1952). *The origins of intelligence in children.* New York, NY: International Universities Press.

Pick, L. (2013). Health care disparities in the deaf community. *Spotlight on Disability Newsletter.* Retrieved from www.apa.org/pi/disability/resources/publications/newsletter/2013/11/deaf-community.aspx

Pierce v. District of Columbia, No. 1:2013cv00134 — Document 90 (D.D.C. 2015).

Pinker, S. (1990). Language acquisition. In D. Osherson & H. Lasnik (Eds.), *An invitation to cognitive science* (1st ed., Vol 1: Language, pp. 135–182). Cambridge, MA: MIT Press.

Pintner, R., Elsenson, J., & Stanton, M. (1941). *The psychology of the physically handicapped.* New York, NY: F. S. Crofts.

Pintner, R., & Paterson, D. (1915). The Binet scale and the deaf child. *Journal of Educational Psychology, 6,* 201–210.

Pisoni, D. B., Conway, C. M., Kronenberger, W., Henning, S., & Anaya, E. (2010). Executive function, cognitive control, and sequence learning in deaf children with cochlear implants. In M. Marschark & P. Spencer (Eds.), *Oxford handbook of Deaf studies, language, and education* (Vol. 2, pp. 439–457). New York, NY: Oxford.

Pisoni, D., Conway, C., Kronenberger, W., Horn, D., Karpicke, J., & Henning, S. (2008). Efficacy and effectiveness of cochlear implants in deaf children. In P. Hauser & M. Marschark (Eds.), *Deaf cognition* (pp. 52–101). New York, NY: Oxford.

Pittman, P., Benedict, B., Olson, S., & Sass-Lehrer, M. (2016). Collaboration with Deaf and hard of hearing communities. In M. Sass-Lehrer (Ed.), *Deaf and hard-of-hearing infants, toddlers, and their families: Interdisciplinary perspectives* (pp. 135–166). New York, NY: Oxford.

Plaza-Pust, C. (2014). Language development and language interaction in sign bilingual language acquisition. In M. Marschark, G. Tang, & H. Knoors (Eds.), *Bilingualism and bilingual deaf education* (pp. 23–53). New York, NY: Oxford.

Poeppel, D., Emmorey, K., Hickok, G., & Pyikkänen, L. (2012). Towards a new neurobiology of language. *Journal of Neuroscience, 32*(41), 14125–14131.

Poizner, H., Klima, E. S., & Bellugi, U. (1987). *What the hands reveal about the brain.* Cambridge, MA: MIT Press/Bradford Books.

Pollard, R. Q. (1992–1993). 100 years in psychology and deafness: A centennial retrospective. *Journal of the American Deafness and Rehabilitation Association, 26*(3), 32–46.

Pollard, R. Q. (1994). Public mental health service and diagnostic trends regarding individuals who are deaf or hard of hearing. *Rehabilitation Psychology, 39,* 147–160.

Pollard, R. Q. (2002). Ethical conduct in research involving deaf people. In V. Gutman (Ed.), *Ethics in mental health and deafness* (pp. 162–178). Washington, DC: Gallaudet University Press.

Poulson, A., Hooymans, J., Richards, A., Bearcoft, P., Murthy, R., Baguley, D., Scott, J., & Snead, M. (2004). Clinical features of type 2 Stickler syndrome. *Journal of Medical Genetics, 41*(8), 41:e107 DOI:10.1136/jmg.2004.018382

Powell, R. (2014). Can parents lose custody simply because they are disabled? *GPSolo, 31*(2). Retrieved from www.americanbar.org/publications/gp_solo/2014/march_april/can_parents_lose_custody_simply_because_they_are_disabled.html

Prasad, H., Bhojwani, K., Shenoy, V., & Prasad, S. (2006). HIV manifestations in otolaryngology. *American Journal of Otolaryngology, 27*(3), 179–185.

Preston, P. (1994). *Mother father deaf: Living between sound and silence.* Cambridge, MA: Harvard University Press.

Pringle, C. (2014). Cytomegalovirus (CMV) infection. *The Merck Manual Home Edition.* Retrieved from www.merckmanuals.com/home/infections/viral_infections/cytomegalovirus_cmv_infection.html

Prinz, P. M., & Strong, M. (1998). ASL proficiency and English literacy within a bilingual deaf education model of instruction. *Topics in Language Disorders, 18*(4), 47–60.

Proctor, R. (2002). Eugenics in Hitler's Germany. In D. Ryan & J. Schuchman (Eds.), *Deaf people in Hitler's Europe* (pp. 32–48). Washington, DC: Gallaudet University Press.

Psychology Today. (2015). *Spirituality.* Retrieved from www.psychologytoday.com/basics/spirituality

Punch, R., Creed, P., & Hyde, M. (2006). Career barriers perceived by hard-of-hearing adolescents: Implications for practice from a mixed-methods study. *Journal of Deaf Studies and Deaf Education, 11*(2), 224–237.

Punch, R., & Hyde, M. (2011). Social participation of children and adolescents with cochlear implants: A qualitative analysis of parent, teacher, and child interviews. *Journal of Deaf Studies and Deaf Education, 16*(4), 474–493.

Punch, R., Hyde, M., & Creed, P. (2004). Issues in the school-to-work transition of hard of hearing adolescents. *American Annals of the Deaf, 149*(1), 28–38.

Qi, S., & Mitchell, R. E. (2012). Large-scale academic achievement testing of deaf and hard-of-hearing students: Past, present, and future. *Journal of Deaf Studies and Deaf Education, 17*(1), 1–18.

Qingzin, Z. (2012). Proceedings from the 2012 International Conference on Education Technology and Computer (ICETC2012) IPCSIT 43: *Is there a critical period for second language acquisition?*. Retrieved from www.ipcsit.com/vol43/059-ICETC2012-T3163.pdf

Quigley, S., Steinkamp, M., & Jones, B. (1978). The assessment and development of language in hearing impairment individuals. *Journal of the Academy of Rehabilitative Audiology, 11*(1), 24–41.

Quigley, S. P., Steinkamp, M. W., Power, D. J., & Jones, B. W. (1978). *Test of syntactic abilities: Guide to administration and interpretation*. Beaverton, OR: Dormac.

Quirk, R., Greenbaum, S., Leech, G., & Svartivik, J. (1972). *A grammar of contemporary English*. White Plains, NY: Longman.

Quittner, A., Smith, L., Osberger, M., Mitchell, T., & Katz, D (1994). The impact of audition on the development of visual attention. *Psychological Science, 5*(6), 347–353.

Raifman, L., & Vernon, M. (1996). Important implications for psychologists of the Americans with Disabilities Act: Case in point, the patient who is deaf. *Professional Psychology: Research and Practice, 27*, 372–377.

Raimondo, B. (2013). It's the law! A review of the laws that provide Americans with access for all. *Odyssey, 14*, 4–8.

Raimondo, B., & Yoshinaga-Itano, C. (2016). Legislation, policies, and role of research in shaping early intervention. In M. Sass-Lehrer (Ed.), *Deaf and hard-of-hearing infants, toddlers, and their families: Interdisciplinary perspectives* (pp. 105–134). New York, NY: Oxford.

Raporport, L. (1970). Crisis intervention as a mode of treatment. In R. W. Roberts & R. H. Nee (Eds.), *Theories of social casework* (pp. 265–311). Chicago, IL: University of Chicago Press.

Rashid, K., Kushalnagar, P., & Kushalnagar, R. (2010). How deaf adult signers experience implants: Some preliminary conclusions. In R. Paludneviciene & I. W. Leigh (Eds.), *Cochlear implants: Evolving perspectives* (pp. 56–70). Washington, DC: Gallaudet University Press.

Rée, J. (1999). *I see a voice*. New York, NY: Metropolitan Books.

Reesman, J., Day, L., Szymanski, C., Hughes-Wheatland, R., Witkin, G., Kalback, S., & Brice, P. (2014). Review of intellectual assessment measures for children who are deaf or hard of hearing. *Rehabilitation Psychology, 59*(1), 99–106.

Reichman, A., & Jacoby, S. E. (n.d.). *A lifetime of learning and earning*. Laurent Clerc National Education Center. Retrieved from www.gallaudet.edu/Documents/Clerc/VR_Galluadet_Stringer.pdf

Reisler, J. (2002). *Voices of the oral deaf*. Jefferson, NC: McFarland.

Remmel, E., & Peters, K. (2009). Theory of mind and language in children with cochlear implants. *Journal of Deaf Studies and Deaf Education, 14*(2), 218–236.

Rinaldi, P., & Caselli, M. C. (2014). Language development in a bimodal bilingual child with cochlear implant: A longitudinal study. *Bilingualism: Language and Cognition, 17*(4), 798–809.

Rinaldi, P., Caselli, M. C., Di Renzo, A., Gulli, T., & Volterra, V. (2014). Sign vocabulary in deaf toddlers exposed to sign language since birth. *Journal of Deaf Studies and Deaf Education, 19*(3), 303–318.

Rizzi, M., & Hirose, K. (2007). Aminoglycoside ototoxicity. *Current Opinion in Otolaryngology & Head & Neck Surgery, 15*(5), 352–357.

Roberson, L., & Shaw, S. (2015). Reflections on deaf education: Perspectives of deaf senior citizens. *Educational Gerontology, 41*(3), 226–237.

Robertson, C., Howarth, T., Bork, D., & Dinu, I. (2009). Permanent bilateral sensory and neural hearing loss of children after neonatal intensive care because of extreme prematurity: A thirty year study. *Pediatrics, 123*(5), 797–807.

Robinson, S. (2006). The extended family: Deaf women in organizations. In B. J. Brueggemann & S. Burch (Eds.), *Women and deafness* (pp. 40–56). Washington, DC: Gallaudet University Press.

Rochester Institute of Technology (2008, April 19). Sign language interpreters at high ergonomic risk. *ScienceDaily*. Retrieved from www.sciencedaily.com/releases/2008/04/080417105449.htm

Rodriguez, Y. (2001). *Toddlerese: Conversations between hearing parents and their deaf toddlers in Puerto Rico* (Unpublished doctoral dissertation). Lamar University, Beaumont, TX.

Rogoff, M. (2003). *The cultural nature of human development*. New York, NY: Oxford.

Rosen, R. (2009). The World Federation of the Deaf. In D. F. Moores & M. S. Miller (Eds.), *Deaf people around the world* (pp. 374–391). Washington, DC: Gallaudet University Press.

Rosenberg, J. (2015). *Deaf business owners overcome obstacles and prejudice*. Retrieved from http://bigstory.ap.org/article/2e65418e122f45b18409dd8bb4af639b/deaf-business-owners-overcome-obstacles-and-prejudice

Ross, M. (1990). Definitions and descriptions. In J. Davis (Ed.), *Our forgotten children: Hard of hearing pupils in the schools* (pp. 3–17). Bethesda, MD: Self-Help for Hard of Hearing People.

Ross, M. (1998). *Dr. Ross on hearing loss/speechreading*. Retrieved from www.hearingresearch.org/ross/aural_rehabilitation/speechreading.php

Ross, M. (2001). Definitions and descriptions. In J. Davis (Ed.), *Our forgotten children: Hard of hearing pupils in the schools* (pp. 11–37). Bethesda, MD: Self-Help for Hard of Hearing People.

Roukema, B., Van Loon, M., Smits, C., Smit, C. F., Goverts, S., Merkus, P., & Hensen, E. (2011). Cochlear implantation after bacterial meningitis in infants younger than 9 months. *International Journal of Otolaryngology, 2011,* Article Id 845879, 1–9. DOI:10.1155/2011/845879

Rubinstein, A., Jerry, J., Saraf-Lavi, E., Sklar, E., & Bradley, W. (2001). Sudden sensorineural hearing loss associated with herpes simplex virus type 1 infection. *Neurology, 56,* 571.

Ruffin, C. V., Kronenberger, W. G., Colson, B. G., Henning, S. C., & Pisoni, D. B. (2013). Long-term speech and language outcomes in prelingually deaf children, adolescents and young adults who received cochlear implants in childhood. *Audiology and Neurotology, 18,* 289–296.

Rymer, R. (1994). *Genie: A scientific tragedy.* New York, NY: HarperPerennial.

Saleebey, D. (1992). *The strengths perspective in social work practice.* New York, NY: Longman.

Sandler, W., Aronoff, M., Padden, C., & Meir, I. (2014). Language emergence: Al-Sayyid Bedouin sign language. In N. Enfield, P. Kockelman, & J. Sidnell (Eds.), *The Cambridge handbook of linguistic anthropology* (pp. 250–284). New York, NY: Cambridge University Press.

Sanna, M., Di Lella, F., Guida, M., & Merkus, P. (2012). Auditory brainstem implants in NF2 patients: Results and review of the literature. *Otology & Neurotology, 33*(2), 154–164.

Sass-Lehrer, M. (Ed.). (2016). *Early intervention for deaf and hard of hearing infants, toddlers, and their families: Interdisciplinary perspectives.* New York, NY: Oxford.

Sass-Lehrer, M., Porter, A., & Wu, C. (2016). Families: Partnerships in practice. In M. Sass-Lehrer (Ed.), *Early intervention for deaf and hard-of-hearing infants and toddlers and their families: Interdisciplinary perspectives* (pp. 65–105). New York, NY: Oxford.

Scheibe, K. (2006). Identity. In N. Salkind (Ed.), *Encyclopedia of human development* (pp. 667–669). Thousand Oaks, CA: Sage.

Scheiber, N. (2015). Fake cover letters expose discrimination against disabled. *The New York Times.* Retrieved from www.nytimes.com/2015/11/02/upshot/fake-cover-letters-expose-discrimination-against-disabled.html?_r=0

Schein, J., & Delk, M. (1974). *The deaf population of the United States.* Silver Spring, MD: National Association of the Deaf.

Schick, B. (2008). A model of learning within an interpreted K-12 educational setting. In M. Marschark & P. Hauser (Eds.), *Deaf cognition: Foundations and outcomes* (pp. 351–386). New York, NY: Oxford.

Schick, B., De Villiers, P., De Villiers, J., & Hoffmeister, R. (2007). Language and theory of mind: A study of deaf children. *Child Development, 78*(2), 376–396.

Schlesinger, H. (2000). A developmental model applied to problems of deafness. *Journal of Deaf Studies and Deaf Education, 5*(4), 349–361.

Schlesinger, H., & Meadow, K. (1972). *Sound and sign: Childhood deafness and mental health.* Berkeley, CA: University of California Press.

Schley, S., Walters, G., Weathers, R., Hemmeter, J., Hennessey, J., & Burkhauser, R. (2011). Effect of postsecondary education on the economic status of persons who are deaf or hard of hearing. *Journal of Deaf Studies and Deaf Education, 16*(4), 524–536.

Schlossberg, N. K. (1981). A model for analyzing human adaptation to transition. *The Counseling Psychologist, 9*(2), 2–18.

Schorr, E. (2006). Early cochlear implant experience and emotional functioning during childhood: Loneliness in middle and late childhood. *Volta Review, 106*(3), 365–379.

Schott, L. (2002, January). Sexual abuse at deaf schools in America. In *The FAED Eagle* (pp. 5–6). Gastonia, NC: The FAED Eagle Newsletter.

Schroedel, J., & Geyer, P. (2000). Long-term career attainments of deaf and hard of hearing college graduates: Results from a 15-year follow-up survey. *American Annals of the Deaf, 145*(4), 303–314.

Schuchman, J. (1988). *Hollywood speaks: Deafness and the film entertainment history.* Urbana, IL: University of Illinois Press.

Schwartz, N., Mebane, D., & Mahony, H. (1990). Effects of alternate modes of administration on Rorschach performance of deaf adults. *Journal of Personality Assessment, 54,* 671–683.

Schwartz, S. (Ed.). (2007). *Choices in deafness* (3rd ed.). Bethesda, MD: Woodbine House.

Seaborn, B., Andrews, J. F., & Martin, G. (2010). Deaf adults and the comprehension of Miranda. *Journal of Forensic Psychology Practice, 10*(2), 107–132.

Sebald, A. (2008). Child abuse and deafness: An overview. *American Annals of the Deaf, 153*(4), 376–383.

Section 504 of the Rehabilitation Act of 1973, Pub. L. No. 93-112, 87 Stat. 394 (Sept. 26, 1973).

Seligman, M. (2008). Positive health. *Applied Psychology: An International Review, 57*, 3–18.

Seto, M. (2008). *Pedophilia and sexual offending against children: Theory, assessment, and intervention*. Washington, DC: American Psychological Association.

Shapse, S. (2015). *When a test is not a test: Tests without forensic validity.* Retrieved from www.hg.org/article.asp?id=7704

Shaver, D., Marschark, M., Newman, L., & Marder, C. (2014). Who is where? Characteristics of deaf and hard-of-hearing students in regular and special schools. *Journal of Deaf Studies and Deaf Education, 19*(2), 203–219. DOI: 10.1093/deafed/ent056

Sheridan, M. (1995). Existential transcendence among deaf and hard of hearing people. In M. D. Garretson (Ed.), *Deafness: Life and culture II: A Deaf American monograph* (pp. 103–106). Silver Spring, MD: National Association of the Deaf.

Sheridan, M. (2001). *Inner lives of deaf children.* Washington, DC: Gallaudet University Press.

Sheridan, M. (2008). *Deaf adolescents: Inner lives and lifeworld development.* Washington, DC: Gallaudet University Press.

Sheridan, M., White, B., & Mounty, J. (2010). Deaf and hard of hearing social workers accessing their profession: A call to action. *Journal of Social Work in Disability and Rehabilitation, 9*(1), 1–11. DOI: 10.1080/15367100903524091

Shultz Myers, S., Marcus, A., & Myers, R. (2010). Hearing children of deaf parents: Issues and interventions within a bicultural context. In I. W. Leigh (Ed.), *Psychotherapy with deaf clients from diverse groups* (pp. 109–135). Washington, DC: Gallaudet University Press.

Sieben, C. (2014). *Working toward improving the writing skills of deaf children in secondary school* (Unpublished master's thesis). Lamar University, Beaumont, TX.

Siedlecki, T. (1999). Intelligent use of the Rorschach Inkblot Technique with deaf persons. *JADARA, 33*, 31–46.

Siegal, M. (2008). *Marvelous minds: The discovery of what children know.* New York, NY: Oxford.

Siegel, L. (2008). *The human right to language: Communication access for deaf children.* Washington, DC: Gallaudet University Press.

Simms, D. (2009). *NTID Speechreading CID Everyday Sentences Test.* Rochester Institute of Technology, Rochester, NY. Retrieved from www.rit.edu/ntid.

Simms, L., Baker, S., & Clark, M. D. (2013). The standardized Visual Communication and Sign Language Checklist for Signing Children. *Sign Language Studies, 14*(1), 101–124.

Simms, L., Rusher, M., Andrews, J., & Coryell, J. (2008). Apartheid in deaf education: Examining workforce diversity. *American Annals of the Deaf, 153*(4), 384–395.

Simms, L., & Thumann, H. (2007). In search of a new, linguistically and culturally sensitive paradigm in deaf education. *American Annals of the Deaf, 152*, 302–331.

Sinai Health System and Advocate Health Care. (2004). *Improving access to health and mental health for Chicago's Deaf community: A survey of Deaf adults. Final Survey Report,* Retrieved from www.sinai.org/sites/default/files/Improving%20Access%20to%20Health%20and%20Mental%20Health%20for%20deaf.pdf

Singletary, P. (2005). New hurdles: The impact of recent federal mandates on the assessment of deaf and hard of hearing teachers and teacher candidates. In J. Mounty & D. Martin (Eds.), *Assessing deaf adults* (pp. 156–168). Washington, DC: Gallaudet University Press.

Singleton, J., & Morgan, D. (2006). Natural signed language acquisition within the social context of the classroom. In B. Schick, M. Marschark, & P. Spencer (Eds.), *Advances in the sign language development of deaf children* (pp. 344–375). New York, NY: Oxford.

Singleton, J. L., Supalla, S., Litchfield, S., & Schley, S. (1998). From sign to word: Considering modality constraints in ASL/English bilingual education. *Topics in Language Disorders, 18*(4), 16–29.

Singleton, J., & Tittle, M. (2000). Deaf parents and their hearing children. *Journal of Deaf Studies and Deaf Education, 5*(3), 221–236.

Skinner, B. F. (1957). *Verbal behavior.* New York, NY: Appleton-Century-Crofts.

Sleeboom-Van Raaij, I. (2015). Psychopharmacological treatment of deaf and hard of hearing people. In A. B. Estrada & I. Sleeboom-Van Raaij (Eds.), *Mental health services for deaf people* (pp. 15–39). Washington, DC: Gallaudet University Press.

Sligar, S., Cawthon, S., Morere, D., & Moxley, A. (2013). Equity in assessment for individuals who are deaf or hard of hearing. *JADARA, 47*(1), 110–127.

Smith, D. H. (2012). Deaf adults: Retrospective narratives of school experiences and teacher expectations. *Disability & Society, 28*(5), 674–686.

Smith, D. H., & Andrews, J. F. (2015). Deaf and hard of hearing faculty in higher education: Enhancing access, equity, policy, and practice. *Disability & Society, 30*(10), 1521–1536. DOI:10.1080/09687599.20151113160.

Smith, J., & Wolfe, J. (2016). Should all deaf children learn sign language? *The Hearing Journal, 69*(2), 18–24.

Smith, R., Shearer, A., Hildebrand, M., & Van Camp, G. (2014). Deafness and hereditary hearing loss overview. In R. A. Pagon, M. P. Adam, H. H. Ardinger, S. Wallace, A. Amemiya, L.J.H. Bean, T. D. Bird, C-T. Fong, H. C. Mefford, R.J.H. Smith, & K. Stephens (Eds.), *GeneReviews* (Internet). Seattle, WA: University of Washington, Seattle. Retrieved from www.ncbi.nlm.nih.gov/books/NBK1434/.

Social Security Administration. (2015). *Disability evaluations under social security.* Retrieved from www.socialsecurity.gov/disability/professionals/bluebook/

Sonnenstrahl, D. M. (2002). *Deaf artists in America: Colonial to contemporary.* San Diego, CA: DawnSign Press.

Sousa, D. A. (Ed.). (2007). *How the special needs brain learns.* Thousand Oaks, CA: Corwin Press.

Spangler, T. K. (1988). Exploration and the relationship between deaf children's attachment classification in the Strange Situation and effects of parents' success in grieving and coping. *Dissertation Abstracts International, 49*(1–B), 244.

Spark Policy Institute. (2011). *Standards of care for serving deaf and hard of hearing clients.* Denver, CO: Daylight Project, Mental Health Center of Denver, and Colorado Commission for the Deaf and Hard of Hearing.

Spencer, P. E. (2010). Play and theory of mind: Indicators and engines of early cognitive growth. In M. Marschark & P. Spencer (Eds.), *The Oxford handbook of Deaf studies, language, and education* (Vol. 2, pp. 407–424). New York, NY: Oxford.

Spencer, P. E., & Marschark, M. (2010). *Evidence-based practice in educating deaf and hard-of-hearing students.* New York, NY: Oxford University Press.

Sroufe, L. A. (2005). Attachment and development: A prospective, longitudinal study from birth to adulthood. *Attachment and Human Development, 7*(4), 349–367.

Sroufe, L. A., Egeland, B., Carlson, E., & Collins, W. (2005). *The development of the person: The Minnesota study of risk and adaptation from birth to adulthood.* New York, NY: Guilford.

St. John, R., Lytle, L., Nussbaum, D., & Shoup, A. (2016). Getting started: Hearing screening, evaluation, and next steps. In M. Sass-Lehrer (Ed.), *Deaf and hard-of-hearing infants, toddlers, and their families: Interdisciplinary perspectives* (pp. 169–197). New York, NY: Oxford.

State v. Rewolinski, 464 N.W.2d 401, 159 Wis. 2d 1 (1990).

State v. Wright, 768 N.W.2d 512, (S.D. 51 2009).

Stein, M., Barnett, S., & Padden, C. (2001). Parental request to withhold a hearing test in a newborn of deaf parents. *Journal of Development and Behavioral Pediatrics, 22*(2), S77–S80.

Steinberg, A., Loew, R., & Sullivan, V. J. (2010). The diversity of consumer knowledge, attitudes, beliefs, and experiences. In I. W. Leigh (Ed.), *Psychotherapy with deaf clients from diverse groups* (pp. 18–38). Washington, DC: Gallaudet University Press.

Steiner, A. (2015). Award recognizes state efforts to make mental health care available to all deaf Minnesotans. *MinnPost.* Retrieved from www.minnpost.com/mental-health-addiction/2015/11/award-recognizes-state-efforts-make-mental-health-care-available-all

Stevenson, V. (2015). Protesters say school appointment is tone deaf. *Toronto Star.* Retrieved from www.thestar.com/yourtoronto/education/2015/11/09/protesters-say-school-appointment-is-tone-deaf.html

Stewart, D. (1991). *Deaf sport.* Washington, DC: Gallaudet University Press.

Stewart, L. (1992). Debunking the bilingual/bicultural snow job in the American deaf community. In M. Garretson (Ed.), *Viewpoints on deafness: A deaf American monograph* (pp. 129–142). Silver Spring, MD: National Association of the Deaf.

Stewart, N. (2015, December 23). Inquiry shows struggles of disabled New York students and their families. *New York Times.* Retrieved from www.nytimes.com/2015/12/24/nyregion/inquiry-shows-struggles-of-disabled-new-york-students-and-their-families.html

Stinson, M. & Kluwin, T. (1996). Social orientations toward deaf and hearing peers among deaf adolescents in local public high schools. In P. C. Higgins & J. E. Nash (Eds.). *Understanding deafness socially: Continuities in research and theory* (2nd ed., pp. 113–154). Springfield, IL: Charles C. Thomas.

Stinson, M., & Kluwin, T. (2011). Educational consequences of alternative school placements. In M. Marschark & P. Spencer (Eds.), *The Oxford handbook of Deaf studies, language, and education* (2nd ed., Vol. 1, pp. 47–62). New York, NY: Oxford.

Stoffel, S. (Ed.). (2012). *Deaf-blind reality*. Washington, DC: Gallaudet University Press.

Stokoe, W. C. (1960). Sign language structure: An outline of the visual communication systems of the American deaf. *Studies in Linguistics, Occasional Papers* (No. 8), Buffalo, NY: University of Buffalo.

Stokoe, W. C. (2001). *Language in hand: Why sign came before speech*. Washington, DC: Gallaudet University Press.

Strong, M., & Prinz, P. (2000). Is American Sign Language skill related to English literacy? In C. Charmberlain, J. Morford, & R. Mayberry (Eds.). Language Acquisition by Eye (pp. 131–141). Mahwah, NJ: Lawrence Erlbaum.

Stuart, M., Stainthorp, R., & Snowling, M. (2008). Literacy as a complex activity: Deconstructing the simple view of reading. *Literacy, 42*(2), 59–66.

Sue, D. W., & Sue, D. (2015). *Counseling the culturally diverse* (7th ed.). Hoboken, NJ: Wiley.

Supalla, S. (1991). Manually Coded English: The modality question in signed language development. *Theoretical issues in sign language research, 2,* 85–109.

Supalla, S. (1992). *The book of name signs: Naming in American Sign Language*. San Diego, CA: DawnSign Press.

Supalla, S. J., & Cripps, J. H. (2011). Toward universal design in reading instruction. Bilingual Basics, 12(2), 1–13.

Supalla, T., Hauser, P. C., & Bavelier, D. (2014). Reproducing American Sign Language sentences: Cognitive scaffolding in working memory. *Frontiers in Psychology, 5,* 859.

Sussman, A. (1974). *An investigation into the relationship between self concepts of deaf adults and their perceived attitudes toward deafness* (Doctoral dissertation, New York University, New York). Retrieved from Dissertation Abstracts International (34, 2914B).

Sussman, A., & Brauer, B. (1999). On being a psychotherapist with deaf clients. In I. W. Leigh (Ed.), *Psychotherapy with deaf clients from diverse groups* (pp. 3–22). Washington, DC: Gallaudet University Press.

Swain, J., French, S., Barnes, C., & Thomas, C. (Eds.). (2005). *Disabling barriers-enabling environments*. London, UK: Sage.

Swanepoel, D., & Louw, B. (2010). *HIV/AIDS related communication, hearing and swallowing disorders*. San Diego, CA: Plural Publishing.

Swearer, S., & Hymel, S. (2015). Understanding the psychology of bullying: Moving toward a social-ecological diathesis-stress model. *American Psychologist, 70*(4), 344–353.

Szymanski, C. (2010, November). An open letter to training directors regarding accommodations for deaf interns. *APPIC E-Newsletter,* 1–3.

Szymanski, C. (2012). Managing behavior by managing the classroom: Making learning accessible for deaf and hard of hearing students with autism spectrum disorders. *Odyssey, 13,* 26–31.

Szymanski, C., Brice, P., Lam, K., & Hotto, S. (2012). Deaf children with autism spectrum disorders. *Journal of Autism Development Disorder, 42*(10), 2027–2037.

Tajfel, H. (1981). *Human groups and social categories*. Cambridge, UK: Cambridge University Press.

Task Force on Health Care Careers for the Deaf and Hard-of-Hearing Community. (2012). *Building pathways to health care careers for the deaf and hard-of-hearing community: Final report*. Retrieved from www.rit.edu/ntid/hccd/system/files/FINAL_REPORT_Building_Pathways_March_2012.pdf

Taylor, B. M., Anderson, R. C., Au, K. H., & Raphael, T. E. (2000). Discretion in the translation of research to policy: A case from beginning reading. *Educational Researcher, 29*(6), 16–26.

TDI World. (2015). 21st TDI Biennial Conference proves historic! *TDI World, 46*(3), 10–13, 16–18, 22–26. Retrieved from https://tdiforaccess.org/resources/tdi-publications-archive/tdi-world/

Theunissan, S., Rieffe, C., Netten, A., Briaire, J., Soede, W., Schoones, J., & Frijns, J. (2014). Psychopathology and its risk and protective factors in hearing-impaired children and adolescents: A systematic review. *JAMA Pediatrics, 168*(2), 170–177.

Thomas, L. (2014). *The impact of youth camp experiences on the self-efficacy, identity, and social skills for deaf and hard of hearing adolescents: A mixed method study* (Unpublished doctoral dissertation). Lamar University, Beaumont, TX.

Thomson, N. R., Kennedy, E., & Kuebli, J. (2011). Attachment formation between deaf infants and their primary caregivers: Is being deaf a risk factor for insecure attachment? In D. Zand & K. Pierce (Eds.), *Resilience in deaf children* (pp. 27–64). New York, NY: Springer.

Tiersma, P. (1999). *Legal language*. Chicago, IL: The University of Chicago Press.

Titus, J. (2009). Gender differences in victimization among youths with and without hearing loss admitted to substance abuse treatment. *JADARA, 43*, 7–33.

Titus, J. (2010). The nature of victimization among youths with hearing loss in substance abuse treatment. *American Annals of the Deaf, 155*(1), 19–30.

Tolan, C. (2015, September 28). *Deaf Mexican immigrants are declaring asylum in the U.S.—and winning*. Retrieved from http://fusion.net/story/205119/deaf-mexican-immigrants-declaring-asylum-us/

Toriello, H., & Smith, S. (2013). *Hereditary hearing loss and its syndromes* (3rd ed.). New York, NY: Oxford.

Torre, P., Hoffman, H. J., Springer, G., Cox, C., Young, M. A., Margolick, J. B., & Plankey, M. (2015). Hearing loss among HIV-seropositive and HIV-seronegative men and women. *JAMA Otolaryngology–Head & Neck Surgery, 141*(3), 202–210. DOI: 10.1001/jamaoto.2014.3302.

Torres, A. (2009). *Signing in Puerto Rican*. Washington, DC: Gallaudet University Press.

Traxler, C. B. (2000). The Stanford Achievement Test: National norming and performance standards for deaf and hard-of-hearing students. *Journal of Deaf Studies and Deaf Education, 5*(4), 337–348.

Traxler, M. (2012). *Introduction to psycholinguistics: Understanding language science*. Malden, MA: Wiley-Blackwell.

Trezek, B., Wang, Y., & Paul, P. (2011). Processes and components of reading. In M. Marschark & P. Spencer (Eds.), *The Oxford handbook of Deaf studies, language, and education* (2nd ed., Vol. 1, pp. 99–114). New York, NY: Oxford.

Trumbetta, S., Bonvillian, J., Siedlecki, T., & Haskins, B. (2001). Language-related symptoms in persons with schizophrenia and how deaf persons may manifest these symptoms. *Sign Language Studies, 1*, 228–253.

Tucker, J. (2010/2011). Child first campaign. *The Maryland Bulletin, CXXXI*(2), 3.

Tucker, J. (2015, Spring). 2015 ICED. *Maryland Bulletin*, 12.

Tugg v. Towey, 864 F. Supp. 1201 (S.D. FL. 1994).

Turner, G. (2005). Toward real interpreting. In M. Marschark, R. Peterson, & E. Winston (Eds.), *Sign language interpreting and interpreter education* (pp. 29–56). New York, NY: Oxford.

Ulibarri v. City & County of Denver, No. 07-CV-1814-ODS (D. Colo. July 20, 2012).

Undercoffer, D.G. (1983, April). An interview with Michael Graves. *Visual Merchandising & Store Design*, 114, 68D.

United Nations. (2006). *Some facts about persons with disabilities*. Retrieved from www.un.org/disabilities/convention/pdfs/factsheet.pdf

University College London. (2015). *Creating neuropsychological assessments and services for Deaf patients with neurological impairments*. Retrieved from www.ucl.ac.uk/impact/case-study-repository/neuropsychological-assessments-for-the-deaf

Usami, S., Abe, S., & Shinkawa, H. (1998). Sensorineural hearing loss caused by mitochondrial DNA mutations: Special reference to the A1555G mutation. *Journal of Communication Disorders, 31*, 423–435.

U.S. Census Bureau. (2010). DataFerrett [Data analysis and extraction tool]. Retrieved from: http://dataferrett.census.gov/.

U.S. Census Bureau, Population Division. (2012). *Table 4. Projections of the population by sex, race, and Hispanic origin for the United States: 2015 to 2060* (NP2012-T-4).

Vacco v. Mid Hudson Medical Group, P.C., 877 F. Supp. 143, 149 (S.D.N.Y 1995).

Valente, J., Bahan, B., & Bauman, H-D. (2008). Sensory politics and the cochlear implant debates. In R. Paludneviciene & I. W. Leigh (Eds.), *Cochlear implants: Evolving perspectives* (pp. 245–258). Washington, DC: Gallaudet University Press.

Valentine, G., & Skelton, T. (2008). Changing spaces: The role of the internet in shaping Deaf geographies. *Social and Cultural Geography, 9*(5), 469–485.

Valli, C. (1995). *ASL poetry* (DVD). Available from www.dawnsignpress.com.

Valli, C., Lucas, C., Mulrooney, K., & Villanueva, M. (2011). *Linguistics of American sign language: An introduction* (5th ed.). Washington, DC: Gallaudet University Press.

Van Cleve, J. V. (Ed.). (1993). *Deaf history unveiled.* Washington, DC: Gallaudet University Press.

Van Cleve, J. V., & Crouch, B. (1989). *A place of their own: Creating the deaf community in America.* Washington, DC: Gallaudet University Press.

van Gent, T. (2015). Mental health problems in deaf children and adolescents: Part II—Aspects of psychopathology. In B. Estrada & I. Sleeboom-Van Raaij (Eds.), *Mental health services for deaf people* (pp. 167–191). Washington, DC: Gallaudet University Press.

van Gent, T. Goedhart, A., Hindley, P., Treffers, A., & Phillip, D. (2007). Prevalence and correlates of psychopathology in a sample of deaf adolescents. *Journal of Child Psychology and Psychiatry, 48,* 950–958.

van Gent, T., Goedhart, A., & Treffers, P. (2011). Self-concept and psychopathology in deaf adolescents: Preliminary support for moderating effects of deafness-related characteristics and peer problems. *Journal of Child Psychology and Psychiatry, 52*(6), 720–728.

Vasishta, Madan. (2011). *Deaf in D.C.* Washington, DC: Gallaudet University Press.

Vazquez, M.-P. (2014). Treacher Collins syndrome. Orphanet. Retrieved from www.orpha.net/consor/cgi-bin/OC_Exp.php?Lng=GB&Expert=861

Vermeulen, A. M., Van Bon, W., Schreuder, R., Knoors, H., & Snik, A. (2007). Reading comprehension of deaf children with cochlear implants. *Journal of Deaf Studies and Deaf Education, 12*(3), 283–302.

Vernon, M. (1965/2005). Fifty years of research on the intelligence of deaf and hard-of-hearing children: A review of literature and discussion of implications. *Journal of Deaf Studies and Deaf Education, 10*(3), 225–231.

Vernon, M. (1969). *Multiply handicapped deaf children: Medical, educational, and psychological considerations.* Reston, VA: Council of Exceptional Children.

Vernon, M. (1970). The role of deaf teachers in the education of deaf children. *Deaf American, 23,* 17–20.

Vernon, M. (2009a). ADA routinely violated by prisons in the case of deaf prisoners. *Prison Legal News, 20*(7), 14–15.

Vernon, M. (2009b). The horror of being deaf and in prison. *American Annals of the Deaf, 155*(3), 311–321.

Vernon, M., & Andrews, J. (1990). *The psychology of deafness: Understanding deaf and hard of hearing people.* White Plains, NY: Longman.

Vernon, M. & Andrews, J. (2011). Basic legal issues in handling cases of defendants who are Deaf. *The Champion, XXXV*(2), 30 37.

Vernon, M., & Andrews, J. (2012). Individuals with disabilities and the issue of false confessions. *The Champion, 36*(6), 34–42.

Vernon, M., & Daigle-King, B. (1999). Historical overview of inpatient care of mental patients who are deaf. *American Annals of the Deaf, 144*(1), 51–61.

Vernon, M., & Greenberg, S. F. (1999). Violence in deaf and hard-of-hearing people: A review of the literature. *Aggression and Violent Behavior, 4*(3), 259–272.

Vernon, M., & Leigh, I. W. (2007). Mental health services for people who are deaf. *American Annals of the Deaf, 152*(4), 374– 381.

Vernon, M. & Miller, K. (2001). Linguistic competence to stand trial: A unique condition in some deaf defendants. *Journal of Interpretation, 11,* 99–120.

Vernon, M., & Raifman, L. J. (1997). Recognizing and handling problems of incompetent deaf defendants charged with serious offenses. *International Journal of Law and Psychiatry, 20*(3), 373–387.

Vernon, M., & Rich, S. (1997). Pedophilia and deafness. *American Annals of the Deaf, 142*(4), 300–311.

Vernon, M., Steinberg, A. G., & Montoya, L. A. (1999). Deaf murderers: Clinical and forensic issues. *Behavioral Sciences & the Law, 17*(4), 495–516.

Vernon, M., & Vernon, M. (2010). *Deadly charm: The story of a deaf serial killer.* Washington, DC: Gallaudet University Press.

Vesey, K., & Wilson, B. (2003). Navigating the hearing classroom with a hearing loss. *Odyssey, 4,* 10–13.

Visual Language and Visual Learning Science of Learning Center. (2011, May). *Visual attention and deafness* (Research Brief No. 3). Washington, DC: Elizabeth Hirshorn.

Volterra, V., & Erting, C. J. (1998). *From gesture to language in hearing and deaf children.* Washington, DC: Gallaudet University Press.

Vygotsky, L. S. (1978). *Mind in society: The development of higher psychological processes.* Cambridge, MA: Harvard University Press.

Waddy-Smith, B. (2012). Students who are deaf and hard of hearing and use sign language: Considerations and strategies for developing spoken language and literacy skills. *Semin Speech Lang, 33,* 310–321.

Walker, E., & Tomblin, J. B. (2014). The influence of communication mode on language development in children with cochlear implants. In M. Marschark, G. Tang, & H. Knoors (Eds.), *Bilingualism and bilingual deaf education* (pp. 134–151). New York, NY: Oxford.

Wampler, D. (1971). *Linguistics of visible English.* Santa Rosa, CA: Early Childhood Education Department, Aurally Handicapped Program, Santa Rosa City Schools.

Wang, L., Andrews, J. Liu, A., & Liu, A. (2016). Case studies of multilingual/multicultural Asian deaf adults: Strategies for success. Paper accepted *American Annals of the Deaf, 161*(1), 67–88.

Watkins, S., Pittman, P., & Walden, B. (1998). The Deaf Mentor Experimental Project for young children who are deaf and their families. *American Annals of the Deaf, 143*(1), 29–34.

Watson, D., & Taff-Watson, M., Eds. (1993). *A model service delivery system for persons who are deaf-blind* (2nd ed.). Fayetteville, AR: University of Arkansas.

Wauters, L., & Knoors, H. (2008). Social integration of deaf children in inclusive settings. *Journal of Deaf Studies and Deaf Education, 13*(1), 21–36.

Wax, T. (2010). The evolution of psychotherapy for Deaf women. In I. W. Leigh (Ed.), *Psychotherapy with Deaf clients from diverse groups* (pp. 65–84). Washington, DC: Gallaudet University Press.

Weick, A., Rapp, C., Sullivan, W. P., & Kisthardt, W. (1989). A strengths perspective for social work practice. *Social Work, 34*(4), 350–354.

Weinberg, G. (2006). Meningitis in children. *The Merck Manual Home Edition.* Retrieved from www.merckmanuals.com/home/childrens_health_issues/bacterial_infections_in_infants_and_children/meningitis_in_children.html

Wenger, E. (1999). *Communities of practice: Learning, meaning, and identity.* New York, NY: Cambridge University Press.

White, B. (1999). *The effect of perceptions of social support and perceptions of entitlement on family functioning in deaf-parented adoptive families* (Unpublished doctoral dissertation). Catholic University of America, Washington, DC.

The WHOQOL Group. (1998). The World Health Organization Quality of Life Assessment (WHOQOL): Development and psychometric properties. *Social Science and Medicine, 46,* 1569–1585.

Whyte, A., Aubrecht, A., McCullough, C., Lewis, J., & Thompson-Ochoa, D. (2013). Understanding Deaf people in counseling contexts. *Counseling Today.* Retrieved from http://ct.counseling.org/2013/10/understanding-deaf-people-in-counseling-contexts/

Wilkens, C., & Hehir, T. (2008). Deaf education and bridging social capital: A theoretical approach. *American Annals of the Deaf, 153*(3), 275–284.

Williams, C., & Mayer, C. (2015). Writing in young deaf children. *Review of Educational Research, 85*(4),630–666. DOI: 10.3102/0034654314564882

Williamson, C. (2007). *Black deaf students.* Washington, DC: Gallaudet University Press.

Willis, R., & Vernon, M. (2002). Residential psychiatric treatment of emotionally disturbed deaf youth, *American Annals of the Deaf, 147*(1), 31–37.

Wilson, J., Guthmann, D., Embree, J., & Fraker, S. (2015). Comparing outcomes from an online substance abuse treatment program and residential treatment programs for consumers who are deaf: A pilot study. *JADARA, 49*(3), 172–184. Retrieved from http://repository.wcsu.edu/jadara/vol49/iss3/3

Winefield, R. (1987). *Never the twain shall meet: Bell, Gallaudet, and the communications debate.* Washington, DC: Gallaudet University Press.

Winn, S. (2007). Employment outcomes for people in Australia who are congenitally Deaf: Has anything changed? *American Annals of the Deaf, 152*(4), 382–397.

Winston, E. (2005). Designing a curriculum for American Sign Language/English interpreting educators. In M. Marschark, R. Peterson, & E. Winston (Eds.), *Sign language interpreting and interpreter education* (pp. 208–234). New York, NY: Oxford.

Witte, T., & Kuzel, A. (2000). Elderly Deaf patients' health care experiences. American *Journal of the American Board of Family Practice, 13*(1), 17–22.

Witter-Merithew, A. (July 29, 2003). *The anatomy of an interpretation: An examination of decision-making during the interrogation of a police interrogation.* Paper presented at the RID National Conference, Chicago, IL.

Wolbers, K. A., Dostal, H. M., Graham, S., Cihak, D., Kilpatrick, J. R., & Saulsburry, R. (2015). The writing performance of elementary students receiving strategic and interactive writing instruction. *Journal of Deaf Studies and Deaf Education, 20*(4), 385–398. DOI: 10.1093/deafed/env022

Wolf, M. (2007). *Proust and the squid: The story and science of the reading brain.* New York, NY: Harper Collins.

Wolfe, J. (2014). Ten advances in cochlear implant technology and services. *Plural Publishing.* Retrieved from www.pluralpublishing.com/wp/?p=2135

World Health Organization. (2014). *Deafness and hearing loss.* Retrieved from www.who.int/mediacentre/factsheets/fs300/en/

Worsøe, L., Cayé-Thomasen, P., Brandt, T., Thomsen, J., & Østergaard, C. (2010). Factors associated with the occurrence of hearing loss after pneumococcal meningitis. *Clinical Infectious Diseases, 51*(8), 917–924.

Wright, M. H. (1999). *Sounds like home: Growing up black and deaf in the South.* Washington, DC: Gallaudet University Press.

Wu, C., & Grant, N. (2010). Asian American and Deaf. In I. W. Leigh (Ed.), *Psychotherapy with Deaf clients from diverse groups* (2nd ed., pp. 210–236). Washington, DC: Gallaudet University Press.

Wu, C., Lee, Y., Chen, P., & Hsu, C. (2008). Predominance of genetic diagnosis and imaging results as predictors in determining the speech perception performance outcome after cochlear implantation in children. *Archives of Pediatric Adolescent Medicine, 162*(3), 269–276.

Xie, Y.H., Potměšil, M., & Peters, B. (2014). Children who are deaf or hard of hearing in inclusive educational settings: A literature review on interactions with peers. *Journal of Deaf Studies and Deaf Education, 19*(4), 423–437. DOI: 10.1093/deafed/enu017

Yoshinaga-Itano, C. (2013). *Joint Committee for Infant Hearing position statement, 2013.* Retrieved from www.audiology.org

Yoshinaga-Itano, C. (2014). Principles and guidelines for early intervention after confirmation that a child is deaf or hard of hearing. *Journal of Deaf Studies and Deaf Education, 19*(2), 143–175.

Yosso, T. (2005). Whose culture has capital? A critical race theory discussion of community cultural wealth. *Race Ethnicity and Education, 8*(1), 69–91.

Young, A., & Tattersall, H. (2007). Universal newborn hearing screening and early identification of deafness: Parents' responses to knowing early and their expectations of child communication development. *Journal of Deaf Studies and Deaf Education, 12*(2), 209–220.

Young, A., & Temple, B. (2014). *Approaches to social research: The case of Deaf studies.* New York, NY: Oxford.

Young, A., Green, L., & Rogers, K. (2008). Resilience in deaf children: A literature review. *Deafness and Education International, 10*(1), 40–55.

Young, A., Monteiro, B., & Ridgeway, S. (2000). Deaf people with mental health needs in the criminal justice system: a review of the UK literature. *Journal of Forensic of Psychiatry and Psychology, 11*(3), 556–570.

Zaidman-Zait, A. (2014). *Parenting stress among parents of deaf and hard-of-hearing children. Raising and educating deaf children: Foundations for policy, practice, and outcomes.* Retrieved from http://raisingandeducatingdeafchildren.org/parenting-stress-among-parents-of-deaf-and-hard-of-hearing-children

Zaidman-Zait, A., Curle, D., Jamieson, J., Chia, R., & Kozak, F. (2015). Cochlear implantation among deaf children with additional disabilities: Parental perceptions of benefits, challenges, and service provision. *Journal of Deaf Studies and Deaf Education, 20*(1), 41–50.

Zand, D., & Pierce, K. (Eds.). (2011). *Resilience in deaf children.* New York, NY: Springer.

Zand, D. H., & Pierce, K. (2013). Self-reported life events among deaf emerging adults–An exploratory study. *Journal of the American Deafness & Rehabilitation Association (JADARA), 46*(2).

Zemedagegehu v. Arthur, No. 1: 15cv57 (JCC/MSN) (E.D. Va. April 28, 2015).

Zhang, X., Anderson, R. C., Morris, J., Miller, B., Nguyen-Jahiel, K., Lin, T., . . ., Hsu, J. (2015). Improving children's competence as decision makers: Contrasting effects of collaborative interaction and direct instruction. *American Educational Research Journal, 53*(1), 194–223. Advance online publication. DOI:10.3102/0002831215618663

Zodda, J. (2015). Condom use among deaf college students. *JADARA, 49*(2), 86–101.

Index

Information in figures and tables is indicated by page numbers in italics.